# PRACTICE
*of*
# NATUROPATHIC
# MEDICINE

# PRACTICE
*of*
# NATUROPATHIC MEDICINE

*in their own words*

Edited by Sussanna Czeranko, ND, BBE
Foreword by Shirley Snow, ND, DNB, HMD

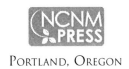

Portland, Oregon

Managing Editor: Sandra Snyder, Ph.D.
Production: Fourth Lloyd Productions, LLC.
Design: Richard Stodart

Cover illustration: An artist's rendition of the buildings and facilities of
Drs. Benedict and Louisa Lust's Health Resort, Yungborn,
in Butler, New Jersey at the turn of the century.
Back cover photo: Dr. E. K. Stretch

Published by NCNM PRESS
National College of Natural Medicine
49 SW Porter Street
Portland, Oregon 97201, USA
www.ncnm.edu

NCNM PRESS gratefully acknowledges the generous and prescient financial
support of HEVERT USA which has made possible the creation and
distribution of the *In Their Own Words* historical series.
The HEVERT COLLECTION comprises twelve historical compilations which
preserve for the healing professions significant and representational works
from contributors to the historical Benedict Lust journals.

Printed in the United States of America

ISBN: 978-0-9771435-8-0
0-9771435-8-9
Library of Congress Control Number: 2015939366

Precious and remarkable to honor, a century later, the ingenuity and innovation that the early Naturopaths brought to their mission of building our medicine in North America.

# Table Of Contents

# FOREWORD

Only one who hasn't strayed from her path can tell Mother Nature's story with as much enthusiasm, consistency and truth as Dr. Sussanna Czeranko, ND, BBE. Our colleague has brought discipline and genius to this huge project, reflected in her deep research and organization of these twelve volumes. Five of them are now complete, capturing the history of our medicine in the very words of its creators. So far, we have: 1, the origins of; 2, the philosophy of; 3, dietetics; 4, the principles of; and 5, this current issue, the practice of.

Our naturopathic elders, in their own words, brought forward to us again in these books, best describe the Naturopathic Way: knifeless, bloodless, dopeless, scientific—the practical realization and application of all that is good in Natural Science, philosophy, and spirituality.

The most beneficent reformatory health movement was inaugurated in 1843 by Priessnitz in Gräfenberg, Germany, a small village in the Silesian Mountains. This man had a genius for healing. His pharmacopeia consisted not of pills and potions but in plenty of exercise, fresh mountain air, water treatment in the cool, sparkling brooks; and simple country fare, consisting of wholesome black bread, vegetables, and fresh milk from animals fed on nutritious mountain grasses. The results were extraordinary! Priessnitz's home in Gräfenberg was surrounded by a Sanatorium where the sick came for cure from every part of the world. Doctors came to Gräfenberg too, where they eagerly learned about Priessnitz's healing methods. Nature cure spread rapidly across Germany (the Fatherland of Naturopathy) and throughout the civilized world.

Benedict Lust, one young man with a dream, strengthened by his faith in God, followed the course of several European Naturopaths like Priessnitz and found the way back to health by all natural processes and treatments. It was the priest-Healer Sebastian Kneipp, via Water Cure, who restored to Lust the soundness of mind and body.

It is said, "To whom is given much is expected."

Benedict Lust was commissioned by Kneipp to bring the Kneipp Water Cure to America. The young Lust arrived in America in late 1892 from Michelbach, Germany, a small burg near Gaggenau. Grounded in Natural Healing Methods, he visited health institutions and spread his discoveries. Lust received a D.O. degree from the University Osteopathic College of New York and a medical degree from the N.Y. Homeopathic Medical College; he also held medical doctor licensure in the state of Florida.

In 1901, Dr. Benedict Lust acquired the name Naturopathy, first coined in 1895 by Dr. John H. Scheel, a Homeopathic physician of German extraction, who operated Badekur, a large Sanitarium located at 121 E. 83rd St. in New York City.

Dr. Lust became known as the "Father of Naturopathy" in the USA. In 1897, he founded The American Naturopathic Association (ANA) and was the first to publish a national magazine for Naturopaths.

Dr. Lust was the originator of health food stores in America. Throughout his immensely productive career, Dr. Lust hailed the pioneers of Nature Cure:

> The Kneipp cure (water cure system),
> The Kuhne Theory of Unity of Disease,
> The Ricki Atmospheric Cure,
> The Priessnitz Austrian Water Cure,
> The Schroth Theory of Moist Heat,
> The Just Theory of Favorability of Acute Disease,
> The Jenning Doctrine of non-Treatment (let Nature Heal),
> The Hahnemann Doctrine of the Law of Similars,
> The Lindlahr Philosophy of Naturopathy,
> The Hippocratic Oath formulated by Hippocrates.

No "YES" man, he was opposed to all unnatural systems of immunization. Among many other such positions predicated on a devotion to the *Vis* he was also opposed to vivisection; to the administration of drugs and narcotics; to the use of alcohol; to the use of tobacco; to the pasteurization of milk; to the processing of foods; and to experiments on inmates in prisons. Moreover, he was opposed to legislation that prevented a family from attending to its own ills. He was opposed to the use of herbicide and insecticide sprays.

October 1922 at the 26th Annual Congress of the ANA at Washington DC, Dr. Lust said, "The time is coming when Naturopathy will be recognized universally; to accomplish this, the Naturopaths must cooperate and give to their cause the true and honest support that conforms with MIRACULOUS POWERS nature had given into their hands." Almost a quarter century later, on August 30, 1945 at the 49th Congress of the ANA came Dr. Benedict Lust provided his answer to a powerful question of that day and of our time too: "What is the future of Naturopathy?" He said:

> I can give my opinion in very few words. For fifty years, I have been in the thick of the fight to bring to the American people true Naturopathy; a simple, effective healing system composed of all the Natural forces our God has given to us in abundance. During that period of time, I have had the opportunity to judge

what Naturopathy has done and what it can accomplish. I see the gradual recognition of this true healing art, not only due to the conscientious practitioners but because of the bungling asinine mistakes by orthodox medicine—[to cite one, the fiasco of the sulfa drugs as emphasized disastrously in our armed forces is just one straw in the wind] creating a public distrust in all things medical. The increasing lack of confidence in the infallibility of modern medicine will eventually make itself felt that the man on the street will turn to these self-constituted oppressors and not only demand but FORCE a change! I may not be here to witness this revolution, but I believe with all of my soul that it is coming! Yes! The future of Naturopathy is indeed bright! It merely requires that each Naturopath carry on to his/her best ability.

Exactly five days later Dr. Lust departed from this earth leaving deep, deep footprints in the sand.

I feel humbled and privileged to have been a small, but also a big part of this mode of health care for more than forty years. Over the years I have utilized the Water Cure, Bloodless Surgery, Atmospheric Cure, Naturopathic Manipulation, Kinesiology, locating electrical interference fields, CRA (diagnostic scan), Theory of Ionization, Brain Hemispheric Balancing, Tenscam (Crystals), Gem Healing, Syntonics, Iridology-Sclerology, Zone Therapy, Acupressure, Acupuncture, Essential Oil Therapy, Mud Baths (Thalgo), Foot Baths (herbal), Hair Analysis, addressing the uniqueness of the individuals' nutritional needs, Herbology, Natural Pharmaceuticals, Bach Remedies, Bio Chemical Theory (Cell Salts), HBO, Detox Therapy, Yoga, Nature Walks, Hardening, and more.

To those who may ask where or how long have I practiced Naturopathic Medicine, may I say, respectfully, using a "pat" answer: "I have never PRACTICED my ART nor will I ever. Rather, I KNOW what I am doing!" To quote Isaac Newton "If I have seen further, it's by standing on the shoulders of GREATS".

As Naturopathy goes forward, and in our time THE POWERFUL HEALING FORCES of Nature are increasingly utilized in their simplicity by our present and future doctors and by the scientist of the future, it will, as P. Wendell put it, thanks to the sacrifices of the past, present and future BENEDICT LUSTS.

Shirley S. Snow, ND, DNB, HMD<br>
Manchester, New Hampshire<br>
April 2015

# Preface

*Practice of Naturopathic Medicine*, the fifth book in the *Hevert Collection*, brings together a sampling of therapies that the early pioneering Naturopaths used to help their patients restore health. These articles, chosen from the Benedict Lust publications spanning from 1899 to 1923, show the eclectic scope of their vision of what was possible therapeutically using what Nature provided. The essentials: air, water, sun, earth, diet, exercise and breathing never failed to be the mainstay of the early Naturopaths armamentarium as they added new methods alongside the old. There are therapies that did not survive for good reason, yet there are others that quietly vanished in North America with absolutely no rational or comprehensible explanation. *Practice of Naturopathic Medicine* does not include hydrotherapy and its various applications, nor herbal medicine, mind-body medicine or physical exercise. These therapies will have their very own books to highlight their contributing wealth of information.

We can glean from these pioneering Naturopaths their fervent belief that Nature was orderly, intelligent and purposeful. As I write this last sentence, the quiet and measured voice of Dr. Jared Zeff comes to mind. There are other voices too; those of Father Kneipp, Adolf Just, Louis Kuhne and others, who left an indelible mark upon the emerging Naturopaths as they forged ahead creating natural, healthy and viable alternatives for medical care in America. The women and men who followed in these men's footsteps took care to replicate and model therapies in North America that would endure and offer the very best in health care. The operative word is "health" which was the unnegotiable goal for these early Naturopaths. Guiding sick people towards health meant the abandonment of toxic substances such as drugs, vaccines and other medical interventions that did harm rather than support the body to restore health.

Such remarkable elders are still among us, keeping the flame of Naturopathy alive in all the quarters of America. Dr. Shirley Snow, who has practiced naturopathic medicine in its many manifestations for more than 40 years. Her service to the naturopathic profession goes beyond the ordinary, and her contributions are many. Legendary on the East Coast for her advocacy for naturopathic licensure, she was instrumental in achieving licensure in New Hampshire and for years of continuous lobbying to reinstate the "sunsetted" Florida naturopathic legislation. While simultaneously juggling a busy practice, she served on the boards of Pacifica College of Naturopathic Medicine in California, and Southwest College of Naturopathic Medicine in Arizona.

An outspoken proponent of Nature Cure, Dr. Snow continues her traditional naturopathic practice to this day out of her beautiful home office in
Manchester, New Hampshire. Her love and work for the good of Naturopathy are truly worth emulating. We are blessed to have Dr. Snow as
one of our own.

The practice of Naturopathy of our forbearers was undertaken with
conviction and the knowledge that the body had the capacity to heal.
What becomes quickly apparent in these articles is that the early Naturopaths were steadfast in their beliefs about how the body healed and in
their commitment to support the body's own healing mechanisms with
appropriate therapies. Their eagerness to help patients recover from illness energized their exploration and use of therapeutic options.

The attraction to new, emerging therapeutic tools never ceased for the
Naturopaths. They were early adopters of electro therapeutics, for example, not hesitating to combine the new with the old. One such innovation was the Violet Ray, perfected by the brilliant Nicola Tesla. Another
example of openness to new approaches were diagnostic tools such as Iridology, embraced enthusiastically by Henry Lindlahr but criticized by the
Regulars as lacking in scientific rigor. However, hasty skepticism abated
for our early forebears after they read, as a case in point and typical of the
writing in this collection, Lindlahr's compelling account of the management of a severely ailing patient. (pp. 248-249)   As we witness currently,
our detractors still discount as unworthy or illegitimate Naturopathy as
a medical system, not recognizing its grounding in medical science in our
era of progressive research activity and publication in epidemiological and
basic science studies and clinical trials at centers such as NCNM's Helf-
gott Research Institute, Bastyr University and the Research and Clinical
Epidemiology Department of CCNM.

The A.M.A., from its inception in 1845, has focused its sanitizing
mandate on eradicating any and all competing medical systems. A half
century later it was persistently dogging other medical groups such as
Naturopathy, Chiropractic and Osteopathy. By 1904, though, Osteopaths, even though under assault, had not yet been assimilated. One
of their leaders characterizes the tensions of the period. C. W. Young
admonished medical professionals to keep an open mind and to not
"make the ridiculous mistake our learned medical friends have made in
calling Osteopathy vile," and urged his colleagues to eschew "many other
opprobrious epithets before they had investigated " (Young, 1904, 68).
He cautioned, "We have much to learn and much to listen [to]. Science is
advanced by accumulating facts and by demonstration and not by hurling
epithets." (Young, 1904, 68)

The role that science has played in medicine pivots on objectivity and the quest for truth. The scientific foundation that medicine sits on has always carried with it a wide range of opinions whose continuum ranges from blind allegiance to ethical doubts about self-serving motives. The censorious name calling that has been hurled at Naturopaths from the period of these articles to the modern period is that we practice quack medicine based on quasi science. Biomedicine, also known as allopathic medicine, has no monopoly on scientific inquiry. In fact, medical science itself has a vulnerable underbelly. John Ioannidis, in this connection, reported his findings in *Scientific American* of the false and exaggerated results in peer-reviewed scientific studies. He notes, "The problem is rampant in economics, the social sciences and even the natural sciences, but it is particularly egregious in biomedicine. Many studies that claim some drug or treatment is beneficial have turned out not to be true." (Ioannidis, 2011, 16) Invariably, and with equal applicability to the field of medicine, noisily appropriating science has not precluded medical disasters, from calomel to thalidomide, from shocking chronicity levels in North America to the hijacking of the U.S. national treasury to the tune of 18% of its GDP.

The writers here remind us that the early Naturopath's trust in Nature with its immutable laws has provided a solid foundation that would endure, while western medical science would often falter with each new discovery, forcing new text books and clinical recalibrations to accommodate the updated and constant changing truth. A pioneering, contemporary naturopathic leader, Dr. Joe Pizzorno, has made this point very clearly, "Conventional medicine says every ten years, 50% of what they thought is wrong. That doesn't happen to us. Our medicine is rooted in the truth of Nature." (Pizzorno, lecture at NCNM, 2013).

The lexicon of our forebears does not reflect the familiar latinate jargon of contemporary scientific terminology. Their language can be rediscovered in these pages. It is a terminology which affects our understanding of their messages, phrases and descriptors which accompanied the therapies which was vital for the correct and effective implementation of the various applications about which they wrote so prolifically. Much of the early Naturopathic lexicon is gone, unfortunately, and with it, valuable tools to understand how to use forgotten or underused therapies. In an upcoming book, *Hydrotherapy of Naturopathic Medicine,* I will be exploring such forgotten words that gave meaning to the many therapies that we have abandoned. Once the words have been lost, an inevitable accompanying consequence is the diluting and even obfuscating of the therapies themselves. The convenience of highly monetized drug and surgical regimens and strategies which excuse the patient from a responsibility for his or her own health, concomitantly eroding the primacy of prevention in health promotion, is reflected in the words our patients hear from us, and in the universe of discourse of the medical professions themselves. One might keep in mind the curious disconnects and accompanying meanings of contemporary terms such as "complementary", "alternative" and "integrative". Complementary and alternative to what? Integrating what with what? The very words of the medical professions make meaning and convey assumptions which have a strong bearing on the nature and effectiveness of the medicine itself.

Making sense of this shifting lexicon of definitions, terminology and descriptors is one very good reason, then, to sift through the archives which comprise our history. Hmmm, we may conclude in our reading of materials from a century ago that the human body has not morphed as quickly as our gadgets and concoctions. We might be less persuaded about the social contract which has accorded allopathic medicine a dominative position in North American and even global medicine. These articles will remind us again, as if for the first time, that one thing *is* very certain in an uncertain universe, and that is that the old Naturopaths listened and trusted the counsel of Nature. Given the choice for the quick fix of drugs and vaccines, they steered their patients to choose natural means of acquiring and regaining health. We might be quick to dismiss the old books as antiquated and having had their day, but trust me, they convey a wealth of clinical pearls that we would be best to revisit, re-embrace, and celebrate anew.

The library housed at NCNM is unique and impressive. Dr. Rick Severson, former NCNM librarian, calculated that no more than 36% of the NCNM collection can be found in 10 or fewer other libraries, and that 16% of the our collection or 2,349 titles, is unique to the NCNM library. "That means we are the only library in the country that owns those things." (Severson, 2012) The NCNM library routinely attracts visitors from the medical community in search of lost and forgotten books. It would not surprise the writers of the articles in this present volume to witness Allopaths in full circle, in search of the very therapies some of which we use less, and have even discarded. That biomedicine professionals are just now co-opting therapies, concepts and protocols long safeguarded by Naturopathic Medicine may feel hypocritical, but it is also indicative of the power of Nature, a central tenet in our philosophy since the very beginning.

I want to thank everyone who has breathed life into this volume, fifth in the Hevert Collection series, *Practice of Naturopathic Medicine*. Behind the glossy cover are hundreds of typed pages which were patiently transcribed by many, magnificent students at NCNM. In fact, so far there are over 1000 articles typed manually, selected after much reflection and deliberation, from the Benedict Lust publications to become the essential content of this volume, the preceding volumes and the upcoming volumes of the *Hevert Collection*. There are many more articles still in the queue as this series emerges and is propelled toward completion.

Let me acknowledge every NCNM student who typed or proof read articles while navigating their intense course loads and juggling their personal lives. Huge heaps of enduring gratitude to *Adam Dombrowski, Anemone Fresh, Avishek Saha, Craig Merhmann, Delia Sewell, Delores Stephens, Elizabeth Wade, Erin Conlon, Fiona Campbell, January Bourassa, Jennifer Samson, Karis Tressel, Kirsten Carle, Lauren Geyman, Lucy-Kate Reeve, Megan Hammel, Misty Story, Olif Wojciechowski, Rebecca Jennings, Tristian Rowe,* and all those whom I am inadvertently missing here. Their work is an essential element in the substance of this book. The words and images when captured by our imagination and our commitment to Naturopathic Medicine mean that we can wander into the past century to rediscover our roots, to anchor ourselves for the present era.

I am indebted to the painstaking hours that *Adam Dombrowski* spent carefully scanning images from the Benedict Lust' journals. Thank you Adam. And, as this book project continues, my appreciation for the invaluable organizational help that I had received from *Dr. Karis Tressel* at the commencement is a daily reminder that book making is an undertaking of an entire community. Karis continues to be my diva of anti-chaos as this conveyer belt speeds along. She has unfailingly helped with technical details that often elude me. I am deeply grateful for her profound love of traditional Naturopathy and her loving tenacity with this project.

Indeed, I so much enjoyed working with each and every student who sacrificed scarce, precious study and leisure time for the hard work of meticulous research and transcription. As you launch yourselves into the Naturopathic profession, never forget how special and important your work has been. You have chosen a path of sacred work. You will be loved and cherished by your patients because you listen and truly care. Remember to trust Nature's power of healing! Pay careful attention to your patients and they will feel enlivened to have found their way to you.

I am very grateful for the encouraging support of the Hevert Corporation here in America and in Germany. Thank you and my most gracious accolades to Americana and Wolf Aulenbacher in America and to Mathias and Marcus Hevert in Germany for believing in the impossible. Yes, we can create 12 books that are an exquisite testimony to the power of Naturopathy. Much gratitude, as well, to the unwavering, behind-the-scenes support of the Board of NCNM, Dr. Sandra Snyder, Susan Hunter, and Jerry Bores who understood from the beginning the importance of this project. I especially would like to thank Kathy Stanford, Director of Human Resources at NCNM for her caring and perceptive observation that my small postage stamp desk was not ideal for a working space with so much paper, so many piles, and so many interconnecting parts. I thank you for providing me with a work station which moves in resonance with the work at hand. Now, in mid project, I'm hitting a stride which includes more than enough space to keep the avalanche of materials and people organized.

I applaud and pay homage to the Fourth Lloyd Productions, Nancy and Richard Stodart, our designers and coaches extraordinaire, who guided NCNM Press and me with alacrity every dance step of the way. To Nancy, I am indebted for her dedicated stance on excellence in every realm. Thank you, Nancy for your constant attention to perfection, your encouragement and insights. From you Nancy, I have learned the art of orderliness that has opened up a new vista of possibilities. It is indeed feasible to keep hundreds of papers organized and accessible at all times. I am awed too by Richard's delicate renditions, converting faded images into artistic manifestations. Richard has transformed century old scanned images into art over and over again. Indeed, the number of pictures increased dramatically in *Practice of Naturopathic Medicine* and with your patience and love of perfection to detail, the illustrations have brought the therapies to life.

This book would be completely irrelevant if it were not for the thousands of Naturopaths working in their communities day after day and year after year, keeping the practice of our medicine alive. Your work and dedication are a testament that Naturopathy is worth doing, that Naturopathy is critical to the health of the planet and its people.

Lastly, I want to thank my dear and loving husband, David Schleich, who has the patience of a saint. Without your daily inspiration and attention, I would not be able to see just ahead, a few thousand pages from now, the sweet taste of crossing the finish line. Daily my woes and concerns blur, but he guides me to a sane refuge, hears me out, listens with genuine curiosity and offers me the wisdom to carry on. "One eye on the manuscript in front of you; one eye on the future," he often says. Without your support, I would not have found my way to the end of this book, the fifth of a dozen. Taking an idea for a writing project and manifesting it in books which line doctors' and students' shelves takes a lot of energy. I am deeply grateful that David shares my love of history and listens to my stories with appreciation, wonder and awe. When I get stuck, say, in 1900, he always helps me find my way back to the present.

You may find that some of the sentences in the writing of our fore-bears can be a mile long or embellished with words no longer in our current vocabulary, but this is on purpose. Stay the course. These articles have been carefully transcribed and edited to ensure that you are escorted safely in an era precious in our formation. So, settle back in a comfortable chair with some green tea, and enjoy these articles chosen from the past and from our elders *in their own words*.

Blessings,
Sussanna Czeranko, ND, BBE

*Here removed from the bustle and turmoil incident to large cities, one finds an alleviating balm spiritually and physically in the unsurpassed bounty of nature, which goes a great ways towards recuperation of health, particularly if, as is the case at "Bellevue", such hygienic surroundings are supplemented by a common-sense diet, cooking being done in such a manner that food is not only prepared to please the taste, but upon scientific principles, which insures the best results nutritively.*

—Louisa Stroebele, 1899, 141

*Health is the foundation of all happiness; man can enjoy all earthly pleasures only in the measure of his health.*

—Adolf Just, 1903, 45

*Many thought it very strange and could not understand how it was possible to get the feet warm by cold water or snow. But it is not only that, such treatment also hardens altogether and prevents many diseases, which is quite natural.*

—Sebastian Kneipp, 1904, 38

*People ought to understand that a physician can never cure but only support the natural powers of the patient.*

—Benedict Lust, 1908, 2

*The most noble object of the Nature Cure is to prevent all diseases. If diseases and all the evils of the body are to be prevented each individual must first of all begin to live a more natural life. Almost everybody is guilty of transgression against Nature.*

—Benedict Lust, 1908, 82

*If we stop for a moment to consider that the body is not an assembled machine but a growth from one cell, we will realize that every part of the organism is related to every other part, and related in such a way that no one part can become disordered without affecting every other part.*

—William Freeman Havard, 1920, 235-236

*Our efforts in treating the sick should be directed in assisting Nature in her efforts at restoration. All changes in the human body, whether it is in life of death, are governed by natural laws. We do not break natural laws; they break us.*

—Charles H. Duncan, 1923, 774

## INTRODUCTION

As Naturopaths we discover many sensational therapies. There are some remarkable ones, though, which we may well have missed on our journey because they have slipped into the shadows over the years. *Practice of Naturopathic Medicine* is all about rediscovering those pearls. This book is a collection of articles carefully selected from among the abundance of writing found in Benedict Lust's journals, in particular those published from 1899 to 1923. Here you may be surprised to discover old therapies that feel completely new. Sadly, some of these simply vanished without a trace, not only in the practice repertoire of thousands of contemporary Naturopaths, but also and alarmingly in the didactic and clinical curricula of our accredited schools. Many of these therapies are in the shadows not because they did not work for the patient. On the contrary, their place in the early Naturopathic armamentarium was prominent precisely because they *did* work, and they worked when patient care options were limited and often ghastly. The question of their disappearance from our repertoire isn't rhetorical; it's historical. My hope is that there will be some therapies described in these pages with which you are familiar, after all, or which you will want to know more about. It is my hope too, that the actual words of our forebears will pique your curiosity and make you eager to reintroduce them into your practice.

As I mentioned, even though some of these old therapies appear to have vanished into thin air here in North America, these same therapies can still be found in active use by Naturopaths and medical doctors alike, in other parts of the world. In Europe and Asia, for example, I have happily come across people who are still able to choose key elements of their own health care. They are not corralled by insurance health plans and public health policy into an allopathic cascade. These patients and their health care providers see wisdom and have long experienced results using such therapies. Sadly, though, such places are everyday fewer than before, in the face of biomedicine's highly monetized, invasive, drug- based frameworks and approaches.

The unassuming simplicity of the early Naturopathic therapies may raise the concern that what may have been good a hundred years ago could well be less relevant today. In this regard, some argue that we live in a completely different world which requires different health strategies, a world in which the cumulative effect of multi-generation vaccination regimens, drug therapies, debased food sources and degraded environments constitutes a new normal. In that world we worry a lot that our patients also face a vastly different cultural milieu a century after our founders, a landscape where the popular culture excels at weaning toddlers on iPads and pablum, and exposes them to every imaginable combination of processed food, marketed as wholesome options, but in actuality at high cost to their health. In the stressed, fast culture in which the contemporary Naturopath practices, we worry too about the escalating consequences of sedentary life style choices, with its accompanying obesity crisis, its long list of accompanying chronic diseases, the cumulative effect of all of which is the threat of severe harm to health and economies, even in developed countries. Naturopathic doctors today watch exponential growth in autism levels and other calamities among our young, rampant chronicity among our elderly, and the unnecessary hijacking of almost twenty percent of our GDP by the biomedicine complex.

And never mind the poor in North America and elsewhere, who struggle to get and sustain the simple necessities, such as clean potable water and adequate food for their families and their extended communities. In such a terrain, there has never been a more dire need for the practices of Naturopathic Medicine to be implemented in our communities and embedded in our health care policies. It may well be time, then, to revisit many of the wise therapies our elders practiced with such success in their equally turbulent times. Reviewing the Benedict Lust journals and studying the problems our Naturopathic forebears faced a hundred years ago, I am awed by their bravery and confidence, whether guiding patients toward wise lifestyle choices or treating disease head on. It is not the case that the conditions and diseases that Naturopaths faced were easier. These articles exude their confidence in what they considered to be solid tools of naturopathic practice. Some of the best of those tools you will find in these pages.

The early literature reveals unequivocally that our early elders did not endorse drugs, in the main because they considered them dangerous, but also because drugs were then, as now, not compatible philosophically, or in many cases, pragmatically, with naturopathic teachings and patient care. Today in my corner of North America, we can prescribe pharmaceuticals, but into the bargain we risk migrating away from our philosophical roots. At one time our tools offered certainty and success which kept us aligned with those principles. The terrain of our practice today, though, has been affected by an allopathically determined set of standards of care with which, in those states where the regulatory framework accords us primary care status, we are obligated to comply. This compliance, though, can easily be accompanied by a dilution of confidence in the traditional therapies and approaches of our forebears. With all of the heroic tools at our fingertips, we drift from our traditional therapies in the exchange. It would be one thing if the old therapies did not work; it is quite another, because they do and always have.

There is an irony afoot these days, in that the biomedicine community is steadily co-opting many such traditional tools and ideas. However, it is not an irony which belongs only to the early twentieth century. Ten decades ago Henry Lindlahr himself was enraged that he was censured for his use of natural therapies when treating infected wounds; censured, in fact, by the very Allopaths who often commandeered such natural methods. He reported more than once, when a particular therapy was successful, that it was assimilated by medical doctors with impunity, as if they were its inevitable and natural custodians, responsible for its discovery and success all along. Lindlahr recounts, for example, "Ever since I publicly began to teach and practice Nature Cure, I have maintained in lectures and writings and demonstrated in daily practice, as examples in point, that the natural and most efficient treatment for wounds and open sores consists in exposure to air and light, and that the best of all antiseptics is lemon juice diluted with water." (Lindlahr, 1918, 124)

A lengthy citation is worth a moment here; it points out this unfortunately all too common occurrence faced by Naturopaths of his era, and familiar to us today. I am reminded of the enthusiasm of modern day Allopaths whose 'integrative medicine' pronouncements repeat pointedly that their profession will invade, where convenient, the very spaces our profession held, under duress, for decades. He writes, citing a specific circumstance:

> Some time ago, Chicago dailies announced in a leading article, "The Most Recent Wonderful Discovery of Surgical Science". They related that, thanks to the discovery of a prominent surgeon in one of the great West Side hospitals, wounds were now being treated with uniform success without antiseptics and germicidal agents, and that this revolutionary treatment consisted solely in exposure of the wounds of light and air. The article concluded by saying that such a revolutionary discovery could be made only by a great and learned surgeon. ... Until recently I was in danger of arrest and trial for malpractice for teaching and practicing this very "recent wonderful discovery of surgical science". (Lindlahr, 1918, 124-125)

When we have confidence in the healing power of Nature, and when we rediscover the profound value of Nature's bounty, our practice accumulates into case histories with stunning results. As we read these early accounts of naturopathic practice in the late 19th and early 20th centuries, we must remember to read between the lines "in their own words" the accounts of these early champions of Naturopathic Medicine to grasp their passion and earnest desire to choose the bounty of nature (earth, air, water, nutrition) as the platform of their treatments for patients, above all else. What I love about the actual words of these men and women in

Practice of Naturopathic Medicine is that they invite us to revisit the wisdom and record of their practice.  We encounter our naturopathic elders with a professional intimacy which familiarizes us with the therapies they used to combat disease and which gives us pause to marvel at their heroic attempts to guide their patients back to health.  Their words are rich pearls for us to this very day.

What tools did the early Naturopaths contain in their *armamentarium?*  Let us begin with Louisa Stroebele, whom Lust within a few short years married.  The first article in *Practice of Naturopathic Medicine* comes from one of the first English articles published in the *Amerikanischen Kneipp-Blätter (1896 – 1899)* edited by Benedict Lust.  Long before she met Lust, Louisa Stroebele had created a mountain air resort in Butler, New Jersey, modelled after the work of Father Sebastian Kneipp and Arnold Rikli, both of whom advocated fresh air, sunshine and water therapies.  In addition to her article, Miss Stroebele placed a full page ad for her **Bellevue Retreat Center**.  She was the sole proprietor of this health establishment which would soon be transformed into a "Jungborn" after she and Benedict Lust formed one of the most enduring and championing partnerships that Naturopathic medicine would ever witness.  Their union on June 11, 1901 cemented not only their marriage, but also a unified vision for "Jungborn", and for a new profession, *Naturopathy*.  The catalytic accomplishments of Benedict and Louisa Lust across their lifetime set into motion a health movement, the genesis of Naturopathy.

In this article, we learn about some of the core therapies employed by the early Naturopaths as they enthusiastically embraced Nature and Health.  In 1899, the rudimentary therapies used included an open air swimming pool, air-, sun- and Turkish steam baths, as well as healthy food based upon sound dietetics.  The number of therapeutic offerings would multiply quickly within a couple of years after the appearance of this article.  Stroebele had previously acquired training in dietetics in England, which would become her strong focus while working with Benedict Lust.  She is emphatic here in her description of the importance of healthy food: "At Bellevue, such hygienic surroundings are supplemented by a common-sense diet, cooking being done in such a manner that food is not only prepared to please the taste, but upon scientific principles, which insures the best results nutritively." (Stroebele, 1899, 141)  Bellevue was a mecca for early healthy Dietetic practice, among the dense forests and exquisite hills of the Ramapo Mountains.

Another interesting historical tidbit to be found in this early testament to these two people who were so central to Naturopathy's launch and early growth is the address at the bottom of the page.  The very last line on the page subtly references their cooperation, directing Bellevue patrons from New York to "the City Office: 111 E. 59th St., New York." (Stroebele,

1899, 141)  This was the address of Benedict Lust's first Kneipp Health Store and where he began practicing as an "Hydropathic Physician", one of the very first indications of their collaboration.  Sadly, this building no longer stands.  In its stead we find a large multi-story office building ironically housing today a Botox Clinic on the ground floor.

Stroebele's voice was not solitary.  Women were welcomed as writers and practitioners in the new Naturopathic profession from the very start.  Carola Staden, for example, who practiced alongside her husband Ludwig Staden in their Brooklyn office, writes about a new therapy called the "Thure Brandt system".  Ludwig specialized in pediatrics and hydrotherapy and Carola specialized in gynecology.  The then prevalent use of corsets meant that many women presented in the early 20th century with abdominal and pelvic mutilation accompanied by horrific pain.  The Thure Brandt method of internal massage was developed by an officer in the Swedish Army who later studied at the Central Institute of Massage and Gymnastics of Stockholm. (Staden, 1900, 23)  The Thure Brandt System reminds us of the ancient Mayan abdominal massage, a non-invasive external massage that gently guides the uterus in place for women.  Staden became an advocate of this massage therapy, helping women with uterine displacements and pelvic distress.  She describes the procedure as an "internal massage [in which] Thure Brandt combines a long series of gymnastic movements." (Staden, 1900, 23)  Others such as Henry Lindlahr and the Lusts also embraced this massage therapy for women in their own clinics.

In the third article of this book, we encounter an emerging fascination with electricity as a healing modality in this era.  In 1900 electricity was brand new and the discoveries of Roentgen's x-rays and Marconi's wireless telegraph stimulated interest to extrapolate possibilities for the use of electricity in treating the human body.  As an example of such strong interest is G. H. Schaefer's exuberance for electricity.  He exclaims, "Electricity is present, not only in all the objects of nature about us, but also in every human and animal being; therefore, I maintain that it is this which constitutes the primal cause and preservative force of the life of functions." (Schaefer, 1900, 110)  His enthusiasm overflows with examples of what this new science had to offer the naturopathic health field.  In one, he describes the work of, Jacob von Narkiewiez-Jodko, a Russian, who in 1896 "by means of experiments in the domain of electricity which he conducted for years, succeeded with the aid of photography in getting the results of his examination of the electric phenomena of both healthy and sick people in a permanent form". (Schaefer, 1900, 110)  Narkiewiez-Jodko's photography experiments are quite similar to the Kirlian photographs capturing auras and electrical fields which were discovered later in 1939.

Schaefer was so enamored with the new field of electricity that he could see no wrong in exploring its use. Just as today, we find ourselves worried by the suffering of our patients, our search for a therapy to help them is ever constant. In this regard, Schaefer developed a device in which he had full confidence. He states, "I maintain that every disease, call it what you will, may be cured with my apparatus, provided the organs, structure, tissues and cells are still in a condition to perform the physical and chemical functions necessary to a cure." (Schaefer, 1900, 111) Notwithstanding Schaefer's enthusiasm and enterprise, some of these early electrical devices were fraught with problems such as electrical shocks and were not as harmless as Schaefer maintained. Electrotherapy evolved and in the next couple of decades, we see the progression.

While the field of electricity applied to health devices and protocols captured some Naturopaths' attention, water therapies were consistently their favorite therapeutic tools. In the early days of Naturopathy, the literature shows repeatedly that Father Sebastian Kneipp exerted enormous influence on the treatments used. For example, his theory of *hardening* was central to hydrotherapy. Benedict Lust explains: "By hardening the constitution we mean making it capable of resistance, especially to cold, and of remaining unaffected by unfavorable weather." (Lust, 1900, 152) The use of cold water was an important element in hardening and Lust gives details on how to harden the body. "The best means of hardening the system are, however, short cold ablutions and baths of no longer than a minute's duration." (Lust, 1900, 152) Kneipp had a reputation for applying freezing cold water on his patients; yet, the length of time involved in exposing the body to cold was extremely short. It is worth noting, though, that what the early water cure practitioners perceived as acceptably warm, we would experience in our day as being shockingly cold. Our love affair with hot showers and baths has displaced the neutral or cool waters, characterizing them as intolerable.

Indeed, our aversion to cold temperatures has redefined cool and neutral temperatures as not appropriate for our patients. Cold waters for hardening in multiple forms were the main therapies offered at the early health sanitariums in North America. Earlier, I mentioned Louisa Stroebele's Bellevue health retreat where she and her staff provided baths and good nutritious meals to complement Kneipp and Rikli's water cure and sun cure therapies. In 1901, we see another infomercial describing the therapies now offered at Butler, New Jersey. The name, Bellevue, has been replaced with "Jungborn" and the offerings have multiplied. Another very significant detail in this ad placed by Benedict and now Louisa Lust in July, 1901 is that the former health retreat center has a dual mission of offering courses in Naturopathy as well as being a health haven.

Prior to this date, in fact, the word "Naturopathy" is absent in the

Lust journals. While Sebastian Kneipp is front and center in this ad, we are witnessing a subtle transformation of Kneippianism that dominated the previous Bellevue and the emergence of Naturopathy when we review the list of therapies offered at the Jungborn. The change of the name of the health establishment offers clues about the transformation. *Jungborn* as the new name was a significant and monumental change. First, Jungborn was the creation of Adolf Just, a young German who revolutionized and introduced a consciousness of health with his book, *Return to Nature* in 1896. Lust became a Nature enthusiast following Just's recommendations in his book. It is important to recall that Just's book was published five years after Louis Kuhne's book, *The New Science of Healing* [1891] and that both of these books left an indelible mark on the young men and women pioneers of Naturopathy. In essence, the therapies introduced by Kuhne, such as the "frugivorous diet", the "friction hip bath" and the "steam bath", as well as the earth cures and the vegetarian diet derived from Just's *Return to Nature* had a huge impact on the form and function of Naturopathy, determining much of its future.

Before Kuhne and Just, the Kneippian water cure treatments had dominated the therapies offered by the Kneipp adherents in America, Benedict Lust and Louisa Lust among them. But after the publication of Kuhne's book, shifts and innovations slowly transformed the sanitariums. Just's book was the impetus that opened up the gates to embrace all that Nature had in her bosom. So, as one reads the activities offered at the new Jungborn in Butler, New Jersey in 1901, one can profoundly appreciate the vision and earnest love that Benedict and Louisa Lust had for Naturopathy. The inclusion and expansion of therapies now include "hip baths [Kuhne], ... whole or partial sand baths and ... [and]sleeping in the open air [Just]" (Lust, 1901, 198) When reading their list of therapies offered, who wouldn't want to go there to restore his or her health? The Jungborn was birthed in 1901 and became a center for health enthusiasts from around the world. The reach of the Lusts was quickly that broad.

One of the treatments offered at the Jungborn was massage. What becomes evident is that when new devices were invented and new therapies discovered, Benedict Lust made a point of including articles about them in his journals for others to discover and try. The "massage roller", for example, was quite popular with the early Naturopaths, quickly becoming a useful, new tool to deliver massage therapy in a novel way. New therapies always had an irresistible attraction for Naturopaths, who were consistently eager to try the latest and the newest methods in their quest to help their patients. The Massage Roller was "devised by a New York physician, Dr. W. E. Forest" (Lust, 1901, 245) and could be used by the patient herself or by a practitioner on the patient. Massage rollers still continue to be a consumer item for those who want a convenient fix for pain. These rollers, for example, were touted as being valuable in the treatment every possible condition a patient could present with when walking into a clinic. Lust elaborates: "The Massage Rollers can be used for all functional troubles like dyspepsia, constipation, biliousness, nervous exhaustion, neuralgia, rheumatism, obesity, etc., and used over the entire body they will be found a great promoter of health and muscular elasticity." (Lust, 1901, 245)  Lust offers numerous examples of how to use the Massage Roller.

Physical ailments needing to be treated could easily be addressed by starting off with a home remedy such as the massage roller; however, physical therapies would soon evolve and find expression in other medical systems such as Osteopathy. In his journals, Lust included many articles written by Osteopaths about Osteopathy. In these same early days of Naturopathy's genesis, there was a kinship which grew between the Osteopaths and Naturopaths. Both struggled against the menacing tactics of the Allopaths and both had a respect for Nature. The complete assimilation of Osteopathy as an allopathic medical profession in the modern era would have seemed unlikely in the early days of Naturopathy.

Osteopath George Boller provides an historical account of the rising profession of Osteopathy, ally to Naturopathy in that era. He writes, "Osteopathy was discovered and developed by Andrew Taylor Still, M.D. in 1874." (Boller, 1901, 269)  Boller cites the fundamental principle of Osteopathic therapeutics, remarkably resonating with Naturopathy. He says, "Attention is paid to the general health of the patient, by specific manipulation to the body tissue, so as to promote free circulation of the body fluids, along with attendance to correct hygienic and dietetic rules." (Boller, 1901, 270)  At this time, Osteopathy still had its roots in Nature and had not yet been co-opted by the allopathic paradigm. Boller's conclusion points out this early symmetry and common ground between the two emerging professions: "[Osteopathy] uses all the therapeutic principles, from a standpoint of nature, such as the use of proper hygienic and dietetic principles, and in fact any principle that is in the line of nature or natural laws of the human body." (Boller, 1901, 271)

The Osteopaths of today have moved away from this philosophical core, having migrated to the biomedicine paradigms, therapies and scope reflected by USMLE/LCME frameworks for curriculum and clinical training; a long way from their roots. Naturopaths, however, have remained closer to their roots, despite the so-called *green allopath* or the more recent *integrative* inclinations of some of our colleagues. Certainly, the remarkable statement made by the presence of a Jungborn, with its programs and protocols, would have been stabilizing and reinforcing for our struggling forebears as biomedicine invaded every quarter of health promotion, public policy and health care funding.

Central to the Jungborn, in those early days, was its location in the middle of Nature, with abundant opportunities to get plenty of fresh air and exercise. Richard Metcalfe, reporting from that era, reports that exercise and "a strong love of activity implanted [in people] by Nature" were powerful catalysts for lifelong wellness and enduring vitality. (Metcalfe, 1901, 312)   Exercise was seen as a vital factor to cultivate the conditions of a healthy, strong and supple body and Metcalfe is quick to remind us that we must make our exercise fun and enjoyable. He states, "It is not sufficient to go daily through a fixed and circumscribed mode of taking exercise. Besides becoming monotonous and spiritless, it only puts in motion a certain set of muscles." (Metcalfe, 1901, 312) Metcalfe also had much to say about another growing feature of American life, sedentary habits. The hours of sedentary occupations such as office work were as problematic a century ago as today. Metcalfe comments, "Persons confined to the desk or study frequently suffer from this cause; the few muscles brought into play are overstrained, but the bulk of them, as well as the bones, become weak from disease, and general debility follows." (Metcalfe, 1901, 313)  How miserable to be sitting all day.

In a short and insightful article in the first issue of the first Naturopathic journal, *The Naturopath and Herald of Health,* we again encounter Louisa Lust.  She writes with wit about annoying people and how they impact our lives.  She describes self-righteous, nagging, jealous, complaining people with humorous anecdotal comments, tallying up a long list of such "provokers".  Here is one of her examples: "Of course, there are the jealous people who make life miserable for us.  When it is real, with wholesome blood and thundering jealousy which cuts our throats or burns down our houses, the authorities take it in hand; but there is also a smoldering, slumbering kind with their covert envy, who wish us ill without our knowing it.  That is the deadly kind." (Lust, 1902, 42) Louisa, even though she was generally a quiet person who stood behind her husband, also had a great sense of humor and was willing to share it. She ends her piece with a self-reflection that we could all heed on occasion: "But do you know, I sometimes wonder privately if I am, perchance, a provoking person myself." (Lust, 1902, 42)

Following the advice given by Louisa Lust, we come to an article by Karl Kabisch who shares his wisdom about how natural healing agents work.  Today, we are in an addictive relationship with pharmaceuticals and yet a century ago, the drug culture was in its infancy.  In this era, Kabisch felt that he needed to explain to those who faithfully relied on drugs how Naturopathy worked. Kabisch states, "The majority of people, when they hear the name Natural-Healing or Naturopathy, have no conception whatever as to the multitude of healing agents over which this method disposes, hence they fail to comprehend how a disease can be cured by means, other than medication." (Kabisch, 1902, 65) He lists the therapies that Naturopaths had at their fingertips: water cure, massage, electricity, vibration, and magnetism, to name a few.

Kabisch's article was written in February, 1902, and appears in the second issue of *The Naturopath and Herald of Health*. Naturopathy is just being launched and articles were published to explain what Naturopathy was to a public who had no idea. Cold water was one of the main therapies used by the early Naturopath. It is hard to believe that a simple bath was therapeutic, but in 1902 the leading causes of mortality were the flu and pneumonia. His comment on the flu: "I have treated and am still treating many influenza patients and must say that they and their people usually recover their health and strength with astonishing rapidity, under Naturopathic treatment." (Kabisch, 1902, 67) We are counselled by Kabisch to administer water treatments to ourselves so that we can teach our patients. Kabisch extols the benefits of Naturopathy, writing further, "Another advantage of Naturopathy consists in its pleasant treatment. How bitter and disagreeable is medicine sometimes; and on the other hand, how agreeable and pleasant is a bath, a poultice, a vapor-bath, gargle or inhalation! Finally, I would like to mention as decided advantage of Naturopathy, that it makes us independent." This article written by Kabisch 112 years ago provides wise counsel and good examples to carry back to our own clinics.

In another article in the same 1902 February issue, Naturopath, A. L. Wood writes about the "Influence of Water on Health and Longevity". Wood continues on the subject of how to be healthy. Wood does not claim that health is only achieved with water, and includes fresh air, exercise, rest and mental health. To live a long and meaningful life is far more important than "to simply exist for a great number of years, a burden to yourself and friends, as is too often the case, and both undesirable and unnecessary". (Wood, 1902, 74) On the subject of how much water we should consume, Wood cites Dr. John Nutt, "Very few Americans drink enough water. Eight to ten glasses of water should be taken," (Wood, 1902, 76) Early writers like Wood often focused on counseling people about how to live. Drinking, eating, breathing, exercising, sleeping, working, thinking and living were the topics of Naturopathy a century ago.

If anyone had the ear of Nature herself, it would have been Adolf Just. He was 37 years old when he published *Return to Nature,* an international best seller of his day. He embraced the wonders of Nature and wrote about her gifts of healing. He described in great detail the use of earth cure for a host of diseases. Just declared, "Health is the foundation of all happiness; man can enjoy all earthly pleasures only in the measure of his health." (Just, 1903, 45) To promote and enable what he thought to be genuine health, Just built a sanitarium called the Jungborn [the name imitated by the Lusts in New Jersey some years later] in Germany's Harz Mountains, where he could show others how to live and be healthy. Adolf Just was the first to sing the praises of "earthing" and to call attention to "the earth's vibratory powers for health restoration".

When he was very sick, Just discovered for himself, that sleeping directly on the earth was restorative. In fact, he advocated sleeping outdoors in all seasons. He professes, "We shall thus soon become aware that nature rewards every step that is taken toward her, for it is still more beneficial and healthful to sleep entirely in the open, than in a light-and-air hut." (Just, 1903, 46) The air-and-light houses were adopted by many in their sanitariums including the Lusts' Jungborn in Butler, New Jersey. These ventilated houses allowed people to enjoy extremes of sunshine and air during the day, and "to have protection during the night against rain; during fair weather it is advisable to place the bed outside the cottage and sleep entirely in the open." (Just, 1903, 46) Just exulted the merits of sleeping outdoors in the fresh air to gain mastery of one's health and was passionate about helping others in their search for health at his Jungborn.

With the same conviction Just embraces overall health, stating, "Health is the foundation of all happiness," (Just, 1903, 45) Augusta Vescilius praises music for its "distinct influence upon life and health". (Vescilius, 1903, 152) Musical therapeutics in her view helped to sooth and relax. She suggests that "the influence of certain keys is that they stimulate and arouse, while others soothe and quiet". (Vescilius, 1903, 153) Music as a healing modality can still be found in the work of toning and in the sacred sounds of Tibetan music bowls. As mentioned earlier, the early literature shows that Naturopaths were esoteric in their choice of healing tools, embracing new ideas and techniques often. In their search for therapies and approaches to wellness, it is not surprising that they included the power of healing music and sound.

Indeed, from celestial realms of music to intestinal regularity, the spectrum of Naturopathic care was extensive and eclectic. Naturopaths also viewed the less elegant process of elimination as a powerful factor in retaining health. In this regard, the enema was praised for its ability "to wash out the intestines and stimulate the peristaltic action". (Lust, 1903, 330) Benedict Lust makes clear that the enema needs to be used correctly and provides instructions on its proper administration. In the case of chronic constipation, he advised that "an enema should never be given until a suppository has been inserted into the rectum and taken effect." (Lust, 1903. 330) Such detail as the use of the enema gives us an insight into its methodology and also into the reasoning that the Naturopaths applied to their various therapies and approaches.

In the next very short article, we get a glimpse into how hypnotism was used in a case involving the amputation of a woman's leg. This article must have astonished many at the time, noting that no drugs such as chloroform were used to anesthetize the patient during surgery. The woman undergoing the surgery claimed that all she felt were "pins and needles. The doctor reported that there were absolutely no symptoms of shock, and that her pulse and temperature were normal." (Lust, 1903, 339) Advertisements appearing in the Lust journals revealed that hypnosis was used by several early Naturopaths as one of their many modalities.

Kneipp left behind three books on water cure which continue to be relevant and invaluable for Naturopathy. The next article reminds us that all things "water" were associated in early naturopathic practice with Kneipp, whose chief contribution was his concept of hardening. Hardening was achieved easily using Kneipp's signature treatments, which were the gush and walking barefoot on the early morning grass covered in dew, or in the very extreme, walking in the snow in the winter. Kneipp viewed the benefits of the snow as most valuable in the promotion of health. Kneipp elaborates, "Nothing else can be more recommended to young and old than walking bare-footed in snow." (Kneipp, 1904, 38) Walking on snow drew blood from the head to the feet, relieving people suffering from headaches. Another great benefit from *snow walking* was aiding those who suffered from cold feet. Kneipp comments, "Many thought it very strange and could not understand how it was possible to get the feet warm by cold water or snow." (Kneipp, 1904, 39)

Of course, snow walking came with some guidelines that Kneipp devised to make the treatment more efficacious. Kneipp recounts a case of rheumatism that ended well after using snow as the means to eliminate pain. Our current abandonment of cold and cold water might induce us to think that these men and women got it all wrong. Especially when reviewing the many articles on cold water and their miraculous outcomes, though, we can see that we may well need to explore these extraordinary practice pearls from the past to understand cold in a new way.

In that era, the use of cold water was popular and its benefits stellar. Breathing, however, also had a surprisingly significant place in our therapeutic armamentarium. Other than for relaxation or in certain forms and modulations as a stress relief technique, our current naturopathic practice is almost devoid of breathing exercises as a therapy. The early Naturopaths, though, left behind a profusion of articles on breathing therapies. I have collected articles and have compiled a file over an inch thick just on breathing from these early days. This is a neglected and deserted field that may enhance our practice should we grasp the importance of breathing once again. In one of the many articles on breathing, Benedict Lust introduces the "breathing cure" as "pneumathotherapy". Lust is quick to allude to the number of breathing schools verging on "charlatanism" and reminds us that "the best School of Breathing is a sleeping child". (Lust, 1904, 52) The child demonstrates the perfect breath with his/her diaphragmatic breathing.

Lust leaves with us seven suggestions, some of which are quite important to remember, "Never breathe through the mouth ... [and] remember that posture is a vital point." (Lust, 1904, 53) We must bear in mind that a century ago, we were not as grounded in the basic medical sciences and physiology as we are today. Since the days of the early Naturopaths, the work of Konstantin Buteyko, Claude Lum and others have expanded our scientific knowledge such that we understand that hypoxia and hypocapnia have real consequences; so that our awareness of breathing is essential for patient management and care.

In the following article, we revisit Adolf Just's *Return to Nature* through the lens of an Osteopath, Dr. C. W. Young, whose work we cited earlier and who appeared often in Lust's journals. Just's impact upon the North American Naturopaths also included the Osteopaths, who classified Osteopathy as "an independent therapeutic system, and as such includes within everything natural, excluding everything foreign or alien to the body organisms." (Young, 1904, 66) C. W. Young embraced the same virtues of Nature as the Naturopaths and also became a huge fan of Adolf Just. In a book review published in *The Naturopath and Herald of Health,* Young unfolds the Just story. As a sidebar to this piece, we learn that the book can be obtained from Benedict Lust's office at 124 E. 59th St. in NYC. This new address is Benedict's second office center in New York and was conveniently located very close to Park Avenue. Today, this building has been obliterated and replaced with a GNC store.

In any case, Young asserts, "The most remarkable claims of *Return to Nature* are made respecting the earth power." (Young, 1904, 69) Alluded to in an earlier article in this collection, Just's writing about his therapies of earth also encompassed baths, compresses and a place for sleeping. Sleeping on the earth was extolled by many. Today, there is a movement of "earthing" which simulates sleeping on the earth for its healing frequencies and vibrations. A century ago, Adolf Just originated sleeping on the earth to "receive a sensation of new health, new life and new ... vigor and strength". (Young, 1904, 69) Young says, "Whoever has not himself tried it and convinced himself of it, can have no conception of how refreshing, vitalizing and strengthening the effect of the earth is on the human organism at night during rest." (Young, 1904, 69)

Sleeping on the earth was not limited to the night but was also a part of "heliotherapy", or sun cure. Sun baths were offered as a therapy at the early sanitariums. People would come from the cities to the country retreat centers to take their sun bath, either with loose, porous, or no clothing at all. Lust provides suggestions: "In the hot sun the bath must be modified, perhaps alternating between sun and shade. Direct contact with the earth is essential." (Lust, 1904, 87) The sun baths were also accompanied with air baths, or "aerotherapy". Aerotherapy was a response to the era of confining and awkward clothing styles.

Naturopathy's choices for garments were loose and made of textiles that included a variety of cottons, linen and ramie which were "non-conducting, non-irritating, non-saturable, refreshing, comfortable and clean". (Lust, 1904, 89) Lust provides guidance here around clothing, which may at first seem to us out of the sphere of Naturopathy; however, we must bear in mind that Naturopathy was educating people about healthy ways of living at a time when the social norms were often based upon antiquated traditions that often were uncomfortable and led to irritation and pain. Some examples include ill-fitting shoes, the widespread use of wool under garments, and the hour glass waist lines that women were condemned to achieve with their corsets. Naturopaths offered choices to people with sandals, cotton and loose fitting under wear. Lust stressed that "simplicity in dress [was] the third requirement of Nature". (Lust, 1905, 3) We take for granted that shoes and clothing are comfortable; however, our ancestors were hampered and pained by the clothing and shoe options available to them.

Naturopaths taught their patients that Nature provided all of the factors ensuring good health. Long before the advent of Vitamin D deficiencies, it was so obvious to them that fresh air and sunlight were essentials to good health, yet they knew that their patients, not unlike our own, spent most of their working days indoors. Benedict Lust follows with an absolute truth: "An abundance of Light and Air is the first condition of Life." (Lust, 1905, 3) Lust speaks also of meaningful work as another condition of living well. In the early 20th century, laborers were required to work long days, often 10 to 14 hours daily, with a half a day of rest for every two weeks of work. He states, "Unnatural sedentary habits always bear the stamp of deterioration and weakness, and we therefore honor the attempts to obtain an 8 hour day for those performing sedentary work indoors." (Lust, 1905, 5) The eight hour work day was endorsed very early on by Naturopaths. Along with work, rest was also considered as a necessary factor in health. The Work Cure and the Rest Cure were considered to be central to healthy living.

Work, to be sure, involved different parameters at the beginning of the 20th century than today. Lust, himself worked as a waiter when he first moved to America, putting in long hours with his half a day off every two weeks. It would surprise us, then, to discover that our early forebears had many ways of overcoming the impact of such long work hours on the health of their patients. They evolved therapies to help address some of the physical injuries sustained from over-exertion. Chiropractic was one of these physical therapies, developed by Dr. D. D. Palmer in 1886. "It took years to discover and develop that which was named Chiropractic, which means hand-fixing. A Chiropractor is one who adjusts or repairs with his hands." (Palmer, 1905, 287) B. J. Palmer, the son of D. D. Palmer goes on to describe the mechanism of Chiropractic:

> Chiropractic finds the cause in pinched nerves of the person ailing, and releases that pressure by adjusting some of the 52 articulations of the vertebral column. In doing this, there is no rubbing, slapping, knife, drugs, artificial heat, electricity, magnetism, hypnotism, stretching or mental treatment, in fact nothing but the adjustment of the displaced vertebra. (Palmer, 1905, 287)

Advertisements of Chiropractors and the Davenport Palmer Chiropractic College would appear frequently in the Lust journals. In the beginning there was common ground between the Chiropractors and the Naturopaths, but as each grew in numbers and strength, a falling out occurred, manifesting ultimately in the demise of the single, remaining Naturopathic program in America by mid-century at Western States Chiropractic College in Portland, Oregon.

The early literature shows that each inventor of a new healing modality would profess at one point or another in the introduction and spread of his system, that he had found the panacea for all illnesses. Such was the belief of Adolf Just, for example, who would be associated with Earth Cure. His claims were sincere and rested upon the laws of Nature. Just insists, "If we really care for our health and bodily well-being, we have again to listen to the language of Nature and try to understand it." (Just, 1906, 23) He found that compresses made with earth, rather than the cold water used by Kneipp and Priessnitz, were far superior. His conviction was firm that earth as a remedy may be a "universal panacea for many troubles". (Just, 1906, 23) The earth abdominal compress, as a case in point, had marvelous outcomes. Just avows, "As the damp earth produces such wonderful effects on the abdomen by drawing out heat and strengthening of the digestive organs, its application is of great importance in such diseases as nervousness, insomnia, melancholia, fever and so forth." (Just, 1906, 23) Having used earth compresses for wounds, burns, cuts, bruises, herpes outbreaks, and excruciating pains, I can attest to Just's complete confidence in earth cure.

Today, earth cure has another label: Peloid therapy, which is essentially the use of mud, peat, clay and other earth materials for the purpose of healing. Peloids are being researched and used in Russia, Germany, Hungary, Czech Republic, Israel, Turkey and numerous other countries where healers still retain their belief in Nature and Balneotherapy. Adolf

Just was the first to bring peloid therapies into prominence, and we are grateful for his insights. Just says, "Packs of earth strengthen and cure the limbs or any part of the body; while lying on the earth cures excitements and feverish conditions." (Just, 1906, 24)

Adolf Just's place in the Naturopathic story is much larger than is commonly understood. He loved Nature and Earth Cure and his book which is often cited in these pages, *Return to Nature* (1896) became an essential textbook for the early Naturopaths. Another giant whose contributions to the foundations of Naturopathy is also less well known is Louis Kuhne. His 1891 book, *The New Science of Healing*, was an indispensable and vital book that every aspiring Naturopath owned. Louis Kuhne, who like Just was revered by the early pioneers of Naturopathy, "was the first one to emphasize the unity of all diseases". (Knoch, 1906, 53) Hans Knoch writes of Kuhne: "Disease is the presence of morbid matter or foreign bodies in the organism. Thus, there is only one cause of disease and also only one disease which comes up in different forms, according to what organ is affected." (Knoch, 1906, 53) From Kuhne we inherited a treatment called the Friction Hip Bath. With this bath, administered in a sitz tub, Kuhne treated successfully many forms of diseases. Kuhne's cites in the last chapter of *The New Science of Healing* 133 cases of a diverse diseases treated in his Sanitarium using the friction hip bath. In the article by Knoch, "The Kuhne Cure", we are given all of the details of Kuhne's procedures for his Friction Sitz Bath.

Knoch also writes about the work of Arnold Rikli, who championed the "Atmospheric Cure" in Veldes, Switzerland. Knoch writes, "Arnold Rikli has received recognition and admiration even from his opponents and opened the way for the triumph of the light-and-air baths." (Knoch, 1906, 58) Louisa Lust was a follower of Rikli and opened her sanitarium in Butler imitating Rikli's model of air-and-light baths. Rikli's sanitarium was located in the Swiss Alps and would become the treatment of choice for tuberculosis which ravaged people in the 19th and early 20th centuries.

The early Naturopaths knew the intricate balance between Mind and Body and made room for inclusion of all branches of Mind Culture. An example of how they embraced in their practice this mind body connection was with humor. The "Laughing Cure" was presented by Edward Earle Purinton as the ultimate healing for the soul. Purinton wrote many articles for *The Naturopath and Herald of Health* and was a man of many words. Some of his comments regarding women were crude and unkind and do not bear repeating. Some of his other insights and commentaries, though, were timely and astute. His contemporaries considered him strange, quirky and a savant. Regarding the laughing cure, Purinton states, "Laughter is the universal solvent of human woes." (Purinton,

1906, 271)  He leaves with us a comprehensive list of 13 reasons why laughter is medicine.  His first admonition is that laughter "jiggers the diaphragm and unkinks the solar plexus" and his second, that laughter "mollifies surly stomach and corrects recalcitrant liver". (Purinton, 1906, 271)  You are sure to be entertained by his colourful use of words.  He is determined to make you laugh with him.

Our sense of humor helps to dispel fear and anxiety.  Purinton adds, "A clear laugh, like a ray of sunlight, shows just where cobwebs are." (Purinton, 1906, 273)  Just as laughter is compared to sunlight, the spring season brings to us a new lease on life.  Lust says, "If any season of the year bears a message of good cheer and hopefulness to the sick and suffering, it is the season of Spring." (Lust, 1907, 139)  Our habits during the winter are often plagued with over eating festive and rich foods, lack of exercise, and remaining indoors.  He continues, "The vital spirits are quickened, the dormant cells stirred into activity and, where the body is sick, efforts are made by the organism to cast out its poisons. Sometimes the body succeeds without any external assistance." (Lust, 1907, 139)  The Spring Cleanse, in particular, was a time to restore the body "back to its normal, healthy condition". (Lust, 1907, 139)  Lust and others contributed many articles advocating a diet of spring vegetables to help the body cleanse itself.  And what better place to accomplish all of this, than Jungborn itself.

The Jungborn [or the Yungborn as it was often called] that Benedict and Louisa Lust operated was a perfect venue for people to come to for health restoration.  Lust proudly states, "All modern curative methods known to Naturopathy are employed at the Jungborn and patients have the advantage of mountain climbing and walks for hours in the beautiful private parks belonging to the sanitarium, etc." (Lust, 1907, 140)  Having visited the site where the Butler Jungborn stood, I can attest to the majestic beauty and peace one feels in those woods.  The food served at the Jungborn included "the various kinds of nuts which must be deemed principal ingredients of human food and to the fine fruits and berries that are raised and gathered on the property, there is always found a bountiful supply of imported foreign fruit, such as oranges, figs, dates, mangoes, bananas, etc." (Lust, 1907, 140)

The therapies available during the Spring Cleanse at the Jungborn included earth cure, air and sun baths and, of course, the Kneipp water treatments.  Away from the Jungborn, water and air cure constituted a large part of the Naturopath's tools used in their practice, whatever their location. Despite the familiarity of Nature Cure to Naturopaths, the need to educate the public about what Naturopathy had to offer was an ongoing effort.  In a lecture delivered to the German Nature Cure Society in New York City, Benedict Lust provides the secret to health, "The keynote of Nature-Cure is *without hardening, no strong health.*" (Lust, 1908, 1) He continues, "We partisans of the natural cure live up to our principles: follow Nature." (Lust, 1908, 2) Lust also referenced another key element of Nature Cure and that is, *prevention.* He says, "The most noble object of the Nature Cure is to prevent all disease." (Lust, 1908, 82) The consensus for the early Naturopaths of what constituted health was crystal clear. Lust reiterates what others shared: "Not until humanity has returned to Nature and has begun to obey her laws can the general condition be improved." (Lust, 1908, 82)

An example given by S. T. Erieg on how to live within the laws of Nature was taking a walk in the early morning. Erieg exclaims, "The air at early morning is different than at any other time of the day; it is more invigorating, more life producing; it permeates the body with health and the brain with clearness." (Erieg, 1908, 179) He continues on the importance of walking, "There is no exercise that affords so much pleasure and holds so much in store as the means of walking." (Erieg, 1908, 170)

Another therapy that was embraced by Naturopaths was Homeopathy. Dr. Rudolf Weil expressed his displeasure with his own colleagues and their "great ignorance of the nature of Homeopathy". (Weil, 1908, 297) He adds, "Nothing hinders the art of healing more than narrow-mindedness and stubborn loyalty to a certain principle." (Weil, 1908, 299) He viewed Homeopathy as a kindred complement and entirely harmonious with the water, light and air treatments found in Naturopathy. He states, "After long experience I believe that Homeopathy combined with the natural healing agents will produce the best and speediest results." (Weil, 1908, 299) The clinical successes of Homeopathy found in the Homeopathic Journals during the numerous epidemics that ravaged America are testament to its superiority as a medical system.

Jaquemin's article, next in this collection, stresses the importance of "Climatology" in Naturopathy. Climatology was a branch of medicine begun in the 19th century that studied the influence of climate on health and disease. There is a journal that exists still today that can be viewed online called *Archives of Transactions of the American Clinical and Climatological Association [ACCA].* The ACCA publications began in 1884 and have endured until the present day. We can glean from these invaluable historical documents the dialogue that took place on climate and Balneotherapy even among the early Allopaths before their practice domains became dominated by pharmaceuticals.

In the early 20th century, tuberculosis continued to be a health menace and was the second leading cause of mortality in the USA. Knowing what kind of climate these patients needed and where to send these patients for a cure was investigated with rigor. Jaquemin writes, "Whatever the differences of climate and of the meteorological factors at the various health resorts may be, one thing is demanded of all: air free from dust and smoke." (Jaquemin, 1909, 416) Taking in all of the factors of mountainous altitudes, Jaquemin states, "the climate of high altitudes is highly recommended for consumption, especially in winter". Sanitariums were built for consumption patients in mountainous areas where the air was free from dust and optimal air pressure and humidity were found. At the time, sanitariums were abundant in Europe and lacking in the United States. Jaquemin provides the reader with an analysis of some of the sanitariums found in Switzerland, Germany, and France. He writes with optimism, "We trust that in the United States, the great leader in philanthropic enterprises, there will soon spring up Sanitaria in every state, where the poor may be restored to health." (Jaquemin, 1909, 418)

Whatever the questions raised by Naturopaths regarding what constituted healthy conditions, whether these included climate, exercise, or food, their intent was to find the elements needed to help their patients. For example, Ludwig Staden had a clinic in Brooklyn, NY that he operated with his wife, Carola Staden. Ludwig Staden poses a question that still reverberates amongst Naturopaths: "Are the inorganic salts better and more profitably assimilated from the vegetable or from the mineral kingdom, especially in case of disease, or is there no difference at all in the assimilation from the two kingdoms?" (Staden, 1909, 618) This question hinges on Staden's belief that the foods that we consume are forms of vitalistic energy or 'Prana' as he mentions. His contribution to the discussion of the vital force inherent in organic matter leads us to Schuessler and his twelve mineral salts. Staden endorses highly the Schuessler salts and reminds us that "the same life force is the quintessence of organic and inorganic matter, higher in degree in the vegetable, lower in the mineral, [and thus] we comprehend why we will look in general for the supply of inorganic salts from the vegetable and in special from the mineral kingdom." (Staden, 1909, 619)

The next article returns us to a therapy we encountered earlier in this collection, namely, Earth Cure. Earth Cure, as emphasized before, was prominent a century ago. In Robert Bieri's article on "The Healing Power of Clay", we are enlightened with a little history to demonstrate that earth as a healing modality had been with us long before Adolf Just wrote his pivotal book in 1896. Bieri cites examples from Africa and the Orient of various peoples "using moist earth for their open wounds and all skin diseases". (Bieri, 1909, 620) Bieri also talks of the magnetic qualities of the earth and when we live "in accord in with Nature's laws to regain perfect happiness, [it] does not take us long to see for ourselves that the earth has a most refreshing, invigorating and salutary influence as soon as you come into direct touch with it." (Bieri, 1909, 620)

His subject is clay and he includes examples for us to see how clay is therapeutic. For example, "The action of clay is first of all absorbent, acting as a sponge, capable of extracting uric acid accumulation from any part of our body, and all other poisonous matter which has caused us acute or chronic diseases." (Bieri, 1909, 622)  He includes in his list of poisonous matter, "bacilli, bacteria, microbes … streptococcus" (Bieri, 1909, 622)  We know clay as a powerful adsorptive agent capable of removing from our body's toxins, impurities and arrest the growth and spread of viruses and bacteria. (Arledge, 2008)  Bieri's passion for clay shows up crisply in his writing.

Another leader of this period who studied and practiced with a respect and fervent passion for Nature is Henry Lindlahr.  Both Lindlahr and Lust arrived on the shores of America at the age of 20 and both had sought the help of Father Kneipp to restore them to health.  Lindlahr went with diabetes and Lust with tuberculosis and neurasthenia.  Like Lust, Lindlahr yearned to communicate a deep and wide comprehension of the laws of Nature, with the goal of teaching others, in his case, the practice of what he branded as "Nature Cure".  The importance of diagnostic skills is vital for the Naturopath and no one believed that more full-heartedly than Lindlahr.  He states, "Correct diagnosis is the first essential to intelligent treatment, but there are as many and widely divergent methods of diagnosis as there are systems of treatment." (Lindlahr, 1910, 28)  For his part, Lindlahr was smitten with iridology as a diagnostic tool.  He wrote often on this subject, giving Naturopaths tools of invaluable importance.  Our collection here includes only two of the many written by Lindlahr.

In the first, "The Scurf Rim", Lindlahr introduces valuable insights into the skin and lungs.  The scurf rim is the dark ring found on the outer periphery of the iris.  A dark scurf rim indicates that "the skin is weak, enervated, relaxed and anemic". (Lindlahr, 1910, 263)  Lindlahr verifies, "The scurf rim is therefore a reliable indicator of the normal or abnormal condition of the skin.  This becomes of eminent importance in diagnosis and prognosis when we consider that the skin is the largest and most effective organ of elimination." (Lindlahr, 1910, 264)  Lindlahr addresses factors contributing to defective skin conditions and includes the role that uric acid plays.  He gives an interesting diagnostic test to determine uric acid levels in the body.  "The degree of uric acid precipitation in the surface blood vessels may be accurately determined in the following manner by the reflux test." (Lindlahr, 1910, 265)

Some of Lindlahr's terminology reflects his passion for Hahnemann and Homeopathy.  In the second article, "Itch or Psora Spots", he presents the theory of psora and rolls out the connections between Homeopathy and Iridology.  He explains, "The word psora was adapted by Hahnemann, the father of Homeopathy, from a Greek word signifying "itching", and he applied the name to certain skin diseases which are characterized by intolerable itching." (Lindlahr, 1910, 449) He explains, "The psoric theory claims that age-long persistent suppression of itchy, parasitic skin eruptions and of gonorrheal and syphilitic diseases has encumbered almost the entire human race with three well-defined hereditary taints or miasms." (Lindlahr, 1910, 450)

Lindlahr reveals how suppression of skin symptoms with toxic drugs and treatments prepares the body for cancer. His clinical observations lead him to believe most convincingly that acute disease suppression is the reason for cancer. He states, "The almost uniform appearance of itch eruptions as healing crises, during the cure of cancer cases, is certainly of great significance. It throws new light upon the true causes of these dreaded diseases and wonderfully confirms Hahnemann's theory of psora." (Lindlahr, 1910, 452) This article by Lindlahr is enlightening and deserving of our attention as cancer statistics paralyze our common sense as doctors.

Lindlahr's theories didn't stop with homeopathy and iridology, but also included psychology. His article, "The New Psychology" was written to help establish "our own classification of nervous and mental disorders and to describe their causes, symptoms and cures from our own 'Nature Cure' point of view." (Lindlahr, 1910, 458) His purpose in doing this was to clarify the confusing and unsatisfactory Allopathic classifications of mental disorders.

While we are on this topic of 'Nature Cure', may I proffer insights that are easy to miss in the complex and sometimes confusing history of our profession. When Henry Lindlahr says 'Nature Cure', he is purposeful and specific, referring to his system of medicine. We cannot fault him for wanting to create his own system when there were already hundreds of others working very ardently and energetically to legitimize Naturopathy. Lindlahr had placed a copyright on his articles that he published and made it clear that "Nature Cure" as a concept and a system was his.

Lindlahr had been a business tycoon building an empire along the railroad tracks of the Midwest as they expanded across America. He had acquired a business acumen and entrepreneurial disposition which he transferred to medicine. Empires can also be created in medicine, too, or perhaps he had lived long enough in America to learn that opportunity knocks on every door. For whatever reasons, Lindlahr did not think of himself as a Naturopath; rather, he created his own movement, which he called 'Nature Cure'. Lindlahr wrote a biography outlining how he came to Nature Cure and he does not hide the fact that it was Louis Kuhne's book, *The New Science of Healing* (1891) that was the catalyst for his life and health. When one juxtaposes Kuhne's book with Lindlahr's book, *Nature Cure* (1913), we soon discover that Lindlahr liberally and sometimes inappropriately appropriated many of Kuhne's key concepts as his own. Nevertheless, a century later, we can be grateful for the work of both men and also credit Henry Lindlahr with the accomplishment of re-formatting the archaic lexicon left by Kuhne.

In any case, in Lindlahr's piece on the new psychology, we can see his effort to distance himself from the Allopaths. Allopathic answers to mental disease have not changed very much; they still rely upon toxic drugs to deaden and paralyze the spirit and Vis of the patient. Calomel or mercury was commonly used even into the time of Lindlahr and its use discontinued only in the early 1960s. Long before the advent of Environmental Medicine, Lindlahr reports, "It takes the mercury from 5 to 16 years to work its way through the bony structures into brain and spinal cord, and then its destructive symptoms begin to manifest." (Lindlahr, 1910, 459) Lindlahr's mission was to know the causes of psychic diseases and remove the causes. He took within his care 'incurables' and treated them with Nature Cure successfully, saving them from the "insane asylums [that] are veritable 'hells on earth', where ignorant and vicious spirits congregate to obsess and vampirize defenseless victims." (Lindlahr, 1910, 460)

Henry Lindlahr held many beliefs about the 'Regulars' that he had no trouble airing. Benedict Lust shared this interest and activity too. In an article, "Is Medicine Behind Time?" we are privy to Lust's accounts of the trends that he was witnessing over a hundred years ago. Lust experienced the wrath of Allopaths and their *Flexner Report*, which decreed that anyone without an allopathic medical education and license was not allowed to practice any kind of medicine, and especially not Naturopathy. However, when a Naturopath was successful with his or her water or air cures, inevitably the Allopaths took notice. Lust speaks, "Such success was preposterous then to the 'regulars' who would only drug the poor patients, as it is ridiculous to them today, when a Naturopath or an Osteopath or a Chiropractor or a Neurologist succeeds with a confirmed chronic, after all medical school fool-doctors with their nasty drugs had failed." (Lust, 1910, 749) When Lust talks of chronic patients, he is referring to the mindset of the time that chronic patients were simply incurable.

What is very interesting about this article are the parallels that we are witnessing in 2015 as Integrative Medicine encircles us and our patients. The trend that we are witnessing today is the conversion of Allopaths to Natural Medicine, described as "integrative", acquiring the training for particular protocols and methodologies in abbreviated sessions. Lust also observed this tread ten decades back:

> Wide awake medical practitioners are realizing the true situation and are quietly or openly adopting the natural methods of healing and treatment for which the people are clamoring. Unless they drop medicine altogether and try to study the laws of nature and free themselves from all medical notions and fallacies about

the nature, cause and cure of disease, their reforming will not amount to much and their efforts of mixing the natural with the unnatural methods of treatment will be more harmful than beneficial to themselves as well as others. (Lust, 1910, 749)

Lust goes on to caution us: "Their previous medical education is usually a detriment and a drawback hard to overcome. Their mere shifting from one system of treatment into another does by no means give them the knowledge and efficiency so essential in their practice and success." (Lust, 1910, 540) Lust saw then what we are witnessing now. History truly repeats itself.

With the Allopaths or 'Regulars' keen on poaching from the Naturopaths what suited their interests, the definition of a Naturopath was of considerable interest to the emerging profession. Dr. Margaret Goettler provides us with the following definition: "The word is a translation of the German *Naturheil-methode*, which means 'the art of healing by and through nature', that is, air, light, water and earth; air, without which nothing can live; light, the greatest disinfectant there is; water, the nourishment of nature itself; and soil, imparting electricity." (Goettler, 1911, 199) The naturopathic profession did not have an easy time coexisting side by side with the Allopaths. Goettler recounts the legacy of struggle in her comments, 'Kuhne, who taught the oneness of disease and made wonderful cures, died with a broken heart, and our men of the present time are not exempt. Dr. Lust of New York has to sacrifice much of his time and money in the courts of that city, and Dr. Carl Shultz, who brought Naturopathy to the western coast, has had an abundance of trials and tribulations." (Goettler, 1911, 200)

Despite the obstacles, the Naturopaths saw merit in their work. Goettler implores her colleagues, "Allow me to urge you to learn to know what naturopathy fully stands for; time not allowing me all that I would like to impress you with. Bear this is mind—Naturopathy does not treat symptoms, but goes to the root and tries to find the cause of mental and physical illness." (Goettler, 1911, 201) She concludes her article with wise words, "Nature can and never will be deceived." (Goettler, 1911, 201)

Naturopaths not only listened to Nature and followed her laws but also knew that the elements of Nature, such as water, earth, sun and air, were essentials for naturopathic treatment. In teaching about air-and-light baths, Benedict Lust lists 15 rules to help Naturopaths administer these baths. Air-and-light baths were available at the Butler Jungborn having two air parks; one for women and other for men. Lust points out, "The air-light bath shall not be applied especially for the sake of causing perspiration, but to promote the influence of light and air upon the naked body." (Lust, 1911, 288) Arnold Rikli was the authority who

Naturopaths referenced in conducting these healthy baths in the open air. Louisa Lust offered these air baths from the very beginning when she opened her Bellevue Sanitarium in 1896.

Air baths were definitely part of the outdoor Sanitarium experience and were also important during sleep. According to Edward Purinton, the number one rule for good sleep was "sleep outdoors, or as near it as possible." (Purinton, 1912, 75) There were ads in Lust's journals with devices to allow people to remain in their beds, yet be contained in a tent that allowed them to have full exposure to the outside air. Keeping bedroom windows open was a must regardless of the season. Purinton's second rule for healthy sleep is to sleep alone. Purinton list 10 rules for good sleep and his final rule is "take an air bath. ... A gentle stream of cool, fresh air blowing directly over the body not only equalizes circulation and relaxes nervous tension but also quiets and renews the soul by the etheric influences of psychic and spiritual origin." (Purinton, 1911, 80-81)

In the next article, "Vibration and Health", T. R. Gowenlock reminds us about Naturopathic fascination in the early days with medical devices. In this piece we are introduced with perhaps over-zealous enthusiasm to his vibrating device. He speaks as if this device was infallible and equates it to the fountain of youth. Gowenlock states, "Yes, electric vibration is the magic wand that is able to wave away our cares and pains and renew our youth again in a great degree. Men have searched for many years for the fabled fountain of life." (Gowenlock, 1912, 713) Gowenlock is earnest in his claims, yet he exaggerates its merits.

When reviewing this article, I was struck by the deduction that vibration improves circulation of lymph and blood. I recently attended a naturopathic conference and visited the exhibit hall and there, on the floor, was a vendor selling a more elaborate device, yet its objective was one and the same: to improve lymphatic and blood circulation. Some things never change. As I indicated earlier, Naturopaths have always had a fascination with new gadgets and new concepts.

A column dedicated to Phrenology was created in *The Naturopath and Herald of Health* early in 1911. Jessie Allen Fowler was the president of the American Institute of Phrenology and was the editor of the column. In an article by Elinor Van Buskirk, M.D., the use of phrenology in medicine is explored. She provides a guiding definition: "Phrenology is a system which teaches that the faculties of the mind are manifested in separate portions of the brain, modified by temperament, the doctrine that the mental powers are indicated by developments of the brain upward, forward and backward from the medulla, which are measured by cranial diameters and distances from the opening of the ear and not from the 'bumps'." (Van Buskirk, 1913, 413)

Phrenologists looked at the shape of a person's head and would be able to deduce his or her strengths, temperament, virtues and other qualities. Phrenology was an obscure mental discipline that its adherents considered science, but its tenets seemed far too metaphysical and occultish. I have included this article by Van Buskirk and there will be others included in a future book of this series, *Mental Culture in Naturopathic Medicine*.

The number of therapies that Naturopaths included within their armamentarium seems vast especially since the Water therapies, Physical Culture (exercises) and Herbs will be covered within this series in their own volumes. Physical and manual therapies certainly had a place in Naturopathy. Dr. Frederick W. Collins was an Osteopath and wrote, "The Science of Kinesiology" defining Kinesiology as "the science of movement". (Collins, 1914, 14) Collins founded the New Jersey Chiropractic College sometime in early 1910's, an initiative not condoned by D. D. Palmer, although Collins had graduated from Palmer via its correspondence chiropractic course. What is most interesting about this article is that the author, Dr. F. W. Collins, an Osteopath and President of the Hudson Osteopathic Association, was nominated by the Constitutional Liberty League in a presidential bid predicated on the drugless platform. Because he threw his hat into the US presidential ring in 1920, there was hope among Naturopaths to counter the suppression of medical freedom that Naturopaths suffered at the hands of the rapidly expanding Allopaths. In the June 1920 issue, Collins published an outline of his platform and his image, straddled with two members of his committee, included Benedict Lust and Dr. Alzamon Ira Lucas. Collins urged his Naturopathic colleagues to come and work together. Collins voiced the Naturopaths' concerns eloquently: "Unless I am greatly mistaken, the great majority of drugless healers and right thinkers will stand behind us and help us go out and give the hosts of oppression a battle which will make them know they have been in a fight." (Collins, 1920, 222)

As an Osteopath, Collins devised a system of 200 moves which were arranged into general treatments. This article is not detailed or comprehensive enough to help us grasp how Collins practiced Kinesiology; I include it here because Collins introduced a therapy that was in practice among Naturopaths and unfortunately, I was unable to find another that was more complete or explicit in the time period of this collection (1899-1923).

Unlike Dr. Collins, who did not explain the practice of Kinesiology with a helpful thoroughness, Dr. William Freeman Havard was very articulate in his description of a different medical system, Homeopathy. His first sentence iterates what every Naturopath today faces when encountering someone new to the natural healing field. Harvard queries, "Every homeopathic physician is constantly receiving requests for information as to the differences between Homeopathy and all other forms of medical treatment." (Havard, 1915, 600) This question still continues to be one of the most commonly posed questions asked of Naturopaths. In "The Science of Cure", Havard answers this age old question and goes on to outline Homeopathy's strengths, elucidating how Homeopathy helps in various disease states. Havard's homeopathic exposé leaves us with a thorough overview of Homeopathy that is as indispensable today as when it was written a century ago.

In the next article following Havard's, we meet another brilliant Naturopath, E. K. Stretch, who specialized in Osteopathy. Its title says it all: "Gynecology minus the knife". Women in the early 20th century endured pain, often suffering at the hands of their surgeons. Dr. E. K. Stretch provides three non-invasive interventions to address dysmenorrhea that include hot packs, traction and concussion. Stretch emphasizes that Osteopaths recognize the misplacement of the uterus and the pain that results, but also "goes a step further and locates the cause of this condition in the spinal area governing these parts." (Stretch, 1916, 40)

Addressing the cause of disease was a key principle that Naturopaths still hold dear and there was a time when Osteopathy shared this principle in their management of disease. Another fundamental consideration for the dysmenorrhea that Stretch includes is the individualized diet. She provides the example, "So you will see that the individual needs must be considered in each case but to those willing to work along these lines I ask that they start with a breakfast of fruit only and with meals and which meat is served to eat a combination salad or raw vegetables instead of potatoes and bread." (Stretch, 1916, 41-42)

Joseph Hoegen's article concludes that dietary indiscretion, along with "lack of exercise in the open air, results in circulatory obstipation or stagnation, imposing a serious and unnecessary burden upon the sanctuary of vitality: the heart." (Hoegen, 1916, 133) Another cause for heart morbidity, in Hoegen's view, was "the failure on the part of the emunctories to rid the body of its waste". (Hoegen, 1916, 61) Hoegen also introduces us to the Nauheim bath which originated in the town, Nauheim, Germany renowned for its carbonic acid mineral waters. The Nauheim Bath was visited by President Roosevelt's father for his heart condition and by his son when he was young boy. Today, the Nauheim baths or the carbon dioxide baths are administered in medical spa settings around the world to treat post myocardial infarctions, diabetes, arthritis, obesity and several other diseases.

The confidence in the Nauheim bath was great, but not every hot spring produced carbon dioxide waters; so the early Naturopaths devised ways of replicating the same conditions of a Nauheim bath in a clinical setting. "Much can be done in the beginning of high arterial pressure with a course of Nauheim Baths of a moderate temperature, combined with strengthening exercises as devised by Dr. Theodor Schott." (Hoegen, 1916, 61)

Having a Nauheim bath is like bathing in a bath tub filled with champagne. The body becomes covered with tiny carbon dioxide gas bubbles and warms up very quickly. Carbon dioxide causes smooth muscle relaxation which results in the dilation of capillaries. The reason Hoegen states is that there is prickling of the gas bubbles, which has proven to be incorrect. Hoegen cites, "The effervescing carbonated bath produces a sensation of warmth to the skin, caused by the prickling of the gas bubbles, and the body of the patient assumes a healthy red color, due to the distention of the cutaneous capillaries." (Hoegen, 1916, 61-62) There will more articles describing the procedure of the Nauheim bath in an upcoming book in this series, *Hydrotherapy In Naturopathic Medicine*.

The subject of inorganic mineral salts was introduced earlier by Ludwig Staden (1909). Richard Peter's article, "The Importance of Nutritive Salts", continues this discussion in an elaborate and convincing presentation for the necessity of inclusion of minerals in the diet. He draws upon the scientific investigations of those scientists in Germany who contributed enormously to this discussion. He provides examples of diseases associated with mineral salt deficiencies and provides the scientific proof. For example, he explains the presence of lime [calcium] in the urine in different conditions. Peters states, "In pathological conditions, especially in chronic malnutrition, an increased lime excretion is found in the urine. On the other hand, an increased lime retention is found in arteriosclerosis." (Peters, 1916, 305) His article provides extensive detail that was uncommon in the articles published in Benedict Lusts journals. Peters provides us with an invaluable perspective that demonstrated a not altogether uncommon rigor in the work of the early Naturopaths as they searched for meaning and struggled to rise to the social, economic and legal levels of their Allopathic colleagues.

That allopathic influence on health at the time is captured in the following article, "Narcotics and the Osteopath". What makes the inclusion of this article on drugs interesting is that first, it appears in 1916 in the Lust journals and second, it was written by an Osteopath indicating that there were still ties between the Naturopaths and the Osteopaths, even though Osteopaths were increasingly defecting to the Allopathic ranks. The Osteopaths and Naturopaths, after all, were both in a parallel struggle for survival following the rollout of the Flexner Report [1910]. By just after mid-century their paths had completely diverged; however, at this stage, the estrangement had been gradual, but consistently incremental. Nevertheless, this 1916 article shows us that Naturopaths and Osteopaths were still learning from each other.

As they expanded their formularies and engaged in some use of pharmaceuticals, the early Naturopaths were keen to grasp how drugs worked and to understand their function. Lawrence Kaim, in this regard, provides a list of narcotics and the organ that each acts on, also explaining mode of action. Kaim explains, "I spoke of the poisonous effects of absorption of the poison and absorption implies solution, therefore, the more soluble the compound, the more speedy the effect." (Kaim, 1916, 391) Some of the drugs mentioned have long since been censured from use, such Calomel, mercury chloride, which was the golden standard of treatment and used as a panacea. Unfortunately, the dangers of some of these drugs were not fully understood and were eventually banished from the pharmacopeia altogether. Kaim introduces the need to administer doses appropriate to children and provides the Rule of Young. Sadly, Kaim unwittingly recommends increasing dosage for children for "purgatives, diaphoretics and diuretics must usually be given to children in larger doses and narcotics in smaller doses than called for by the "Rule of Young"." (Kaim, 1916, 391)

While hind sight can be expediently wise when viewing the literature of our therapeutics, one voice stands out for his critical assessments of the various manual therapy practices: William Havard. Before Havard presents an analysis of various manual and mechanical methods, he begins with the observation that many practitioners do not take the time to thoroughly assess the patient. He states, "A spinal examination for the location of a "lesion" is not sufficient to enable the physician to establish a cure." (Havard, 1916, 479)

Havard was keen to understand the true cause of disease and carefully outlined how the removal of symptoms was not necessarily a cure. He cautions, "If we do not thoroughly understand the action and reaction of the body we are likely to mistake signs and symptoms of disease for the disease itself." Having a comprehensive knowledge of the etiology of disease helps the practitioner to use the right form of therapy. Havard is referring to the underlying causes such as "the accumulation and retention of foreign matter and morbid waste products in the body" (Havard, 1916, 480) so often missed because our focus is on the symptom or lesion. The outcome of not really addressing the true cause of disease results in "systems of manual and mechanical treatment correct only secondary or contributory causes of disease and symptomatic conditions with the exception of traumatic cases." (Havard, 1916, 480) Havard's article is filled with clinical insights as invaluable today as when he wrote them a century ago.

Neuropathy was a favourite manual therapy used and Havard provides insights as to its application. He notes, "From a chart of the nervous system showing the location of the vaso-motor and viscera-motor centers in the spinal cord, one can determine what mechanisms are involved in the disorder. For example, if your reflex shows hyperactivity of the dilators, the region controlling the activity of the stomach is in a state of inflammation." (Havard, 1917, 151) Palpation of the erector spinae in terms of heat, hyperesthesia, hypertonicity, hypotonicity, passive congestion, atonicity and atrophy were essential features. (Havard, 1917, 151)  The laws of action and reaction are given that explain how the body compensates when attempting to meet any interference to the body's homeostasis.  In a detailed account, Havard explains how the body compensates in the distribution of blood in the arteries in the case of inflammation.  He clarifies, "Consequently, where one part of the body is inflamed, the blood vessels of some other part must be constricted.  Where such compensation fails, the heart is called upon to maintain the blood pressure circulation by increasing the rate of its beat." (Havard, 1917, 153)  His examples and explanations of physiology in disease and within the theories of Neuropathic diagnosis are welcome at a time when we are so quick to treat symptomatically which he attests "is that in about 99% of cases proves to be suppressive". (Havard, 1916, 482)

Naturopaths also advanced therapeutics in the use of light and various types of lamps.  Early Naturopaths were staunch believers in the power of sunlight which was "the best sterilizing, disinfecting and hygienic agent we have, but also one of the best means of restoring functional activity". (Nelson, 1918, 470)  Per Nelson gives an account of the properties and uses for three lamps: Arc lamp, Finsen lamp and Incandescent or Leucodescent lamp.  The Arc lamp mimicked sunlight and was used in "all diseases where increased oxidation was desired and of course, in conditions where the bactericidal effect is sought." (Nelson, 1918, 470)  Dr. Finsen, a Danish doctor, invented the Finsen light which produced an ultra violet ray.  The Finsen light was renowned for its efficacy for a skin condition called lupus.  The third lamp, the incandescent, was used in cabinets designed to promote sweating.  Nelson was leery of the light cabinets used solely for inducing perspiration.  Nelson cautions, "Practitioners of this branch of the healing art should always remember that prolonged and frequently repeated treatments by light or any other powerful stimulant may tend to overwork and thus weaken or destroy the delicate sweat-glands." (Nelson, 1918, 472)  Nelson corroborates from Henry Lindlahr's *Nature Cure Philosophy And Practice* that light cabinets which cause "forced sweating, cannot be called natural means of cure. ... [Light cabinets] irritate the organs of elimination into forced activity, without, at the same time, arousing the cells in the interior of the body to natural elimination." (Nelson, 1918, 472)  Henry Lindlahr's opinion mattered and it is worth noting that Naturopaths would make reference to Lindlahr's work.

Acute diseases were recognized by both Allopaths and Naturopaths as self-limiting.  Benedict Lust adds, "Treatment can either assist or hinder the recovery, depending on whether it conserves or lowers the patient's vitality." (Lust, 1919, 166)  We must keep in mind that Lust wrote this piece in 1919, shortly after the Spanish Flu that had decimated the world with over 40 million deaths. His reference to patient care during this epidemic was quite polar: the Naturopaths lost less than 1% while the Allopaths had a dismal record varying from 28% to as high as 70% of their patients. Lust states, "The history of the "flu" epidemic bears out our contention that allopathic treatment is gross interference with nature's methods of cure, for almost without exception: cases recovered without any particular treatment, cases recovered under natural treatment, but a large proportion of cases died under allopathic treatment." (Lust, 1919, 166)

Lust was not the only Naturopath who viewed Allopaths with great suspicion. Gilbert Brown saw that the Allopaths enjoyed absolute indemnity, regardless of their errors and misjudgments. Their treatments employed almost exclusively drugs that were more often than not poisonous, and their history was tarnished with unforgiveable deeds of bloodletting. Gilbert laments, "It is a deplorable fact that drugs killed more people than bullets ever did." (Gilbert, 1919, 441) Although Gilbert's article is more appropriate for its historical significance, he expressed the Naturopaths sentiments against the Allopaths political maneuverings to eradicate the Naturopaths from medical practice of any kind.

There were differences between the theories of practice of Naturopaths and Allopaths. William Havard explains that Allopaths or "the 'Old School' of medicine had accepted the theory that disease was caused by the presence of germs within the body." (Havard, 1920, 234) The germ theory instigated a pharmaceutical monstrosity that would soon dominate disease care and every facet of American life. Havard contends, "Naturopathy pays little or no attention to the germ because it recognizes him as a product of disease rather than a cause." (Havard, 1920, 235) Naturopaths, rather than focused on symptomatic treatment, choose to place more confidence in removing disease by removing its causes: the accumulation of waste matter in the blood.

He gives an example of heart failure and the scientific solution to administer a heart stimulant to the patient. He rationalizes, "But if we stop for a moment to consider that the body is not an assembled machine but a growth from one cell, we will realize that every part of the organism is related to every other part, and related in such a way that no one part can become disordered without affecting every other part." (Havard, 1920, 235-236) In describing the process of organ repair, Havard reminds us, "There is no therapeutic procedure that can take the place of rest for a fatigued organ or fatigued body." (Havard, 1920, 237)

Not all of the early Naturopaths had the common sense of William Havard. One such person was George Starr White whom we could describe as a non-conformist, eccentric, or even as a "New Age" thinker.

White was smitten and fascinated with Chromotherapy. Chromotherapy or color therapy was another tool used by the early Naturopaths and recognized as significant as sunlight. One of the first people promoting Chromotherapy was Edwin D. Babbitt, as evidenced by his rousing 1878 book, *The Principles of Light and Color.* It became a guiding force for those who followed. White wrote on this subject of Chromotherapy with fervor and his style of writing incorporated a phonetic system of spelling, some examples of which are as follows: wer [were], exampl, hav, negativ, oxigen, robd, littl, cigaret in his original article. The temptation to leave his writing alone was great; however, in the interests of clarity, I capitulated and spelt his words as one would find in a dictionary.

White leaves with us directions on how to use color therapeutically and what each color signified. For example the color red was "indicated in tuberculosis, anemia, physical exhaustion, paralysis and all debilitated conditions". (White, 1921, 181) The properties of each color are given and he provides instructions on how to make frames for the coloured silk screens. He preferred silks to glass for his screens emitting the colored light onto the patient. Silks impart a softness that glass does not when using artificial lights. (White, 1921, 182) White was not the first or last to use Chromotherapy. Henry Sperbeck who was a Chiropractor gave clear instruction in the use of color which we will see in his article in 1923. Chromotherapy continues to attract followers and it may require more pursuit into its applications as we solidify the scientific basis of naturopathic therapies old and new.

The fascination with electricity and gadgets for the early Naturopaths, reported earlier in this book, comes through with the types of therapies that they endorsed. E. A. Martin writes "Some few years ago when electricity was discovered, it was so little understood that it was accredited with all kinds of power or force and some medical men went so far as to state that "electricity was life" and their assumption was consequently carried to extremes, this being too much to expect." (Martin, 1921, 442) One such therapy, that has almost been lost and forgotten, is the Violet Ray. With the exception of a very, very few Naturopaths today such as Dr. Letitia Dick-Konenburg, few continue to use this remarkable device. Behind the Violet Ray stands a historical giant in the scientific community, Nickola Tesla, who brought safety to the pioneering of electrical medical devices. Martin recounts Tesla's findings: "To overcome danger of shock Tesla also found it was necessary to give electricity in very small doses (homeopathically it might be expressed), and therefore, he reduced the amperage to practically a negative quantity in the Tesla coil with which the Violet Ray is equipped." (Martin, 1921, 443)

The Violet Ray stimulated blood circulation and nerve function.

Martin describes the machine, "... the many ions of electricity discharged in the vacuum tube bombarding molecules within the tube are most predominant and result in the phenomena of exhibiting a Violet light. That is why a High Frequency instrument is called Violet Ray." (Martin, 1921, 443)    Martin summarizes fourteen effects of the Violet Ray upon the human body.    While Martin extols the virtues of the Violet Ray, he also cautions that the Violet Ray has its place and states its limitations.    Martin attests, "It must be thoroughly understood that while Violet Ray treatments are beneficial in a great number of afflictions or diseases because of the fact that it is a powerful nerve and fluid movement stimulant, due to the tremendous amount of vibrations it is capable of producing, nevertheless it is by no means a cure-all." (Martin, 1921, 449)

Another form of treatment utilized by Naturopaths was magnetism; i.e. using magnets and the human natural magnetism found in laying-on of hands.    In "Animal Magnetism, Curative Magnetism", Benedict Lust recounts some history relating magnetism, that "hidden power" in humans to Paracelsus who reintroduced the science. (Lust, 1922, 168) Lust describes how the magnet works: "The magnet is placed on the affected part of the body for from fifteen to thirty minutes, the part affected being at the same time turned toward the north, while the south pole of the magnet is placed in such manner that its north pole is directed towards the north." (Lust, 1922, 168)

Human magnetism was either acquired at birth or cultivated by "a strong will and mental powers, religious feelings, benevolence and love in harmonious combination". (Lust, 1922, 169)    Magnetizers were deeply spiritual and endowed with purist and highest intentions.    Lust states, "The healer must be inwardly convinced of his calling and his healing powers, the highest and best work of his life.    Only a pure-minded magnetiser can impart a pure magnetism." (Lust, 1922, 169)    Lust describes the magnetic treatment and how to offer a magnetic session both on a patient and on water.

Hands-on treatments often comprised the majority of therapeutic interventions used as the Naturopaths were forging their new profession.    In the early years when the lines among Naturopathy, Chiropractic and Osteopathy were blurred and blended, one finds many articles on the subject of physical and manipulative medicine.    The vertebral spine was manipulated and also concussed to impact the spinal nerves and the organs that they enervated.    In "Spinal Concussion" written by Benedict Lust, we learn how to concuss each cervical nerve to exact an outcome. Lust states, "Concussion is always better if applied after the spine has received proper adjustments." (Lust, 1922, 526)    He describes how to determine the origin of the nerve with its position on the vertebrae of the spine.    This article can be a refresher for those of us not accustomed to manipulative therapies.  Lust provides a detailed account of each of the spinal nerves and the purpose for concussion.  For example, Lust states with respect to the 12th thoracic vertebra, "A most important segment for concussion, as enlarged prostate will reduce very rapidly from it.  Old cases of enlarged and painful prostate gland will become normal in size and function in so short a time as to amaze you." (Lust, 1922, 528)  He leaves us with a wealth of knowledge in treating the body with a simple tool of spinal concussion.

The benefit of a Spinal Concussion was not without its dangers.  Henry Sperbeck noted that spinal adjustments had similar effects as a spinal concussion and counsels, "No one can work on the spine with any degree of intelligence without knowing the spinal reflexes". (Sperbeck, 1923, 63)  He illustrates with an example, "Suppose the appendix was much inflamed and a thrust was given on the second lumbar the organ might be ruptured.  To ignore the spinal reflexes may lead to such bad results as to exhaust them and so make the patient a helpless invalid." (Sperbeck, 1923, 63)

Sperbeck was a Chiropractor who called himself a Drugless Therapist using several modalities that included Chiropractic, Chromotherapy, Massage and Light Therapy.  He offers protocols for the multidiscipline treatments of several disease conditions which give us an idea how these modalities were used in conjunction.

Physical therapies used by Sperbeck and others were often accompanied with hydrotherapies.  The Blood Washing Method was one such hydrotherapy treatment that for a very brief time in the formation of Naturopathy swept through the profession like a wild fire.  Benedict Lust had learned of this therapy from its inventor, a young Greek, Christos Parasco and Lust went on to compile a small booklet describing this bath.  The Blood Washing Method was essentially a very long shower of eight hours long with the shower head raised to the height from 8 to 14 feet high.  Lust's recommendations for the Blood Washing protocol included, "Start by showering the lower parts of the body, the lower joints, the knees, then going upwards all over the body, front, back and sides, from the toes up to the top of the head, then the same showering all over again and again." (Lust, 1923, 524)  Lust continues, "Forty percent of the showering more or less is to be applied upon and around the stomach and the intestines, also upon the sexual parts, the rectum and surroundings." (Lust, 1923, 524)

The Blood Washing Method was one of those therapies that cannot be justified in today's global water shortages; however, I must relate a story of Dr. Betty Radelet. "Reading the testimonials written a century ago was echoed by Dr. Betty who shared with me her experience of the neglected Blood Wash.  I asked her what therapy she found exceptional amongst all of the therapies used in Naturopathy. As I listened to her story, I caught the gleam in her eye and could only imagine the life changing experience that she had taking this unique shower." (Czeranko, 2009, 27).

The second final therapy included in this book is Massage. Benedict Lust's article, "The Physiology of Curative Movements" has imparted all of the essential details of massage and mechanopathy. Lust states, "Massopathy is a manipulation of the tissues of the body by movable pressure in the form of stroking, rubbing, pinching and kneading. Massopathy, whether active or passive, counteracts atrophy of the tissues, increases the circulation, promotes the absorption of pathological elements and improves the general nutrition." (Lust, 1923, 648) Lust continues, "The purpose of massage is that of reinforcing and regulating the nutritive activities whereby functional power is maintained." (Lust, 1923, 652) Mechanopathy was a more vigorous form of massage using a machine to generate a mechanical vibration.

Lust's love of history never fails to find a place in his narrative to connect the past with his topic. He cites, "Hippocrates practised massopathy 400 years B.C. Asclepiades was the father of mechanopathy, and Galen, the most eminent doctor of the Roman Empire, was a great authority for the use of passive exercises." (Lust, 1923, 649)

The methods used in massage are given in detail and we are left with a considerable amount to assimilate. We know today that our lives have drifted into a sedentary waste land as we sit in front of computers or televisions far longer than is deemed healthy. Although we know better, we continue to sit. Inactivity has become the new smoking epidemic. Lust knew this a century ago, "Sedentary life is hard on muscles, heart and lungs. Mental as well as physical ills follow physical restraint and inactivity. It is better to live an active life and be poor than to grow wealthy in a sedentary occupation." (Lust, 1923, 647)

Our final article is another forgotten therapy called Autotherapy. Based upon Homeopathy, the principle of Autotherapy was using the patient's own "unmodified poisons within his body peculiar to and corresponding with his disease". (Duncan, 1923, 775) Autotherapy sounds much like Isopathy where a product of disease [nosode] in a diluted, attenuated dose is given. Fear of contracting communicable diseases has an immense influence on public health both in Canada and United States. The media's ability to mélange fear and terror is palpable as we witness the surge of compulsory vaccination threats. The theory of immunity found in Autotherapy brings the two opposing camps one step closer to those of the Allopaths and their theory of vaccination.

There were so many brilliant Naturopathic women and men who made huge contributions in advancing Naturopathy. Their legacy lives on in their many articles written for the Lust publications. Some of these therapies risk not rising from the pages of books into active clinical practice; yet, as the history of our profession and its practice reveal, so many are worth revisiting.

Sussanna Czeranko, ND, BBE

# 1899

## Mountain Air Resort "Bellevue", Butler, N.J.

### Louisa Stroebele

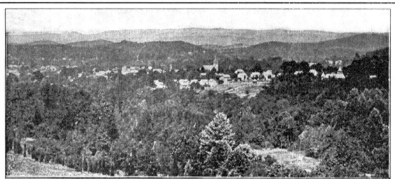

Louisa Stroebele placed this English ad in 1900 in *The Kneipp Water Cure Monthly* which marks the beginning of collaboration between her and Benedict Lust.

# Mountain Air Resort "Bellevue", Butler, N.J.

**by Louisa Stroebele**

*Amerikanische Kneipp-Blätter, IV (5), 141. (1899)*

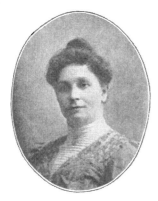

Louisa Stroebele Lust.

Most romantically situated on the top of a hill, about ten minutes' walk from the depot, "Bellevue" comprises thirty acres of woodland, laid out with shady walks along a picturesque brook of clear water, known as Trout-Brook, and with its beauty spots in the shape of quiet nooks, sheltered from the sun, its numerous springs along the hillside, its grand view into the Ramapo Mountains, is an ideal summer-resort for lovers of nature.

The view from the celebrated "Kick-Out" Mountain, one mile from "Bellevue", is beyond description, and at once reminds the spectator of the Alps in Switzerland. It is only of late that this northern part of New Jersey, with its mountain ranges and its attractive sceneries, has become a favorite spot of the people of New York and neighboring cities as a mountain air resort, being recommended for its pure, bracing, and invigorating air by numerous prominent physicians of New York City.

The mountains are from 1,100 to 1,400 feet high. A number of lakes, as Greenwood Lake, Echo Lake, Pompton Lake, and others are within reach for a day's outing, and may be approached either by private conveyance or by railroad.

Many who formerly spent the summer months in the Catskill Mountains give now the preference to these regions, finding the air here as pure as there, with the advantage of being here nearer to their homes and to the seashore. Butler being only thirty miles from New York City, parties wishing to spend a day for a change on the latter place can leave Butler by a morning train and return in the evening, the fare for the trip both ways being only $1.00 by using the so-called ten-trip tickets.

"Bellevue" also offers the advantage of having an open-air swimming-bath grounds, besides the Turko-Russian baths in the building, and the air and sun baths in tents especially arranged for the purpose. Here removed from the bustle and turmoil incident to large cities, one finds an alleviating balm spiritually and physically in the unsurpassed bounty of nature, which goes a great ways toward recuperation of health, particularly if, as is the case at "Bellevue", such hygienic surroundings are supplemented by a common-sense diet, cooking being done in such a manner that food is

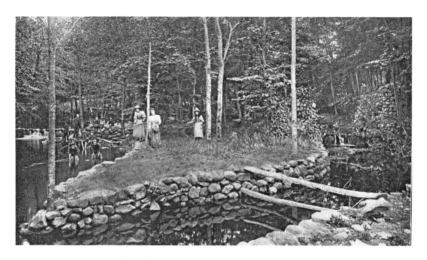

Trout-Brook Island, "Bellevue", Butler, New Jersey.

not only prepared to please the taste, but upon scientific principles, which insures the best results nutritively.  Aside from carefully selected food in the way of cereals, meats, fish and fowl, and vegetables in large variety, the table is abundantly supplied with rich milk and fresh butter, also with fruits at all seasons.

Butler is a station on the New York, Susquehanna & Western Railroad.  The Railroad Company is constantly improving its train service, there being at present fourteen trains to and from New York on week days, and four on Sundays.  It has also been stated that the Electric Railroad Company having now a line from Hoboken to Singac (only six miles from Butler) will before long continue the line through Pompton Plains to Butler and Greenwood Lake.

Expenses at the "Bellevue" are $15.00 per week, baths included, to be paid in advance.  Children under twelve, half price.  Parties desiring carriage on their arrival, for which there will be a reasonable charge, should give notice beforehand.  For circulars and other detailed information address: Miss L. Stroebele, Bellevue, Butler, New Jersey or the city office: 111 E. 59th St. New York City.

*Butler being only thirty miles from New York City, parties wishing to spend a day for a change on the latter place can leave Butler by a morning train and return in the evening, the fare for the trip both ways being only $1.00 by using the so-called ten-trip tickets.*

## The Thure Brandt System
### Carola Staden

---

## Natural Therapeutics And Electricity
### G. H. A. Schaefer, M. E.

---

## Hardening
### Benedict Lust

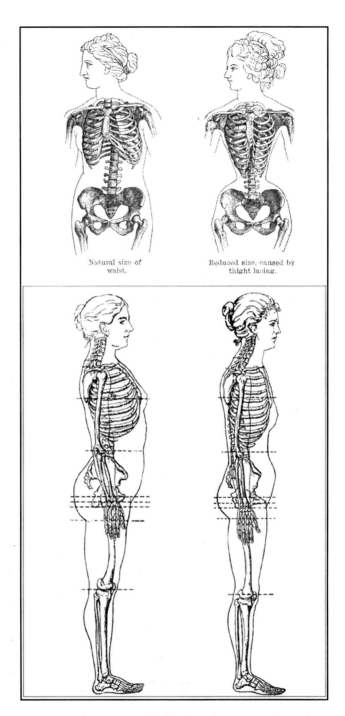

Natural size of waist.

Reduced size, caused by thight lacing.

The contrast between a well-developed woman and one who is corset-deformed.

# THE THURE BRANDT SYSTEM

**by Carola Staden**

*The Kneipp Water Cure Monthly, I (2), 23. (1900)*

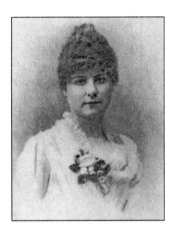

Carola Staden, Brooklyn.

Amongst the innumerable treatments in the great domain of Natural Methods of Healing, the Thure Brandt method is the most unique; being used only for the treatment of female pelvic diseases and displacements.

These cases are becoming alarmingly numerous, especially in the United States. It is stated by the prominent physicians with the wide experience that about seventy percent of the women of this country are afflicted with disorders of the pelvis. Consequently the following instructions will be of practical benefit to nearly every woman who reads them.

Unfortunately, the Thure Brandt system of internal massage is almost unknown in this country and strange as it may seem, the discoverer, Thure Brandt, is not a physician, but has been a soldier, (an officer in the Swedish Army). Indeed, it is a remarkable fact that the principal methods, used in the practice of Natural Healing, have been discovered by a layman.

Thure Brandt left the army in the prime of life, to devote himself to the amelioration of suffering of humanity. He took his degree as Masseur and Gymnast at the Central Institute of Massage and Gymnastics of Stockholm. Like all men of genius he was a keen observer and an original thinker. Powers which the mere possession of a diploma is unable to guarantee. He remained always a student, observing and practicing until he organized an entirely new method of correcting disorders of the organs of the body. He united with a fresh strong mentality an amiable, modest benevolent disposition, which won the confidence and respect of all the women whom he treated.

While treating a case of prolapsus recti one day, he succeeded in permanently replacing it by a certain grip. After his success in replacing the rectum, he concluded from this the possibility of replacing a prolapsus uteri by a similar movement.

After one and a half years of observation and experiment he finally succeeded in doing this.

Together, Carola and Ludwig Staden operated the first light and water cure clinic in Brooklyn, New York.

It was the foundation of his great reputation as a gynecological specialist. For he attracted the attention of renowned doctors and professors, especially those of Stockholm, Jena, etc., and through them was enabled to make thousands of female pelvic examinations, with the result that he cured almost every one he ever treated. The Thure Brandt internal massage is given in the following manner: the patient reclines in a half lying position, the operator holding the fore-finger quietly and motionless against the cervix of the uterus, whilst the other hand, through the peritoneum massages the inner organs. Therefore, the internal massage is manipulated by the outside hand, the inner hand acting as a support only for the organ, and helps to place it. Along with the internal massage, Thure Brandt combines a long series of gymnastic movements, the selection of which requires a nice discrimination that is left to the masseur. They consist of movements which carry the blood to an organ or from it. Also, there are passive and active movements, also movements of resistance. The passive movements of course are given by the masseur. The movements of resistance are used to elevate the uterus also for the distension of the ligaments and of those muscles adjoining the pelvis. While giving these movements, the masseur counts the beating of the coccygeal region which supplies the blood to the pelvis. With some of the exercises a gymnastic apparatus is used, but a piece of furniture will answer in the absence of the apparatus. Thure Brandt recommended water treatment with the massage, such as sponge-baths, sitting-baths, etc.

The Thure Brandt system of internal massage, unlike what is ordinarily called massage, requires deep study and responsibility of the manipulator and a faculty of diagnosing the case in hand, for great harm can be done by a wrong manipulation.

Dr. Reibmayer gives the following reasons for the slow spread of a science that should be universally adopted for the above cases. He says,

"For the ordinary physician, it requires too much hard physical work. Besides the lack of appreciating the necessity of the gymnastics after the internal massage. Again, the dearth of women physicians who practice the Natural Methods of Healing, although the originator was a man, few men are endowed with the delicacy of touch and magnetism of Thure Brandt, so that it offers a particularly fine field for women of fine intelligence and nobility of character."

Dr. Walser, the author of *The Natural Method of Healing* states,

"This redeeming massage would be a Godsend to womankind if female physicians would only practice it. Indeed women with the inclination, intelligence and ability for the medical profession need not put off its practice until after they have received their diplomas. Indeed all the necessary instruction to practice this new science can be had by the teachings of the Natural Method of Healing. Knowledge and experience alone make a physician a true physician, and not the diploma."

We hope and pray that this beautiful massage of Thure Brandt will not drop into oblivion, for it is the healing par excellence in its domain. May it rapidly spread over the entire world carrying benefit and blessings to thousands and thousands of suffering women.

---

*It is stated by the prominent physicians with the wide experience that about seventy percent of the women of this country are afflicted with disorders of the pelvis.*

*The Thure Brandt internal massage is given in the following manner: the patient reclines in a half lying position, the operator holding the fore-finger quietly and motionless against the cervix of the uterus, whilst the other hand, through the peritoneum massages the inner organs.*

*Along with the internal massage, Thure Brandt combines a long series of gymnastic movements.*

*We hope and pray that this beautiful massage of Thure Brandt will not drop into oblivion, for it is the healing par excellence in its domain.*

## NATURAL THERAPEUTICS AND ELECTRICITY

### by G. H. A. Schaefer, M.E.

*The Kneipp Water Cure Monthly, I (7), 110-111. (1900)*

Nothing in modern science causes us so much amazement as electricity, the sovereign ruler of all, Roentgen's epoch making discovery and Marconi's system of wire-less telegraphy are but two manifestations of the mystery whose thick veil has been raised by learned investigators to enable us to catch a glimpse of the magnificent heritage which, in time, we may expect to receive from this wonderful kingdom.

The progress made by experimental physics during the past decade proves, beyond all doubt, the long accepted theory of science, that electricity, ever present, is the mainspring of all the forces of nature that "life" itself is nothing more than active electric force. Experiments have proved that the use of electricity in growing vegetables causes them to thrive most vigorously. Look at the flowers, the very blossoms turn toward the electrifying rays of the sun.

The source of electricity is found in the composition and decomposition of matter by which the requisite amount of heat is produced. What is it but electricity where the sun's rays draw up the water of the ocean so that it may again fall to the earth in the form of rain and dew?

The electric fluid is, as every beginner in the study of physics knows, present in everybody in the universe. Every molecule of matter has a certain amount of electricity which varies with the individuality of the body in question. Electricity is present, not only in all the objects of nature about us, but also in every human and animal being; therefore I maintain that it is this which constitutes the primal cause and preservative force of the life of functions. Endeavors to discover the phenomena of electricity in the human body with the help of photography are not new. The most important results in this field, in recent years were obtained by the Russian savant Jacob von Narkiewiez-Jodko. By means of experiments in the domain of electricity which he conducted for years he succeeded with the aid of photography, in getting the results of his examination of the electric phenomena of both healthy and sick people in a permanent form, which proves incontestably the correctness of the theory which he had advanced. The theories that the human body is an electric battery, so to speak, formed the basis of his conception. The human body contains a great number of human cells in which electricity is present. These cells act as galvanic elements and are neither more or less than the groups of nerves, which, by means of the nerve fibres transmit the current through an unbroken line and lead, exactly like an electric wire to the main battery, the brain.

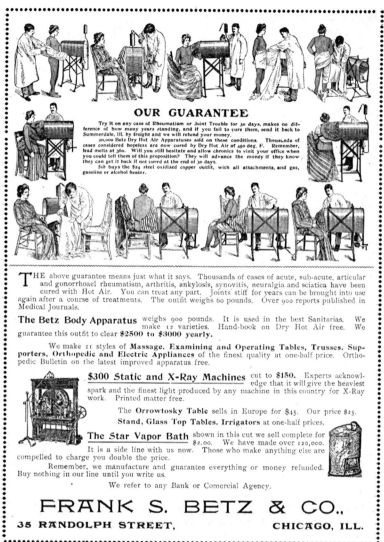

An example of an advertisement that promoted one of many medical electric devices available at the turn of the 20th century.

Just as changes may be produced in an electric battery by making and breaking the current so the nerve cells present different phenomena when they receive an electric current, succeeded with the aid of photography in obtaining a picture of the healthy condition of the nervous system.

As soon as an electric current passes through a given body there is a discharge and a spark leaps from the skin to the pole, the electrode. It is this spark which the Russian scholar photographed. From the picture of the spark Herr von Jodko was able to discover the pathological condition of the subject. By his system he succeeded in photographing a hand the fourth finger of which was seen to be quite weak. The finger was, as investigation showed, lame, so that as the cells of the finger were abnormal, no current could pass and there was no spark.

By means of experiments conducted for years on invalids I have found that Herr von Jodko's theories could be adopted with great benefit in treating the sick. According to my entire experience in the field, persons with weak nerves and those with the gout, during the first stages of the electric treatment show but little change and precisely for the reason that they themselves have too little electricity and in this condition the human body offers too great resistance.

The electric treatment of diseases is not new. In the seventeenth century a Bohemian priest, Prokop Diwisch, affected some notable cures by means of electricity. Diwisch was the first to affirm that which we call strength was reducible to electricity. "The electric fire", said Diwisch, "permeates all bodies, including that of man. If the electricity leaves man, he dies." I think, this statement is correct. Believing that life itself was based on electricity and that in disease the supply of personal electricity was insufficient, Diwisch determined to endeavor, by the application of weak electric currents, to restore the normal amount of the electric fluid to the patient. By the use of weak currents Diwisch succeeded in effecting some notable cures. The consequence was a bitter attack on the part of physicians. In court, Diwisch showed that his use of electricity had nothing to do with the art of medicine and also that he had treated only patients who had already been given up by both physicians and apothecaries. On the theory that the electric treatment was not within the domain of the schools of medicine and that it had nothing in common with the physician's art, Diwisch was allowed to continue his cures unhindered. Some of the greatest cures that have thus far been affected by the electric treatment were made by two Austrian physicians. These gentlemen applied mild electric currents to the body. According to their view electricity is the ruling healing principle.

As electricity itself is a motive force so it works as much in the human body. Bloodless parts are supplied with blood since electricity empties the congested parts and drives the blood to those which need it. This can easily be shown as patients who suffer from cold feet find their feet are warm after the electric treatment. On the other hand, electricity also causes decomposition. Just as electricity is produced by the decomposition of certain combinations zinc and carbon so, by the application of electricity, all matter which causes disease is rendered soluble and is eliminated in the urine, perspiration, faeces, etc. The application of electricity affects astonishing changes in the digestion.

Patients, who have suffered for years with constipation, generally find relief with the electric treatment. On the other hand, the most difficult cases of diarrhoea are cured by this simple treatment. The electricity brings about a healthy action of the stomach and intestines. In short after a brief electric treatment, the organs begin to perform their functions better. And since numerous ills are due to disturbances in the nutrition of the organism (over-nutrition belongs to this class, for example, gout,) it will be readily understood how patients suffering from various diseases are benefited. A weak woman may by improper nourishment become gouty. That in such cases electricity works wonders, I have myself found in innumerable instances. In the application of electricity to the human body it is of the utmost importance that special apparatus be used, constructed with a view to the individual needs of the patient. It is moreover, wholly unnecessary, in fact it is harmful, to use strong currents as certain practitioners do. Static as well as faradic electricity are in my opinion, not adopted for my treatment. Frequently I have been asked whether harm may not result from too frequent use of my apparatus; and whether the system will not become dependent upon electricity. To which I reply that it is impossible to injure the human organism with my apparatus no matter how often it is used; and while the system may become dependent upon drugs, it never does upon electricity. Furthermore I maintain that every disease, call it what you will, may be cured with my apparatus, provided the organs, structure, tissues and cells are still in a condition to perform the physical and chemical functions necessary to a cure or improvement, and the patient himself is curable or capable of improvement.

With deep sorrow I often see some young life destroyed by diphtheritis, pneumonia, typhus, etc., in spite of the best care and medical treatment. Had the electric treatment been followed, I feel safe in saying that fully ninety-nine out of every hundred cases would have been cured. Since, however, most physicians have only a shrug of the shoulders for this new curative method, many a human being must die of a curable ailment before it wins its proper place, and is universally recognized as the safest curation method known. Science is still far from having said the last word regarding electricity. There are many things that have not yet been proved to the bottom, but the throbbing loom of time constantly yields new discoveries in this field and brings us one step nearer each day to a solution of this mysterious riddle, and as man a hundred years ago characterized those who endeavored to find a healing power in the secret forces of nature, as "charlatans", so many at the present time feel only contempt for those who do not rigidly follow rules of the regular schools of medicine but they will perhaps after the lapse of fifty years remember with gratitude those who now are unable to see infallibility in the practice of the schools.

## HARDENING

### by Benedict Lust

*The Kneipp Water Cure Monthly, I (9), 152-153. (1900)*

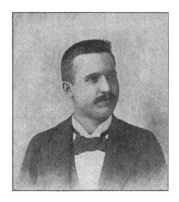

Benedict Lust.

By "hardening" the constitution we mean making it capable of resistance, especially to cold, and of remaining unaffected by unfavorable weather.

In commencing a hardening treatment, however, the patient's age, sex, habits of life and above all, the conditions of his nervous system must be taken into consideration.

### TREATMENT

The desired degree of hardening will be attained by daily cool or lukewarm ablutions and rubbing of the whole body if persevered in for some length of time, or by baths, together with the use of a moderate amount of clothing and bed-covering, taking constantly into consideration the constitution and nervous system of the patient. The best means of hardening the system are, however, short cold ablutions and baths of no longer than a minute's duration.

1. Commence with lukewarm ablutions, gradually reducing the temperature till the water is cool. In the case of individuals not suffering from weak nerves, the whole body may be rubbed with water of the same temperature.

2. Baths (91° F.) [33° C.] at the beginning, with cool affusions to be taken two or three times a week.
   Swimming baths of at least 71° F. [22° C.] may be recommended, also river baths of the same temperature in summer, duration two to four minutes. The bather should move vigorously all the time he is in the water.

3. It is not necessary to rub one's self dry after these baths. Exercise should be taken in the sunshine or in warm air until all moisture has evaporated from the body.

4. Walking barefoot is a simple and natural means of hardening the system.

Children should always walk barefoot. Anxious parents who are afraid to follow this advice should, at any rate, see that their children wear boots and shoes which admit fresh air coming in contact with the skin.

Children who can already stand and walk know how to help themselves. They throw away the troublesome and uncomfortable shoes and stockings without the slightest compunction and are quite happy immediately, especially in spring, when they are allowed to romp about as they please. Poor children are rarely interfered with in this pleasure. Less fortunate are the children of the rich. Prudent parents residing in towns and not possessing gardens should allow their children to walk barefoot at certain times and in certain room or passages, so that their feet may at times be quite free from covering and exhale properly; may absorb fresh air and move about in it like the face and hands.

Grown-up people of the poorer classes often walk about in the country barefoot, and do not grudge the richest dweller in the town the instruments of torture which he calls his boots, however, elegantly the latter may be fashioned and polished.

Grown-up dwellers in towns should walk up and down in their rooms from ten minutes to half an hour at a time immediately before retiring to rest or after rising in the morning, and in order that no discomfort may be experienced from commencing this practice too suddenly, at first in stockings, afterwards with bare feet. Before taking these walks the feet should be dipped for a few minutes in cold water up to the ankles.

Before walking barefoot, also before walking in water or on grass, care must be taken that the feet are thoroughly warm. If they are cold, they must be warmed by rubbing or by a short warm foot-bath. During the cold season these applications should be continued only for a short time, two minutes at the commencement.

A specially beneficial kind of barefoot walking is walking in wet grass. The wetter the grass, the longer and more often repeated the exercise, the greater will be the benefit derived from it. As a rule, the duration of one of these walks should be about a quarter of an hour.

After the walk, any sand, grass or dirt should be at once removed or washed from the feet, and dry shoes and stocking put on while the feet are still wet. Then a walk should be taken, starting off at a rapid gait which may be gradually reduced. The duration of this walk will depend on the rapidity with which the feet get dry and warm and should not exceed a quarter of an hour.

5. Walking on wet stones has an effect somewhat similar to that of walking in wet grass. A larger or smaller piece of stone paving will be found somewhere or other about every house. One can run rapid backward and forward in a long passage: on a small piece of paving one can tread the stones as the vintner treads the grapes or the baker's apprentice treads the dough in many places. The essential thing is that the stones should be wet and that one should not stand still on

them but walk or run with tolerable rapidity. A jug or watering-can can be used and a fair amount of water employed in making as broad and long a path as space may allow, and the water should be spread by the feet.

When used for curative purposes the duration of these applications should not exceed three to fifteen minutes. As a rule, from three to five minutes will be sufficient. Patients suffering from cold feet, throat troubles, catarrhs, tendency of blood to the head with consequent headache, should take these "wet stone walks" frequently.

6. A still more powerful effect will be obtained walking in fresh snow for half a minute.

7. Walking in water. It may appear a simple matter to walk in water reaching to the calves; this nevertheless is an excellent means of hardening the body. The patient may commence with moving about in a large bath with water enough to cover the ankles. The action is more powerful if the bath be filled with water reaching to the calves, and still more so when the water comes up to the knees. In the case of feeble patients it is best to commence with lukewarm water and gradually reduce the temperature till the water is quite cold.

8. For hardening the extremities (arms and legs) the following process is recommended by Kneipp. The patient should stand in cold water reaching up to or over the knees, not longer than a minute. After putting on his shoes, he must next bare his arms to the shoulders and hold them for a minute in the water. If possible both these processes should be performed at the same time, which presents no difficulty if the bath be long enough. A convenient plan is to stand with the feet in the vessel on the ground while the bared hands and arms are put in a wooden tub resting on a chair. A necessary condition of this application is that the body should be warm.

9. The knee-affusion as well as other "Kneipp" affusions is well adapted for hardening.*

10. On going out of a warm room into cold air in rough or cold weather it is a good thing to drink cold water, in order to strengthen the respiratory organs and make them capable of resisting the effects of cold air. Many colds may be avoided in this way both with children and adults. Breathing should be performed through the nose.

11. Vigorous exercises, such as gymnastics, swimming, etc., are conducive to the hardening and strengthening of the body.

Infants and small children may be strengthened by pouring a jug of

---

*The Kneipp knee affusion refers to the knee gush that was administered with a simple garden watering can or a hose and became Kneipp's signature water therapy. —Ed.

water over them on the conclusion of their daily bath, the water from the jug being a few degrees colder than that used in the bath (96° to 91° F.) [36° to 33° C.]. This, however, must not be done till a fortnight after birth and the temperature must be somewhat higher at the first and gradually reduced. Dr. Baumgarten, of Wörishofen, advises that children, after the first week of their life, should be dipped for a moment in water of 82° to 73° F. [23° to 28° C.] after every bath.

Hardening the body must be regarded as one of the most important aids to health and strength and a sovereign means for rendering it capable of resistance to injurious influences. In former times much less was heard of the necessity for hardening the constitution. The reason of this was not merely that little attention was paid in those times to national health and public hygiene, and that little interest was taken in these matters, but that the necessity for drawing attention to the importance of hardening did not exist to the same extent, as the conditions of life in those days were naturally adapted to "harden" people. It will be enough to remind our readers of the method of travelling in the days before the invention of railway trains and steamers. How many men and women, and even children, were employed more or less regularly as messengers, and got the opportunity of hardening themselves by travelling along almost impassible roads, in every kind of weather and often for hours without a halting place! Not only villagers but dwellers in towns were accustomed to long journeys on foot, with only a moderate amount of clothing, and freely exposed to the air, sunshine, and rain. It can be readily understood that laborers whose duties compelled them to walk long distances, and all pedestrians must have had abundant opportunity to harden themselves under such conditions! At a time when workshops were never heated, when there were no double windows, when servants and many others slept in icy cold attics, and when warming pans were used only by elderly people, opportunities for hardening were not lacking. In those times, moreover, the housework, even in families of good position, was much harder than now, so that servants were compelled to get hardened. In those days the popular recipe for the prevention and cure of anaemia and weakness in young girls was plenty of bodily work at home, and the universal medicine was—plenty of open-air exercise in all weathers without any anxiety about catching cold.

Since the conditions of life in the present day do not offer such opportunities in the same measure, the hardening process must be performed systematically by means of baths, wet rubbings, swimming, gymnastics, etc. Notwithstanding this artificial hardening and strengthening, most people have a dread of heat, cold, wind, and rain when they walk abroad, and walk in the country, even with a pleasurable object in view, is too much for them. This is the case not only among the well-to-do classes,

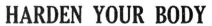
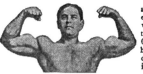
Benedict Lust began the first health food store in NYC selling Kneipp "hardening" products and opened a second store at Yungborn, Butler, New Jersey.

but even among the poor. Nowadays most people have a positive dread of bodily exercise.

Just because the altered conditions of life in the present day exact more brain work than in earlier times, no one should neglect bodily exercise, and give way to laziness and luxurious habits. Only in alternating mental and bodily exercise, work, and repose can a man develop naturally and remain in good health.

> *It is not necessary to rub one's self dry after these baths. Exercise should be taken in the sunshine or in warm air until all moisture has evaporated from the body.*
>
> *Before walking barefoot, also before walking in water or on grass, care must be taken that the feet are thoroughly warm.*
>
> *Walking in water. It may appear a simple matter to walk in water reaching to the calves; this nevertheless is an excellent means of hardening the body.*

# 1901

## PROSPECTUS OF THE NEW YORK NATUROPATHIC INSTITUTE AND COLLEGE AND OF THE SANITARIUM YUNGBORN
BENEDICT LUST

---

## MECHANICAL MASSAGE—HOW IT IS APPLIED
BENEDICT LUST

---

## OSTEOPATHY AND ITS RELATION TO NATURE
GEORGE BOLLER, D.O.

---

## THE VALUE OF PHYSICAL EXERCISE
RICHARD METCALFE

These ads appeared in 1901 in *The Kneipp Water Cure Monthly*. John Scheel was the first to use the term, "Naturopathy".

# Prospectus Of The New York Naturopathic Institute And College And Of The Sanitarium "Jungborn", Bellevue, Butler, New Jersey

by Benedict Lust

*The Kneipp Water Cure Monthly, II (7), 197-199. (1901)*

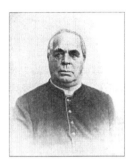

Mgr. Sebastian Kneipp.

The convincing results of Hydro-therapeutics (Water-applications) are evidenced by the fact that a great many medical men of high professional standing have abandoned Allopathic treatment and taken recourse to Hydro-Thermo-Therapy. Hundreds of Institutes for Water-Cure are at present scattered over Germany, one third of them being under the management of Doctors of Medicine.

Within a few years over 100 books on Water-Cure have been written and published in Germany. Some of these have been translated into many foreign languages and sold by the hundred thousands. Water-Cure is at present being introduced in many hospitals and all liberal-minded physicians adopt or recommend it in their practice.

Amongst all names who have furthered the cause of Water-Cure, shines first and foremost the name of that simple and humble Clergyman and physician at Wöerishofen, Rev. Father Kneipp, who, convinced of the superiority and efficacy thereof, inaugurated a new era in this particular department of the healing art by establishing a system of his own, built upon individual and keen observation, which has rapidly gained renown in all civilized portions of this globe, and is universally known as the "Kneipp Water Cure Method".

All the ills that flesh are heir to can (if curable) is treated successfully by HYGIENIC METHODS. When health is lost, it is folly to complicate the case or render it hopeless even, by taking drug poisons.

We do not believe in drug medicines, and we do not give them to our patients. The two systems (drugopathy and Hygeio-Therapy) [sic] do not work together.

When we are sick, the body is loaded with impurities. By taking drug-medicine we add to these impurities, and make the case harder to cure.

Better help the system to heal itself. The depurative organs and these alone, must do all the work of purification, and there are ways to aid them, which have no bad effects.

By treating with the Natural healing methods we assist Nature, and thus do not fill the country with invalids and cripples.

## DISEASES OF WOMEN

We have for many years made a specialty of the treatment of these diseases, and our uniform success in this kind of practice has given the greatest confidence in the methods we employ. Often we treat patients who have been under medical treatment for one, two or three years or even longer without having received any benefit therefrom, and after 60 to 90 days, we send them home well.

In cases of Chlorosis in young girls, painful menstruation, suppression, etc., the natural healing methods not only always give prompt relief, but also affect a speedy and complete cure.

Where there is displacement of the pelvic organs we employ with the best results, what is known as internal massage, "Thure Brandt Massage". This, in combination with ordinary natural treatment, consisting of baths, sun-light- and-air-baths, etc., especially adapted to this class of disorders, as well as to chronic congestions, inflammations of the ovaries, growths, polypi, etc., etc.

Pity it is that women should go under the knife and suffer mutilation at the hands of surgeons, when they could easily and effectually be cured by Natural Healing Methods.

For General Diseases, acute as well as chronic, the natural methods are admirably adapted, and when cured, "no other disorders set in". We do not believe in curing one disease by producing another; we remove the cause of the disease and so get rid of it entirely.

Amongst the disorders we have treated successfully are: Headaches, Vertigo, Constipation, Piles, Jaundice, Enlarged Spleen, Obesity, Congestion of the brain, Erysipelas, Apoplectic tendencies, Epilepsy, Chronic Diarrhoea, Dysentery, Inflammation and Ulceration of the stomach and bowels, Catarrh, Laryngitis, Bronchial affections, Pleurisy, Congestion of the lungs, Asthma, Pneumonia, Consumption in early stages, Hypochondria, Chlorosis, Hysteria, Gout, Rheumatism, Stiff Joints, Dropsy, Kidney Disease, Diabetes, Bright's Disease, Scrofula, Tumors, Abscesses, Eczema, and other disorders too numerous to mention.

## FORMS OF TREATMENT

(a) Application of Water: Full-Baths, Half-Baths, Trunk-Baths, Hip Baths and Partial Baths of the most varied temperatures are applied and there is a Swimming Bath in the Park of the Sanatorium. Full, Three quarter and Half Packs, etc. The Kneipp Wraps and Partial Wraps, Frictions, Slappings, Wetsheets, and Douches of all kinds according to the Kneipp Method.

(b) Application of Steam: Full Vapor Baths in Boxes in the sitting or reclining posture, Partial Vapor Baths, Steam Jets, and Steam Compresses.

(c) Application of Hot Air: Hot Air Baths—whole or partial—Sandbaths.

(d) Application of Light and Air: Sun baths, nude and in wraps, Electric-light baths, Air Baths, Walking Barefoot, Sleeping in the open air (open huts).

(e) Application of Electricity: Galvanic, Faradic, and Inductive Electricity applied with greatest exactitude. Electric Massage. Electric Baths (Faradic and Galvanic).

(f) Massage: of the whole or parts of the body according to approved Systems. Vibratory, Membranous and Internal Massage according to the Thure-Brandt Method.

(g) Gymnastics: Swedish or Resistance Gymnastics (particularly Manual Gymnastics on the Thure-Brandt Method).

(h) Psycho-Therapy: Mental and Suggestive Treatment.

All above applications are made by competent assistants.

## DIET

Mixed Diet, i.e., Meat and vegetables daily—if desired, Vegetarian Diet only. The food prescribed is that which is best suited to the constitution of each individual patient and the disease in question. A special diet is prescribed for patients suffering from any kind of gastronomic ailment under supervision of one of the doctors of the establishment.

The object of the establishment is:

1.  To cure or relieve as much as possible chronic patients of all kinds by the application of Natural Method of Healing by employing only Air, Light, Water, Electricity, Magnetism, Hypnotism, Massage, Gymnastics and Rational Diet.

2.  To reinstate convalescents in full possession of their strength as soon as possible by the application of strengthening treatment.

3.  To instruct (by means of lectures given by the doctors or manager) the patients in the Natural Mode of Living and in our Method of Healing, so that they may be enabled to protect themselves and their relatives at home from disease.

## NOTICE

1.  Application for treatment should be sent in at least one week in advance.

2.  Charges: The regular charges for one week including treatment, room and board is from $16 to $35 according to room and location. Children under twelve, half price.

3.  For extra service, additional board, meals served in rooms, etc., special rates will be charged.

4.  For patients who do not live in the Sanatorium, the weekly charge for treatment is $3 to $10 per week.

5.  Payments are to be made invariably, weekly, in advance.

6.  Consultation: Free, but a charge of $2 for a first examination will be made in every case. All further examination free.

7.  Patients and visitors must conform to the rules of the house.

8.  Any complaints are to be lodged with the manager or one of the Doctors in charge.

9.  All patient will have to furnish their own linen, bandages for water applications, Spanish mantles, wraps, etc., which they can purchase at a moderate charge on the premises.

    Visitors will be received at a charge of $2 per day.
    Single meals: 50 cents each.

Butler is a station on the New York, Susquehanna & Western R. R. [Rail Road]. Trains leave from Pennsylvania R. R. Depots. Time table mailed free on application.

Advice given by mail.

Correspondence in English, French, German and Spanish.

Parties desiring carriages on their arrival in Butler should give notice before hand.

For further information address:

N. Y. Naturopathic Institute, 135 E. 58th St., New York
or "Jungborn" Sanitarium, Bellevue, Butler, N.J.

---

*When we are sick, the body is loaded with impurities. By taking drug-medicine we add to these impurities, and make the case harder to cure.*

*We do not believe in curing one disease by producing another; we remove the cause of the disease and so get rid of it entirely.*

# MECHANICAL MASSAGE—HOW IT IS APPLIED

## by Benedict Lust

*The Kneipp Water Cure Monthly, II (9), 245-248. (1901)*

The great value of massage in the restoration of health is fully recognized, and in all cities and towns there are men and women who make a profession of the application of this form of treatment; physicians prescribe it as they do medicine; patients who can afford it employ these professional masseurs to give the treatment and from one to five dollars an hour is paid for the application of what is known as manual massage, which is given with the hand. This is of great service in many cases. Some find the treatment quite indispensable and it is kept up continually, of course at a good deal of expense. But there is another form of this treatment, known as mechanical massage, and there are institutions where this is applied by expensive machines that are operated by steam or other power, which is found to be very effective.

There has been recently devised by a New York physician, Dr. W. E. Forest, a hand appliance for the giving of mechanical massage, known as Massage Rollers, by which this treatment can be applied by one's self or an unskilled attendant.

The Massage Rollers consist of a series of wheels, about 1½ inches in diameter, each turning separately, on a flexible axle. Around the centre of each is a band or buffer of elastic rubber. This is set in a suitable handle convenient for use, and with these a strong, steady pressure can be brought to bear on the deep tissues and the internal viscera. These are not like a rolling pin, which may give pressure, but it is only by having the wheels turn separately that the peculiar effect, that is so like the human hand, is produced; there is alternate pressure and release, which impels a rapid circulation of the fluids of the body. There is little or no friction on the skin from the fact that the rollers turn, and the treatment may be taken over the underclothing or light bed clothing, without any exposure of the body, a very decided advantage over manual massage in many cases.

The Massage Rollers can be used for all functional troubles like dyspepsia, constipation, biliousness, nervous exhaustion, neuralgia, rheumatism, obesity, etc., and used over the entire body they will be found a great promoter of health and muscular elasticity. They should always be used over the underclothing after the bath, and will be found invaluable on the bare skin in connection with the air bath, that should be taken daily, exposing the skin to the fresh air, giving it a much more healthful condition, opening the pores and allowing them to breathe.

For rheumatism use a No. 1 or No. 2, roll very lightly over the affected part and if in the joint rub thoroughly above and below; if in the back or shoulders roll around the part, and where there is a good deal of inflammation treat the part affected but lightly and roll thoroughly the adjacent parts and over the whole body to stimulate the circulation. For chronic cases treat twice daily, for acute cases every two hours. For stiffness following attacks of rheumatism or sprains roll the part very thoroughly and persistently so as to break up the adhesion of the muscles, which is the cause of this condition.

Those who have to stand much, causing the muscles of the limbs to become tired, will find great relief in the use of the roller. The method of application is shown very well in fig. 2. Either one roller or two may be used.

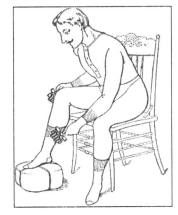

Fig. 2

For paralysis go thoroughly over the affected part with as much pressure as is agreeable at least three times a day, rolling up and down and crosswise, treating mostly the part affected, that the blood and nutrition may be brought there to build up and strengthen the nerves and muscles. Of course recovery will be likely to be slow, but often there is relief from the very first.

In cases of neuralgia such treatment should be given as will take the blood from the congested parts. If in the head and face the movement should be downward over the veins and blood vessels using the No. 3 roller, repeating frequently until relief is afforded, taking as much rest as is possible.

If you wake up in the morning tired, too tired to rise and dress, perhaps lame and sore from unusual exertion—we all have such mornings—and can prevail upon some friend or companion to take the roller, and, while you lie covered with a sheet, go over you vigorously, up and down and across the back and along the thighs, legs and arms, then the chest, and finally a thorough treatment of the abdomen, by that time there will not be a nerve in the body but tingles, and you will feel as vigorous as a well-groomed race horse.

This is a real tonic, not an irritant, to the system; a tonic well fitted to restore energy and life to many a sofa-bound invalid.

Dyspepsia, including all forms of stomach troubles, indigestion, constipation and torpidity of the liver, can be relieved and cured by the use of the Massage Rollers over the stomach and bowels, over the liver and the back.

For indigestion drink as much water as can be taken readily and massage over the stomach thoroughly. Finish with an upward movement from the left to the right over the stomach, so as to empty the stomach and cleanse it of accumulated impurities; then roll over the small intestines a few times, and the breakfast will digest much better. This treatment should be continued until there is relief from the trouble.

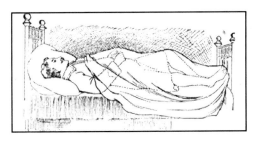

Fig. 3

For constipation it is recommended that the rollers be used thoroughly morning and night by the person lying down, taking the No. 1 or No. 2 roller by the frame in both hands as shown in fig. 3, thoroughly massaging the centre of the abdomen so as to stimulate the action of the small intestines, also treating close to and under the edge of the ribs, the stomach and liver. Then finish by passing the roller up on the right side over the ascending colon, across just below the ribs and down over the descending colon on the left side as much as one hundred times and in severe cases more than this. This treatment should be with as much force as feels agreeable and pleasant—not necessary to use more than this. Sometimes the movement of the gases in the intestine will cause some slight pain or griping, but this should be considered as a favorable

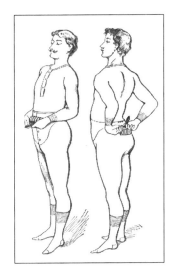

Fig 4. for bowels. Fig 5 for back.

indication showing that results sought for are being accomplished. After rising, the roller may be used over the stomach and bowels the same as when lying, as indicated in fig. 4, and some find better results from taking the most of the treatment in this way. It is also well to roll the back as in fig. 5, reaching up as high as is convenient and down over the hips. The most severe forms of constipation have been relieved by this method of treatment.

The following letter, which bears strong testimony as to the value of the rollers in indigestion, is from a lady who is well known, but naturally prefers not to publish her name in this connection, though almost daily she recommends the rollers to those she meets who would be benefited by their use.

Dear Sirs—For many years I have been a great sufferer with a stomach trouble, which the doctors at last, after dieting and taking all kinds of medicines without more than a momentary relief, pronounced neuralgia of the stomach and bowels, I bought a Muscle Roller in the spring of '97, used it faithfully and regularly, and now for a period of five months I have had no trouble whatever. I eat as I will, and what I will, and nothing causes me any disturbance. The roller has taken away the soreness from the stomach, which was at times extreme. I am grateful for the relief I have received from it, and most unhesitatingly pronounce it something which everyone could use with benefit. It will relieve nervousness, and will rest and give relief to overtired muscles. In my case it has saved doctors' bills and druggists' bills as well, which were a large item of expense before I began to use the roller. Wishing you all success, I am,

       Yours, sincerely,
       L.A.F.
       Boston, Nov. 11, 1897.

In the use of the roller for this and all chronic troubles, it must be done thoroughly. It will not answer to use it only occasionally, or as you may feel like it, but make a business of it, and the sought for result will surely follow. Of course, it is also important to observe proper care as to diet, exercise and all the laws of health and hygiene.

There are two conditions to be avoided in the acquiring of health, strength and comeliness of form or personal beauty; one is the excess of adipose tissue or flesh, the other is the want of it. These conditions depend upon heredity and environment or conditions; whatever the cause may be, something may be done to overcome the results of either condition.

The person who is becoming too fleshy should of course avoid an excess of fat producing foods and take an abundance of exercise. When this can be fully carried out, the desired result will be secured, but often times it may be difficult to regulate the diet properly, and especially for want of time and physical strength to secure the necessary amount of bodily exercise, as this frequently comes with advancing years when there is a lessening of physical force and strength, or is the result of diseased and abnormal conditions, rendering the person weak, and there is not sufficient bodily strength to take the requisite amount of exercise for the accomplishment of the purpose much to be desired.

There is often, especially in advancing years, an accumulation of fatty tissue, particularly over the hips and abdomen that is undesirable from the standpoint of health as well as beauty. Various anti-fat remedies are advertised and used, but these cannot be commended, for if the result is obtained, it is at the expense of health and strength by an impairment of the functions of digestion and assimilation, and a general weakening of the system.

This form of massage has been found very effective for the reduction of flesh by a steady, hard pressure with a long sweeping movement. The soft, often watery cells are broken up, carried into the circulation and so eliminated, and thus the accumulation of fatty tissue, particularly over the hips and abdomen, can be overcome in a very effective and satisfactory manner with a constant increase in vigor, strength and muscular activity. Women can secure a reduction of the hips by rolling with a steady pressure up and down over each side from above the waist to the lower part of the thigh (fig. 6) and on down to the knees and ankles if necessary (fig. 9). Ladies who are not strong may begin this treatment in bed before rising in the morning, over the night dress, on the hips and abdomen and finish it after rising. A favorable time to take it is after the bath; the use of the roller then over the entire body will prevent fatty accumulations and preserve a good form and figure.

This treatment should always be lengthwise of the muscular tissues and not crosswise and should be applied a hundred or more times over each part morning and evening. Where there is special abdominal fullness, it can be overcome by rolling the side of the abdomen just in front of the hip bone (fig. 7) which will tend to a contraction of the muscles, drawing the abdomen back in place. Ladies who have a maid can be relieved of a part of the work by being rolled by her over the hips and thighs while lying on a bed or couch.

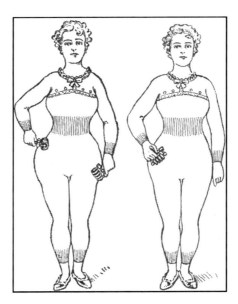

Fig 6. For reducing hip.        Fig 7.

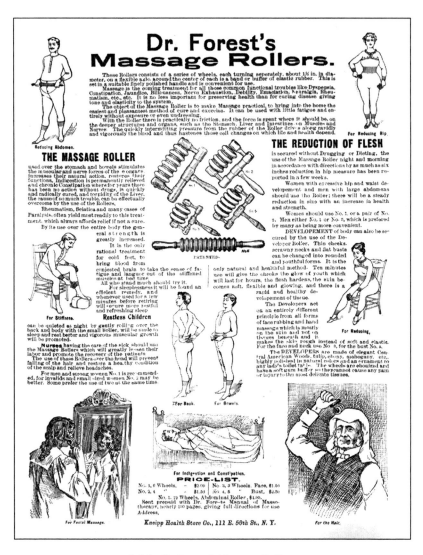

Ad for Dr. Forest's Massage Rollers.

Men who are stout find the most effective results by the use of the No. 5 roller, as shown in fig. 4. and with this roller the waist and abdominal fullness can be reduced with a continuous increase of bodily comfort, health and strength. There should be a firm, steady pressure brought with the roller over the abdomen and over the hips, sides and back, taking the treatment every night and every morning, on retiring and on rising, over the under-clothing.

Wherever there is a tendency to a flabby condition of any part, this will help to restore the muscular strength and activity. While it is not necessary to restrict our diet to certain specific articles, it is well, when there is a tendency to make flesh fast, to avoid food that is especially fat producing.

As developers, the use of the rollers have been found very effectual for a rapid and healthful filling out of the face, neck and bust.

It is often asked how it is possible that the same appliance will both reduce and increase flesh, but a word of explanation will make this plain. In the reduction of the tissues the pressure is made sufficiently hard to break down the fatty cells, which are carried into the circulation and in this way eliminated, while for the building up of any part, treatment is given very lightly and, as far as possible, crosswise of the veins and muscles, so that it brings the blood to the parts, and of course in this way feeds the tissues, which must result in building them up. For the face, the treatment should be made with a somewhat rotary motion over the cheeks, and crosswise of all wrinkles, which will remove these, and around the neck and over the chest both crosswise and up and down, so as to thoroughly stimulate the activity of the absorbents, bearing in mind it must be done lightly. If the breasts are thin and flat, in the morning on rising bathe them in cold water, rubbing briskly; put on the under vest and, with a No. 4 roller, roll from the sides and under the busts towards the centre, in this way building up these parts, rolling lightly but firmly, and as many as a hundred times or more over each part. If the hands are thin and bony, roll them lightly, so as to bring the blood into them and so fill out the tissues. Roll across the arms or limbs to develop these parts. This treatment takes the nutrition from a part of the body that is full to a part that is wanting. If there is general emaciation, the rollers should be used over the stomach and bowels so as to increase nutrition, and over the whole body so as to restore circulation, promote assimilation and secure better nutrition.

For the hair or scalp, a light towel or handkerchief may be put over the head, and then a thorough rolling of all parts of the scalp with a No. 3 roller, as shown in fig. 12. If this is done daily it will tend to a much more healthful condition of the scalp and so of the hair, and will often stop or prevent falling out.

For insomnia, roll with the No. 3 roller downward over the arteries at the side of the neck from three to five minutes. Retire as quietly as possible; relax all the muscles and lie heavily on the bed forcing yourself to think of nothing. Having an attendant with No. 2, roll the side and back up and down gently or as hard as feels pleasant, and over the arms and limbs, turning quietly so as to have the other side treated also; turn on the back that the chest, stomach and bowels may be gently rolled, then on the right side, and lie slightly forward that the back and spine may be rolled from the head downward and over the limbs, and sleep will almost always be secured with much more of refreshing rest. In cases of collapse and swooning away for want of strength, the vigorous use of the roller

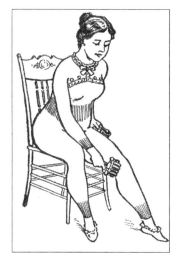

Fig 9. For reducing.

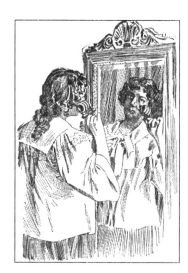

Fig 10. For facial massage.

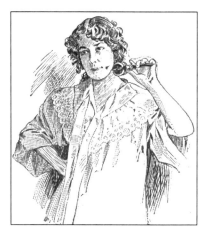

Fig 10. For insomnia.

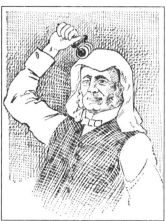

Fig, 12. For the hair.

will restore the circulation and revive the patient. It acts as a tonic and stimulant, from which there will be no reaction.

In general, for stimulating and equalizing the circulation, roll the entire body from head to feet for ten minutes over the underclothing or on the bare skin, in which case the advantage of an air bath is also secured. This in the morning will be found to arouse the circulation, a good preparation for the day, and often much better than the cold water bath, and at night it will equalize the circulation, draw the blood from the brain, and relieve cold extremities. Either No. 1 or No. 2 can be used for this purpose. It is not too much to say there is no morbid condition of the system that will not be helped by a proper application of the massage roller treatment, for the simple reason that it promotes and equalizes the circulation and promotes the building of a new tissue.

*These are not like a rolling pin, which may give pressure, but it is only by having the wheels turn separately that the peculiar effect, that is so like the human hand, is produced; there is alternate pressure and release, which impels a rapid circulation of the fluids of the body.*

*For constipation it is recommended that the rollers be used thoroughly morning and night by the person lying down, taking the No. 1 or No. 2 roller by the frame in both hands as shown in fig. 3, thoroughly massaging the centre of the abdomen so as to stimulate the action of the small intestines, also treating close to and under the edge of the ribs, the stomach and liver.*

*Of course, it is also important to observe proper care as to diet, exercise and all the laws of health and hygiene.*

## Osteopathy And Its Relation To Nature

### by Dr. George Boller, Osteopathic Physician, New York

*The Kneipp Water Cure Monthly, II (10), 269-271. (1901)*

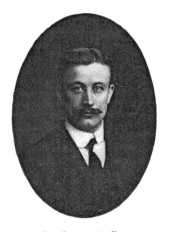

Dr. George Boller.

What is Osteopathy?

Osteopathy is derived from the two Greek words, *Osteon* meaning bone, and *Pathos* meaning suffering, and is now the name of the new scientific method or system of treating diseased conditions of the human body, without medicine or knife.

Osteopathy is nothing more or less than an adjustment of the human body. It aims to correct misplacements of a bone, ligament or muscle, the obstruction of a blood vessel, nerve inactivity, fluid congestion or the collection of diseased germ-laden fluids in the system. In the removal of these obstructions, irritations and hindrances to free activity lies the osteopathic work, the secret of health restoration.

The name Osteopathy was given to the new science on account of the fact, that the displacement of bone occupied the first place in the category of causes or lesions producing disease conditions.

Osteopathy was discovered by Andrew Taylor Still, M.D. in 1874. His reasoning was, "that a natural flow of blood is health; that disease is the effect of local or general disturbance of the blood; that to excite the nerves causes muscles to contract and to compress venous flow of blood to the heart; and that the bones could be used as levers to relieve pressure on nerves, veins and arteries." Dr. Still conceived the idea that the human system is a machine, perfectly framed by its Maker and if kept in a condition of proper adjustment, it is capable of surviving for a long time. He found that manipulations could be made, almost at will, in connection with the skeletal structure, with the result that all the organs could be stimulated to perform their normal functions. Out of this beginning there has developed a system, able to restore all the abnormal structural and functional disorder of the human body.

Osteopathy is based on accurate knowledge of the anatomical structure and physiological functions of the human body or organism. Nature has placed within the body certain vital forces, vitalized fluids, and vitalizing processes and activities, which in harmony with one another maintain the equilibrium of the body-mechanism. Any disturbance of these forces, fluids or processes and any interference with their activity, circulation or distribution involve the absence of harmony and interference of body order. In the removal of these disturbances and hindrances to free activity lies the great secret of Osteopathy. Scientific manipulations are designed to restore these to their normal condition, so that the body may regain its normal functional equilibrium and form. In this way life is revitalized and strengthened by vital forces, vitalizing fluids and processes, disease being removed or overborne by getting rid of functional disorder that produces disharmony in the body and prevents normal activity of body functions.

Osteopathy makes no demands upon the vitality of the patient, but enlists all the curative powers contained within the body, which readily respond when properly appealed to. Its method is purely mechanical and its therapeutic principles might be classified as follows:

1.  Scientific manipulations, that correct displacements in the bony or tissue structure of the body, in its membranes or organs;
2.  Scientific manipulations, that are designed to rectify the disturbances in the circulation of the body fluids and to restore them to their normal condition, especially blood conditions and defects in the blood circulation and distribution; and
3.  Scientific manipulations that utilize the nervous system with its fibres, ganglia and centres, with the view of correcting nervous disorders, toning up the general system, or its local parts, promoting trophic conditions of the nerves and muscles and stimulating a normal correlation of the psychic with the physiological and vegetative functions of the human body.

Osteopathic diagnosis is entirely a new science and involves the idea of a refined and sensitive taction [to touch]. It is based upon the theory of discovering the cause or causes of disease.

Osteopathic symptomatology summarizes diagnostic conditions as follows:

1.  Displacement of bone, cartilage, ligament, muscle, tissue, or organs in the body;
2.  Disturbances in the fluids of the organism, including the blood, lymph and other secretions of the body; and
3.  Disorders or derangements of tension, impingement, thickening, induration, etc., of the nervous system, including its centres, ganglia, plexuses and fibres.

A complete anatomical and physiological knowledge enables the practitioner to properly discriminate between normal and abnormal conditions. Osteopathic examination of a patient by far excels any subjective statement of the case, as facts become the scientific basis of true diagnosis. The osteopathic physician traces the condition of disturbance to its primary cause, through or by the aid of symptoms and secondary conditions. Here, Osteopathy has stepped far ahead of any other science or school of healing.

The first examination of a patient by an Osteopath is with special reference to the normality of the skeleton, for though a luxation* may be but partial, it may be causing a pressure at some point upon a nerve or blood vessel, of which the patient is entirely unconscious and which thus remains unaccounted for, as a barrier to healthy restoration.

That luxations are much more common than supposed, and can be produced by an accident so slight, as to go unobserved, is painfully demonstrated by the thousands of cases that have been overlooked by some of the most eminent physicians. When, had they been searched for from the osteopathic standpoint, they could, no doubt, have been easily reduced, thus removing the cause of many so-called chronic diseases, that often prove so perplexing to the practitioner of the medical science.

Osteopathy does not ignore the fact, that there are many indirect causes that may be classified under the head of predisposing causes, distinguished from the direct causes of diseased conditions. From a sanitary and hygienic standpoint, bacilli of multiform variety, infested germs, come into play in producing disturbances of functions and causing local or general disorder in the tissues of the body. Osteopathy proves that behind these secondary causes is found the real cause of disease; these conditions simply furnishing the means for the action of a perverted function and therefore involving a derangement of the tissue.

Osteopathically, the first fundamental principle of therapeutics, when diagnosis has discovered such structural or fundamental disorder, is to remove the lesion or correct the displacement, whether of bone, cartilage, ligament or muscle. Hereafter, attention is paid to the general health of the patient, by specific manipulation to the body tissue, so as to promote free circulation of the body fluids, along with attendance to correct hygienic and dietetic rules.

A free flow of blood is the remedial agency in the osteopathic treatment of inflammatory processes, their termination by resolution being promoted by relaxation of the structures involved, thus freeing the blood-passages through and from the affected area, whereby the capillaries are flushed with a fresh supply of blood, removing rapidly morphological elements as the circulation is being restored. This method is not only effective in simple processes, but especially so in those where micro-organism is a peculiar characteristic, such as diphtheria or typhoid fever. Osteopathy has for its purpose in the treatment of all such diseases, simply the resto-

---

*Luxation is a complete dislocation of a joint. —Ed.

ration of healthy tissue, as no microbe can inhabit tissues physiologically normal, and only such as have imperfect elimination of waste materials are susceptible to their invasion and are suitable for their development. They are, therefore, the result rather than the cause of pathological conditions.

The greatest physiologists teach that one of the most important offices of the white blood corpuscles is to destroy invading micro-organisms. Undoubtedly they are a powerful microbicide, a remedial agency in these processes, especially provided by nature, and consequently uninjurious to the system.

Osteopathy has discovered that stimulation of the spleen by vibration will increase the corpuscular richness of the blood, thereby aiding in the destruction of the micro-organic germs.

Treating diseased conditions by the vasomotor system, it is possible to keep the circulation of fresh and nutritious blood, so as to check the ravages of the micro-organic germs to such an extent as to promote the destruction of microbes by the action of phagocytes, by stimulating the white blood corpuscles to activity in the destruction of the micro-organism or by the production of chemical compounds that destroy the germs. This renders unnecessary the dangerous injection of serum, on the basis of serum-therapy, including vaccination that inflicts untold suffering and brings death to thousands of ignorant mortals yearly.

The Osteopath looks upon the nervous system of the human body as an immense electrical machine, containing its own batteries, wires and other necessary appliances. It is capable of generating all the force needed and simply requires perfect continuity and coordination by mechanical methods. The brain receives sensory impressions, and transmits motive impulses. The spinal cord conducts them to and from the various wires, which carry the impulses to the most remote tissues of the entire body.

The control of the nervous system over the functions concerned in the motion, sensation and nutrition of the entire body, places it among the leading agencies of Osteopathic therapeutics.

In the spinal cord, the most important part of the human body to the Osteopath, there are localized subsidiary centers, corresponding with the primary brain centers, so that in nervous disorders or diseases of a nervous origin or complication, the operator can reach those centers of vital activity in connection with the vital forces, by manipulation along the spine. It is, therefore, within the power of a skillful Osteopath to produce effects in almost any part of the body, so that by spinal stimulation, neural harmony, neural trophicity* and neural continuity of impulses may be established.

---

*Trophicity is an archaic term for the body's innate mechanisms—i.e., its *physiology*—*by which it replenishes depleted nutrients and restores homeostasis.* —Ed.

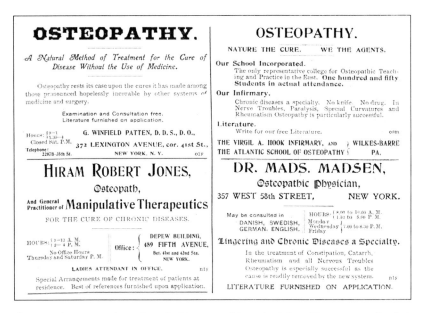

Osteopaths were aligned with Naturopathic principles. These are ads that appeared in 1901 in *The Kneipp Water Cure Monthly*.

The Osteopath, with a thorough knowledge of the many nerve centers and the innervation of the various tissues and organs, is capable to co-ordinate the nerve force of the body, and to increase the nerve-current in almost any part of the being. The practicability of this has been satisfactorily demonstrated in the osteopathic treatment of ataxia, paralysis, anesthetic and hyperesthetic conditions as well as in regulation of the secretory and peristaltic processes in the intestines, the regulation of the action of the heart, controlling the circulatory system, and all inflammatory and febrile conditions.

The old school of medicine made it a study and practice for centuries, to discuss and explore the field of drug-action upon the tissues and organs of the human body, while the Osteopath has been substituting the laboratory of human nature for the medical drug laboratory. This human laboratory, the human organism, is the most wonderful that exists anywhere in the universe. It generates acids, alkalies and all necessary fluids and chemical compounds to wash away accumulations of waste and impurity. The most wonderful chemical results are taking place, every moment of our lives, which form the basis of those normal changes that keep the body in a healthy condition. All bodily disorders are the result of mechanical obstructions to free circulation of vital fluids and forces and harmony of nerve force; they are an interference with the normal action of the human laboratory.

If, for example, a quantity of blood is thrown out by means of rupture, the result is a tumorous condition, resulting in the temporary suspension of vital activity. Such deposits are capable of being removed by nature's means, osteopathically. In the body's chemical laboratory process of compounding, reducing and forming substances of all chemical varieties, lies nature's power to dissolve the most solid substances, so as to prepare for the up-building process.

Osteopathic manipulations, scientifically applied, will throw in the chemical supplies of the human laboratory, where they are most demanded, thus assisting nature in the renovation, by furnishing it with such substances as are needed, so as to remove all hindrances to health, and to supply all that is necessary to normal vitality.

The Osteopath's knowledge of the great natural laws of nerve action, in connection with the human body laboratory, enables him to hold the forces of the body at his finger's ends and to direct them toward the recovery of the natural conditions of health.

Osteopathy began by demonstrating its therapeutic value in the case of alleged chronic conditions. It has branched out in every direction, until to-day it covers the whole field of medicine.

The osteopathic principle is a time-honored one, *similia similibus curantur*, in the sense, that the only rational and scientific method of curing disease is based upon nature. It uses all the therapeutic principles, from a standpoint of nature, such as the use of proper hygienic and dietetic principles, and in fact any principle that is in the line of nature or natural laws of the human body.

Osteopathy gained its results, because it uses natural methods and aids nature. All nature is pregnant with force, and natural force is the most remedial, because it is natural.

---

*Osteopathy is nothing more or less than an adjustment of the human body. It aims to correct misplacements of a bone, ligament or muscle, the obstruction of a blood vessel, nerve inactivity, fluid congestion or the collection of diseased germ-laden fluids in the system.*

*The Osteopath's knowledge of the great natural laws of nerve action, in connection with the human body laboratory, enables him to hold the forces of the body at his finger's ends and to direct them toward the recovery of the natural conditions of health.*

## THE VALUE OF PHYSICAL EXERCISE

### by Richard Metcalfe

*The Kneipp Water Cure Monthly, II (11), 312-314. (1901)*

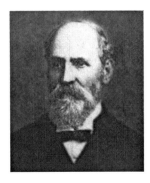

Richard Metcalfe.

The structure of man's body renders exercise absolutely necessary to his health. He resorts to it instinctively, impelled by the strong love of activity implanted in him by Nature for her own wise purposes. By exercising the circulation is promoted, especially in the multitude of minute vessels which ramify through every part of the body, a vigorous action of the lungs is secured, vigor and activity are imparted to all the organs as well as healthful energy to all the functions, and strength, elasticity, and grace developed in the body. Attention to exercise will bring out all the constitutional power inherent in the system, and tend to secure health and longevity.

When any organ is active, blood and nervous energy flow to it in an increased degree; hence increased nutrition and tone, proportionate to the demands made upon the organ in question. When its action is judiciously regulated, being alternated with repose, a permanent increase in the supply of arterial blood takes place, which leads to increased development and vigor of function. This is strikingly illustrated where one arm is vigorously exercised and the other is unemployed. The muscles of the former exhibit a far more powerful development than those of the latter.

Hence the due development and maintenance of the whole system depends on each part's being fully exercised, so that a certain amount of labor or activity of some sort is essential to a man's welfare. Without it he cannot possess the bodily vigor, health, buoyant spirits, and keen sense of enjoyment of which his nature is capable. Every individual ought, therefore to lay himself (or herself) under a necessity to take exercise of some sort. Where it is not had in the ordinary employments, walking, riding, out-door sports, or gymnastics should be had recourse to: It matters not particularly what method is pursued so long as a due amount of exercise be secured.

A most important point is that the mind be exercised at the same time with the body. Exercise in order to be beneficial must be enjoyed. A solitary ride or walk is of infinitely less benefit than the social canter or pedestrian trip, or picnic. Exercise does most good when enjoyment is the immediate object—when all considerations for health are for the moment forgotten, and social health and hilarity inspire every movement.

This is too much lost sight of in the exercises engaged in by many people. The formal walk of the young ladies' boarding school makes the poor creatures an object of pity. How different would be their motions and the benefit derived from them if engaged in active play or dancing! How stirring is the effect of martial music on soldiers wearily trudging along the march; and a South African trudging along on the march; and a South African traveler tells us when he and his party were exhausted with fatigue, as soon as they got a glimpse of the game all their languor left them in an instant. The bright eye and elastic step of exercise, when mingled with mirth, show how great is the power of the nervous stimulus to increase the benefits of the muscular action.

It is not sufficient to go daily through a fixed and circumscribed mode of taking exercise. Besides becoming monotonous and spiritless, it only puts in motion a certain set of muscles, and so fails to affect the purpose which was had in view. There must be variety in exercise. By the means the whole or greater part of the muscular system is brought into play, and each single muscle secures that alternate contraction and relaxation which is the only condition favorable to its perfect development. The action of each set of muscles is, of course, more or less local; thus walking more particularly exercises the muscles of the legs, rowing those of the chest and arms, etc.; so that, if only one description of exercise be engaged in, the benefits derived therefrom are to a considerable extent confined in that part of the system thus brought into action, though there can be no doubt that all the healthful exercise must result in general good to the constitution from the impulse given to the functional activity of the system.

It is contrary to all physiological law that any one set of muscles should be kept long in a state of relaxation or tension, as is the case with the living model of the statuary who must preserve for hours the same attitude. From the same cause much deformity exists among boarding-school girls, from the constrained positions which many of them for hours are compelled to maintain. Persons confined to the desk or study frequently suffer from this cause; the few muscles brought into play are overstrained, but the bulk of them, as well as the bones, become weak from disease, and general debility follows.

How inactivity of the voluntary muscles should impair the general tone of the system will appear when it is considered that their special purpose is to use up the animal fibrin or richest portion of the blood, and that when not doing so some 30 percent of the blood is rendered useless and thrown back into the general circulation. The brain, ganglionic centres, spinal marrow, lungs, heart, and blood vessels thus become filled to repletion, and the functions of the viscera are embarrassed by the stoppage of the chief outlets to waste. Apoplectic or paralytic seizures are consequently rendered imminent. It must be remembered that the voluntary muscles form one entire half of the human frame, that they are extremely vascular, and that in proportion to their activity they demand nutrition. But where no stimulus is, there can be no flexes, and hence internal congestions with their unhappy issues.

It is really surprising, when thus considering its importance both as a preserver of health and preventive of disease, that the exercise should have been so long and so much neglected. But it only affords another instance of the fact, that, in spite of our many advantages, we are still far behind the ancients in many branches of knowledge and art. Even the Chinese, whom we still look upon somewhat in the light of half barbarians, have from time immemorial seen and provided for the necessity of adequate exercise. The humidity of the climate was looked upon as a prolific source of the endemic and epidemic diseases, against which the only effectual preventative consisted in the regular exercise of the body by a description of gymnastic dance; and so all-important was it considered in relation to the welfare of the people that it was under Government regulation.

In addition to this, the Chinese have a system of medical gymnastics, dating back, it is said, to over two thousand years anterior to the present era; and so potent is it in the cure and relief of many diseases that people of every rank resort to it when every other means has been tried in vain. Father Amiot, a Jesuit Missionary who spent some forty-four years in China during the latter half of last century, says: "Volumes might be written of the traditions, stories, and extravagant virtues of the Cong Fou [Kung Fu], which are implicitly believed; even the majesty of the throne not exempting many emperors from a stupid credulity. Notwithstanding the priestly superstitions connected with it (for the priests persuade the people that it is a true exercise of religion), it is really a very ancient practice of medicine, founded on principles, and potent in many diseases."

M. Amiot gives, at considerable length, a description of the methods and principles of this therapeutic system of movements, from which it appears that morning was considered the proper time for treatment. The Cong Fou consisted in placing the body in certain positions and keeping it in each successive posture for some time, great stress being at the same time laid on particular methods of breathing. These methods were chosen and combined according to the disease of the patient.

The ancient inhabitants of Hindustan also practiced many bodily movements of a nature greatly resembling those of the Chinese. One of the most weighty of them was the retention of the air in respiration, it being believed that air has the same effect on the body that fire produces upon metals exposed to its influence—namely, that of purifying it. Similar ideas were entertained among the Greeks. We learn from the narrative of a Greek who visited India in the third century before our era that there was an order of Brahmins who relied chiefly on regimen of diet, together with external manipulations, for the cure of disease; and we know that there is at the present time an order of Brahmins whose principal therapeutic agency is hygienic shampooing.

Little need be said respecting exercises among the Greeks and Romans. Everyone, who has any acquaintance with the history of those peoples, knows what an important part gymnastics played in their educational system, more especially among the former. With the Greeks the gymnasium was the place for both physical and mental culture, the two going hand in hand, and probably no town of importance was without one of these schools. Education began at the seventh year, and consisted of music, grammar, and physical training. It is asserted by some historians that as much time was given to the development of the body as to the culture of the mind. In Sparta physical culture was of paramount importance, polite literature and the arts suffering proportionately in consequence. Even the women were obliged to go through the same exercises as the men; for, said the law givers, "Female slaves are good enough to stay at home and spin; but who can expect a splendid offspring—the appropriate gift of a free Spartan woman to her country—from mothers brought up in such occupation?"

With the Romans there was less appreciation of exercise, as a sanitary or educational means; they being a nation of soldiers, the first and often sole object they had in view was the promotion of physical strength for warlike purposes. They had gymnasiums, but these became perverted, especially in the latter days of the empire, into exhibitions of the most brutal and degrading description.

During the whole of the Middle Ages, exercise, that is, exercise as a system, appears to have been universally neglected; and it was not until Ling called attention to the subject that the modern mind began to appreciate its importance. To him we are indebted for one of the most perfect systems of physiological gymnastics ever invented. It is known as the *Swedish movements*. Dr. Dio Lewis, Mr. Watson, and Dr. Roth have also given their attention to gymnastics and calisthenics, and their systems have met with much favor. Of all four it may be said that they "comprise a great variety of movements calculated to develop the osseous and muscular systems, and so give freedom and ease to the carriage." They may be used by invalids, women, and children without any risk and with considerable benefit.

It connection with this subject of exercise, I must not omit to mention in the hands of Dr. W. Johnson, Mr. Grosvenor, Dr. Balfour, Admiral Henry, and others has almost been reduced to a science. I refer to rubbing and percussion, though to enter upon the subject here in anything like a

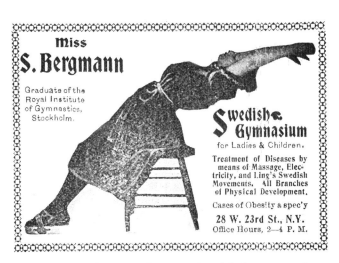
Peter Ling had developed exercises known as Swedish Gymnasium that could be performed using simple equipment such as a chair.

concise form would lead me too far. I must simply be satisfied by referring my readers to Dr. W. Johnson's valuable work entitled, *The Anatriptic Art.*

While thus urging the importance of exercise, it is always with the proviso that it be proportioned to the strength of the patient. Pushed beyond this, it is followed by exhaustion, and the body is weakened instead of being strengthened. Some inconsiderate people, thinking that if exercise be a good thing the more they have of it the better, make an amount of exertion altogether disproportionate to their muscular development or vital stamina, and hence experience a painful sense of weariness and exhaustion, and their sleep is uneasy and disturbed, they having drawn too much on both the muscular and nervous energy. Not only does undue exertion have this effect, but it also alters the constitution of the blood itself by impairing the powers of nutrition. This is noticeable in animals that have been hunted to death, whose blood is found to be in a fluid state, and whose bodies speedily become putrid, and in that of soldiers, worn out with long marches, who, when attacked with fever, seldom recover.

As muscular activity involves waste, and therefore active nutrition, it is evident that food, in proportion to the exertion made, is absolutely necessary. Activity and appetite generally go together, and where the activity goes on, the appetite remains unsatisfied; there is loss of flesh and diminished vital power. This is the state of multitudes of poor people whose vocations compel them to exertion, but whose scanty and unnutritious diet is altogether incapable of adequately supplying the waste caused by it. Hence the pallor, feebleness and disease of debility so common among that class in our large cities; and from this cause it is no doubt that the stimulus of ardent spirits is too often had recourse to.

A sudden bound from an inactive, sedentary life to that of a pedestrian or gymnast would of course be attended with injurious consequences. Everything must have a beginning, and personal habits are in man so influential in modifying his bodily powers that one set cannot be all at once exchanged for another without inconvenience. The transition to be beneficial must be gradual. A person who has been unaccustomed to activity should therefore be careful to graduate his eversions when he does begin them, so that his powers shall never be overtaxed, otherwise he may jump to the conclusion that exercise does not agree with him. Let him go on by degrees from little to much, and he will find that it does, and leads him on "from strength to strength".

The times for exercise ought to be judiciously selected. One grand rule is that is should never be engaged in after a full meal. For the healthy, early morning is the best time, when the stomach is empty and the body refreshed by sleep. Invalids, however—unless their appetite for breakfast is defective, in which case they may take a short stroll in the open air should defer their walking exercise till after breakfast, and always leave off before exhaustion from want of food sets in. The necessity of this precaution also mitigates against the expediency of much walking or other active exercise immediately before a meal. In both cases the blood is diverted from the digestive organs, where it is urgently needed, and digestion is interfered with in consequence. An interval of rest should always precede and follow any meal.

The kinds of exercise which should be resorted to must depend on a variety of circumstances. Walking is most readily had recourse to by most people, and it brings well into play the muscles of the loins and lower limbs. It, however, does not secure sufficient play to the muscles of the arms and chest, and should therefore be diversified by such exercises as rowing, fencing, shuttlecock, bowls, hand-ball, etc., which besides exercising the muscles of the trunk and arms pleasantly stimulate the mind— an advantage which has already been dwelt upon.

Riding is, especially for those of weak lungs, a most healthful exercise, having the advantage of not hurrying the breathing. "It calls into more equal play," says Dr. Combe, "all the muscles of the body and at the same time engages the mind in the management of the animal, and exhilarates by the free contact of the air, a more rapid change of scene. Even at a walking pace, a gentle but general and constant action of the muscle is required to preserve the seat, and adapt the rider's position to the movements of the horse; and this kind of muscular action is extremely favorable to the proper and equable circulation of the blood through the extreme vessels, and to the prevention of its undue accumulation in the central organs. The gentleness of the action admits of its being kept up without accelerating respiration, and enables a delicate person to reap the combined advantages of the open air and proper exercise, for a much longer period than would otherwise be possible. From the tendency of riding to equalize the circulation, stimulate the skin, and promote the action of the bowels, it is also excellently adapted as an exercise for dyspeptic and nervous invalids.

Dancing—when not associated with late hours and hot rooms—is also a most healthful and invigorating exercise, and very well adapted to women and children. Not less useful are the musical gymnastics now much in use both in this country and America. No school should be without some such system for the physical training and development of children.

From the foregoing remarks it will be seen that the importance of exercise, along with other hygienic practice, cannot be overestimated, and that the individual who wishes to remember the motto, *mens sana in corpore sano*, must not neglect one healthful means more than another.

---

*Exercise does most good when enjoyment is the immediate object—when all considerations for health are for the moment forgotten, and social health and hilarity inspire every movement. ... It is not sufficient to go daily through a fixed and circumscribed mode of taking exercise. Besides becoming monotonous and spiritless, it only puts in motion a certain set of muscles, and so fails to affect the purpose which was had in view.*

*Persons confined to the desk or study frequently suffer from this cause; the few muscles brought into play are overstrained, but the bulk of them, as well as the bones, become weak from disease, and general debility follows.*

*The Chinese have a system of medical gymnastics, dating back, it is said, to over two thousand years anterior to the present era; and so potent is it in the cure and relief of many diseases that people of every rank resort to it when very other means have been tried in vain.*

*During the whole of the Middle Ages exercise, that is, exercise as a system, appears to have been universally neglected; and it was not until Ling called attention to the subject that the modern mind began to appreciate its importance. To him we are indebted for one of the most perfect systems of physiological gymnastics ever invented. It is known as the Swedish movements.*

1902

## Provoking People
Louisa Lust

---

## Naturopathy
Dr. Karl Kabisch

---

## Influence Of Water On Health And Longevity
A. L. Wood, M.D.

Benedict Lust moved from his first NYC office location, 111 E. 59th St to 135 E. 58th St in 1902. He then opened his Naturopathic School of Regeneration, later renamed New York Naturopathic Institute.

# Provoking People

**by Louisa Lust**

*The Naturopath and Herald of Health, III (1), 42. (1902)*

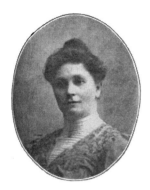

Louisa Lust

We all have our experience with provoking people. They are, as a rule, relatives and sometimes so-called friends, and must be put up with. In the first place, there are those who never see us at our best—... at least they never tell us we are at our best—but let us be at the smallest disadvantage and see how quick they are to mention it. "Isn't it a pity you talked so much the other night?" one said to a lady friend of mine the other day; "I saw Mr. Smith trying to find a chance to say something, but he couldn't get in a word edgewise, poor man."

Then there are the self-righteous people; the I-always-do-so-and-so variety. Their children always have clean hands; their servants never leave, and the snow always drifts away from their side of the street. Then there are the people with imaginary grievances. All seems to be going well and the air is unclouded when we suddenly miss our friend Sophia and go to hunt her up. We find her off in a corner by herself, sulking. All the polite inquiries in the world elicit no information.

This is the sort of people that speak of their extreme sensitiveness and tender feelings; but they never for a moment consider the sensitiveness and tender feelings of anyone else.

I have different desires toward different varieties of provoking people. This kind I feel like slowly torturing.

Of course there are the jealous people who make life miserable for us. When it is a real, wholesome blood-and-thunder jealousy which cuts our throats and burns down our houses the authorities take it in hand, but there is a smouldering, slumbering kind, a covert envy, which wishes us ill without our knowing it, that is the deadly kind. These people flatter and fawn upon us and then when we can no longer be of service to them they turn upon us. This kind makes me wish to forswear the world or become a nun.

Perhaps of all the kinds of provoking people the most provoking are those who never get mad. We feel if they would just give us the satisfaction of answering back once, we could die happy. But they won't. The nagging sort is almost as bad; so is the I-told-you-so species. We dread anything turning out differently from what we expected, even changes in the weather, for fear they may begin to croak. Hanging is too good for them.

In addition to these there are many minor sorts of provoking people. For instance, those who always will make mistakes in the matter of other people's ages. Have you ever noticed that they never err on the side of making us out younger? Men would laugh at this so we won't tell them anything about it—but you and I know whether it is pleasant to be accredited with an extra number of birthdays.

The "harping" kind is still another. They never drop a thing, but keep referring to it long after we thought it was dead and buried. In short, there is no end to the provoking people in the world, and I suppose we must put up with them.

But do you know, I sometimes wonder privately if I am, perchance, a provoking person myself.

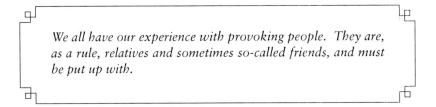

*We all have our experience with provoking people. They are, as a rule, relatives and sometimes so-called friends, and must be put up with.*

# NATUROPATHY

## by Dr. Karl Kabisch

*The Naturopath and Herald of Health, III (2), 65-68. (1902)*

Now, after having treated the history and character of Naturopathy in a general way, it would seem proper to illuminate its advantages over all other healing methods. The majority of people, when they hear the name Natural-Healing or Naturopathy, have no conception whatever as to the multitude of healing agents over which this method disposes, hence they fail to comprehend how a disease can be cured by means, other than medication. Thus they naturally lack faith in this method of healing. Once they are instructed upon the subject they will no longer turn up their noses, but will be forced to timidly admit that we and our method have a certain *raison d'etre*. To be sure our Healing Agents* are not legions like those of Allopathy, nevertheless we can enumerate a goodly number. Let us merely contemplate the various manners and forms in which we apply water. There is cold, tepid, warm, hot water, and finally water in the form of steam. What thorough and versatile use do we not make of air and light, partly so far as it is required in the sick chamber, partly in the shape of light, air and sun baths. Of late electric light baths have been substituted for the latter with great success. Then there are the various subdivisions, bandaging and packings** we employ according to the requirements of each and every individual case. Then, too, we have as healing-agent, massage and its various forms of application.

Altogether exceptional importance has been gained of late by the vibration or shake massage, by means of which we are able to reach and stimulate the finest blood vessels which in turn nourish the nervous system and thus strengthen the entire organism. Indeed, in cases of constitutional disturbances, improper circulation of the blood, rheumatic or gouty affections, indigestion, etc., no other treatment has achieved such splendid results. I myself have seen results with the vibration treatment that, in some cases, bordered on the miraculous.

Again look upon the powerful weapon we possess in electricity! Nor can magnetism and hypnotism escape attention. But especial praise, as a healing factor, must be accorded to gymnastics or athletics which, together with the other methods mentioned, we employ either regularly or irregularly in dealing with the enemies of the human organism. One thing, though, all methods of treatment herein mentioned have in common, namely: they contain nothing that could be directly harmful to the

---

*Dr. Kabisch was German and when writing English used the German practice of capitalizing nouns. —*Ed.*

** Bandaging and packings refers to cold water compresses. —*Ed.*

organism. Is there any other system of healing that can honestly say that much? Certainly not! Therein alone lays the one great advantage of Naturopathy over all other methods of healing. A further advantage not to be under-rated is the fact that in all cases treated in strict accordance with the rules of Naturopathy, recovery takes place considerably sooner and much more certain. It certainly matters a great deal to many people compelled to live from hand to mouth whether they regain their ability to work a few days sooner or later in substantiation of which I could mention no end of cases from my own practice, but will confine myself to one. It happened to me several times last summer that I was treating measles at a house where other just such cases were being treated by one of my local colleagues. In every instance my little patients recovered first. And what did I do with the children? I simply had them given a bath twice daily, during which they were thoroughly massaged in order to stimulate the action of the skin. Immediately afterwards I had them rubbed down "cool", for stronger children "cold" and put to bed without being dried. For the fever symptoms I ordered cold-water applications to chest and back three or four times a day. Success was always immediate. The fever subsided, the eruption developed most beautifully and scaled nicely. If constipated, which is very common in such cases among children, I ordered enemas of lukewarm water, cooling fruit juices and cold milk internally. As diet, aside from milk, I gave cooked fruit, soup, grits or oatmeal. The results were always most gratifying.

While treating these simple diseases of children now I frequently think of my student days when I was, and had to be, a confirmed Allopath. And I ask myself, "Why didn't I let those children bathe that time? Why did I give them Anti-pyrine against the fever; why morphine preparations to calm the irritation of their cough, and why was I satisfied with flannel to the neck, hot milk with honey, gargles of lemon or salt water, or, when the children were too small, with giving it to them by drops in the mouth?" Much has changed since then, and the majority of physicians are using our methods, especially in diseases of children. I am told almost daily, "Doctor so-and-so says, yes, you can give the child a bath or a rubbing."

There is but one drawback: it generally doesn't go further than words, since the gentlemen are too insufficiently familiar with the method of application themselves to show the parents how to do it the first time. Thus many have to depend upon good luck for success, which means many disagreeable complications. Then they abuse Hydrotherapy and say, "If we only had not done it that way"; whereas in reality it is all due to ignorance of the subject.

It is not only in diseases of children, however, but in those of adults as well, that we obtain with Naturopathy in most cases quicker and better results. In this connection I desire to re-emphasize that a theoretically and practically perfect treatment and correct diagnosis of the case at hand is absolutely necessary. When laymen read books on Naturopathy with the report of cases cured thereby, and thereupon attempt to cure diseases, then of course this is altogether wrong. How often am I told, "We have used Naturopathy now for such or such a length of time; but the trouble has been getting worse all the time instead of better." Then if I inquire as to who treated the case I am told, "Oh, we didn't have a physician, we only read in 'Bilz' or 'Kneipp' what it says regarding the disease which is seldom the one—and followed the directions given on that page." Thus I recall a case, where people gave their servant girl, who complained of pains in the stomach, permanent applications of hot water to the abdomen, whereas a careful examination on my part revealed the fact that the girl was pregnant. Those good people had mistaken it for an abdominal swelling of some kind and wanted to allay the inflammation. This case only illustrates how natural treatment when based upon ignorance frequently attains the opposite results.

In what extraordinary manner, for instance, are we not able to cope with the everywhere prevailing influenza? For we treat systematically, that is, we endeavor to overcome the various complaints in turn. Thus we prescribe cold ablutions for increased temperature and wrappings. Internally we give cooling drinks, milk, lemon water, etc. For headache we use deducting foot-baths, cold knee-baths, wet, cold foot-bandages to draw the heat toward the extremities. In throat troubles we order gargles, inhalations, throat-bandages, and hot milk with seltzers or Emser water to drink. Stomach complaints we treat dietetically, that is, we let the patient hunger a few days rather than burden the stomach with anything it is unable to bear. Thus we endeavor to calm the stomach nerves by either cold or warm fomentations. Only after this is accomplished we try porridge or broth gradually followed by a more substantial diet. For constipation we use permanent abdominal poultices, sitz-baths, enemas and small swallows of water hourly. In general debility, which usually manifests itself in peculiarly disagreeable sensations in arms and limbs, we successfully employ rubbings of the extremities and torso every hour. I have treated and am still treating many influenza patients and must say that they and their people usually recover their health and strength with astonishing rapidity, under Naturopathic treatment. Not infrequently I hear the remark, "The last time I had influenza, two or three years ago, I suffered a great deal more and did not recover near as quick."

Thus I could enumerate a whole line of cases I have treated to prove that in the majority of them Naturopathy accomplishes much speedier and better results than any other method. A further great advantage of the Naturopathic treatment is that among families who know and follow our laws, many diseases which would otherwise develop never declare themselves. How frequently does a plain catarrh develop into pneumonia in a single night? True, few people will hasten to consult a physician because of a simple catarrh, which in many cases would be ridiculous indeed; yet those who know the benefit of wet applications to throat, chest or feet in just such cases of catarrh will certainly use them. But how about him who ignores this? He will stick to his catarrh—or rather, the latter will stick to him—and perhaps will be obliged to be out with it in wind and weather besides. His catarrh does not improve, but drags along, entering first the upper and then the deeper finer air-passages, and finally attacks the lungs themselves. Then we have pneumonia with all its evil consequences. This sounds simple and harmless enough, but it is just as true. A further instance may serve as proof. How many people suffer from dyspepsia and lament the fact that they evacuate but every two, three or four days! Quite recently a lady patient told me that her bowels moved but once every eight days. What will all this not give rise to? Generally depression, hemicrania, headache, disinclination to do anything, melancholia, and finally diseases of the intestines and surrounding organs, viz., inflammation of the bowels, appendicitis and calcification of the bowels with its nearly always fatal results, the vomiting of fecal matter. Thus all those who are not informed as to the dangers of retaining the contents of the bowels longer than 24 hours may well figure upon more or less fatal results. How very different with those who have studied the laws of nature! They seek by all possible means to aid nature in asserting her right, by choosing a diet that has a tendency to act upon the bowels, in which connection the drinking of much water, of milk, the eating of vegetables and the avoiding of all constipating food, such as legumes, cocoa, etc., is of great importance. Or else they seek relief in Sitz-baths, abdominal poultices, enemas, all of which seek to mildly and readily dissolve that which has hardened, within the course of time, without irritating the bowels by drastic purgatives. In order to touch briefly upon another subject I will let the enumeration of the foregoing cases suffice.

Naturopathy furnishes us the means of regaining our normal condition in the best and speediest manner possible after recovery from a disease. It furnishes the proper diet, likewise rules for the subsequent modes of living and eventually massage-gymnastics, thus hardening us. For instance, I've obtained magnificent results in convalescents from rheumatism, by means of the vibration-massage, cold douches, etc.

As a further advantage Naturopathy shows us how to protect ourselves against diseases by hygienic modes of living, hardening, abstinence from alcoholic beverages, early habituation of the children to air, light, and water, by sensible clothing, especial avoidance of too tight lacing, then by the sojourn in pure, fresh air, sleeping with open windows, gymnastics, running, swimming, mountain climbing, skating, etc. Every thinking human being should endeavor to seek fresh energy and strength by spending their leisure time and Sundays in God's free Nature instead of passing them in town or in damp, crowded or insanitary places. Why, for instance, are there so many sanatoriums for children being established near the seashore of late? Simply because the children of the poor pass the biggest part of their lives within the unhealthy atmosphere of ill-lighted, ill-ventilated and filthy tenement houses.

Another very material advantage of Naturopathy is the fact that the treatment of a disease is so much cheaper. Expensive cures and the sojourn at private clinics are unnecessary notwithstanding the fact that I occasionally recommend it to those to whom a few greenbacks don't matter. Otherwise all may perfectly well attend themselves at home where they can have their own institution. The one original expenditure connected therewith is a bathtub, a Sitz-bathtub, some swathing clothes, and eventually perhaps a steam apparatus. These will pay, for years to come, the apothecary's and sometimes the doctor's bill for an entire family. On the other hand think what we pay sometimes for a single prescription! Besides, if the latter should not produce the desired result, there will be another the next day. Whereas our receipt is always the same, differing only in it application. Another advantage of Naturopathy consists in its pleasant treatment. How bitter and disagreeable is medicine sometimes; and on the other hand, how agreeable and pleasant is a bath, a poultice, a vapor-bath, gargle or inhalation! Finally I would like to mention as decided advantage of Naturopathy, that it makes us independent. For once a certain disease has occurred in a family, especially among the children, the parents will carefully note what was ordered and will at once know what to do in case of a recurrence of the disease. Nor is it necessary for them, in simple cases, to go for the physician, since the means at their command usually produce good results. Herein again lies another great advantage for many families, especially when the next physician is miles away.

---

*The majority of people, when they hear the name Natural-Healing or Naturopathy, have no conception whatever as to the multitude of healing agents over which this method disposes, hence they fail to comprehend how a disease can be cured by means, other than medication.*

*Naturopathy furnishes us the means of regaining our normal condition in the best and speediest manner possible after recovery from a disease. It furnishes the proper diet, likewise rules for the subsequent modes of living and eventually massage-gymnastics, thus hardening us.*

# INFLUENCE OF WATER ON HEALTH AND LONGEVITY

## by A. L. Wood, M.D.

*The Naturopath and Herald of Health, III (2), 74-78. (1902)*
Read before the 100 Year Club, Hotel Majestic, Central Park West, NY, Nov. 26, 1901.

Some of the members of this Club seem to think it matters not what they eat, or what they drink, or what their other habits of life are; that as long as they *think* they are well and strong they will remain so. If this is the case, I do not see why they should join or attend the meetings of a Club whose object is the study of health and longevity.

I do not question the fact that there is much truth in the saying that, "As a man thinketh so is he", but the thinking is not all. If you take poison into your stomach thinking it will not harm you, you had better have a doctor near with an antidote or stomach pump. Or, if you intend drinking water contaminated with the germs of typhoid fever, you should make your will and prepare for the happy hereafter.

While the subject of this paper is water, I do not wish to convey the impression by what I may say of its importance for health and longevity, that I think water and its right use is the only things that will aid us in attaining a long, useful and happy life. There are many other things of great importance, but the proper use of pure water is perhaps the most important of all.

The question of food, involving the kind, quality, quantity, mode of preparation, time and manner of eating, mental and physical conditions attending digestion, etc., is very closely related to and intertwined with that of drink. So, also is pure air. The three: water, solid food, and air—are all foods which help to build up and keep the tissues of the body in repair and are all absolutely necessary to sustain life. One can live but a few minutes without air, only a few days without water in some form, but men have lived many weeks without food other than air and water. Then there are the other essentials of exercise, rest and sleep, mental and moral conditions, etc.

I wish to say here that I regard long life as desirable only in proportion to the perfection, development and happiness attained by and the usefulness of, that life. To simply exist for a great number of years, a burden to yourself and friends, as is too often the case is both undesirable and unnecessary.

The general use of water as related to health, happiness and longevity is too extensive a subject for one short paper and I shall confine myself to its use within the body.

### INTERNAL CLEANLINESS

Cleanliness of the surface of the body and of the skin is rightly regarded by thinking people as necessary and very desirable for health and comfort. If this is true, and nearly everyone admits its truth while comparatively few practice it to the most desirable extent, how much more important is it to keep the *interior* of the body, the meat within the shell; the bones that support and sustain; the muscles which move and give flexibility, grace, strength, constituting, as they do, about three-fourths of the body; the brain and nervous system which control and direct all; the vital organs and the organs of digestion, assimilation, secretion and excretion; and especially the blood, which nourishes and strengthens all. How much more important, I repeat, to keep all these pure, clean and in perfect working condition? *Pure water* and plenty of it does this, and it can be done in no other way.

Important as is the external bath in promoting the cleanliness and healthful action of the skin, it has much less influence upon health and longevity than this daily bathing of all the blood and tissues of the body in *pure water*. When I say *pure* water I mean that which is absolutely free from all animal, vegetable and mineral substances whatever.

The proper performance of every function of the body, digestion and assimilation of food, the circulation of the blood, the processes of secretion and excretion and the regulation of the temperature of the body, in fact, every vital action is dependent upon the quantity and quality of the water which is daily taken into the system. If water in insufficient quantity, or if of impure quality, is used, every organ is impeded in its action and every function disturbed, the free circulation of the blood through the microscopic capillary tubes of the entire system, one of most important of life's processes, is seriously interfered with, depuration through the various organs and channels of excretion is retarded and consequently a slow but certain poisoning of the system takes place.

Water constitutes nearly three-fourths of the body. This fact alone shows its great importance. The blood is about 80 percent water, the muscles 75 percent, the brain nearly 80 percent, the gastric juice 97.5 percent, the saliva 99.5 percent, and even the bones contain 13 percent and the teeth 10 percent of water.

Water is continually passing from the body and always carries with it more or less of the waste, worn out and poisonous materials constantly being generated within the system, as well as the injurious substances introduced from without. Every expired breath is loaded with watery vapor filled with these impurities. They are constantly being thrown out through the millions of little sewers, the perspiratory ducts of the skin, in the form of insensible perspiration. So, also with the kidneys and other channels of elimination and water is always the vehicle by the aid of which they are disposed of. If they were not thrown out of the body they would soon clog the wheels of life and produce disease and death, as they are doing all over the world.

We will use a sponge as an illustration of this cleansing and purifying process. If the sponge is badly soiled, the first time water is squeezed through it will come out dark and muddy, the second time less so, the third time less still, until at length the water has done its work and issues forth as pure as when it entered. So with the body. It is filled with impurities, and, unlike the sponge, they are constantly being added to by the worn-out particles of the system which are of no further use, but must be disposed of to make room for the new ones capable of furnishing renewed life and vital force. Water is the only medium capable of absorbing and carrying these impurities out of the body without injuring or destroying it. The larger quantity of water squeezed through the sponge the quicker and more effectively it will be cleansed. It is the same with the body; the more water drank, the quicker and more perfectly it will be purified. And again, the purer the water which is used the sooner and the better will the cleansing be accomplished. Any house-wife knows that if she uses clean water to wash and rinse her dishes and clothes the work will be better done and the article washed be purer, whiter and sweeter than if soiled water were used. Yet how few realize the vastly greater importance of using the purest water to wash and keep pure and sweet the caskets which contain their immortal souls.

### QUANTITY OF WATER REQUIRED

The best authorities agree that under ordinary conditions, at least two quarts of water per day should be drunk by the average individual. Laborers and others exposed to a high degree of heat, who perspire freely, require a much larger quantity. I have known men to drink from two to three quarts of water in the hot rooms of a Turkish Bath within an hour and at the end of the bath their weight was less than at the beginning, showing that they had lost through perspiration more than they had drank.

Care should be observed not to drink so much water at a time as to burden the stomach, nor to take it so cold as to chill it. Where the stomach is weak and in some other conditions, warm or hot water should be used. Large quantities drank at meals or soon after interfere with digestion. Most of the water should be taken from half an hour to an hour before meals. Ice-water should not be drunk as a beverage.

In all kinds of fevers and inflammations, defective nutrition, inactivity of the liver or skin, diseases of the kidneys, constipation, rheumatism, gout and all the various diseased conditions caused by uric acid poisoning, the drinking of still larger quantities of pure water is highly beneficial.

Dr. John T. Nutt in a recent publication says, "Very few Americans drink enough water. Eight or ten glasses of water should be taken daily by the average person."

Gould & Pyle's *Cyclopaedia of Medicine and Surgery* says, "At the present day the subject of drinking water involves the interest, attention and welfare of every civilized community. The question of health largely depends upon the water consumed in which may reside the micro-organisms of disease and death."

Prof. George B. Fowler, M.D., of the New York Post Graduate Medical School says, "I venture the statement that the cause of one-fourth the cases of disordered digestion in fashionable life is the lack of sufficient water in the dietary."

Prof. George Henry Fox, M.D., of the College of Physicians and Surgeons says, "It is quite certain that few people drink too much water, and I feel sure that many unpleasant feelings and symptoms of actual disease would quickly disappear if the sufferers only appreciate the value of this best and cheapest of all remedies. The interior of the body needs cleansing as much as the exterior and a liberal supply of pure water in the treatment of our patients will often bring about the desirable results which drugs have failed to accomplish."

Madame Patti, the famous singer, who at the age of 60 is as perfect a specimen of womanhood both in appearance and reality as she was at 30, in telling how you retain youth and beauty, said, "Drink nothing but water or milk—especially drink water—you can't drink too much of it."

In speaking of uric acid causing rheumatism, gout, biliousness, constipation, slow digestion, inactivity of mind, etc., Prof. Wm. G. Thompson, M.D., of the University of the City of New York says, "Water itself, if taken in sufficient quantities, by increasing the fluidity and consequently the solvent powers of the blood, is often an effective remedy in these cases."

To dilute the blood when it becomes thickened and as a consequence circulates with difficulty, water is a quick and the only effective remedy.

## IMPORTANCE OF PURE WATER

Having considered the absolute necessity for water, some of its various internal uses and the quantity required, we now come to the vitally important question of its purity or impurity.

As a rule in Nature, like produces like. Pure food and drink, under favorable conditions, insures purity and health of body and other things being equal purity and health of body gives purity and health of mind and soul. Conversely, impure food and drink produce impure and diseased physical conditions, and these in turn influence all mental and moral states.

If we desire a strong, active, healthy body, free from pain and disease and obedient to our will and one that shall so remain for one hundred years or more; if we wish an active and vigorous brain that shall give us clean, wholesome, energetic thoughts to the end of life, let us see to it that none but the purest and most suitable to our digestive organs, under proper conditions, to make and keep the body and brain clean, strong and enduring. Pure water is the only liquid agent in existence that will do this.

Prof. Simpson, a noted scientist and physician, says, "The complacency with which we swallow the filthy, impure, disease-bearing water which is delivered through poisonous pipes to our homes, affords a spectacle of self-abasement as melancholy as it is disgusting."

Prof. Charles F. Chandler, of Columbia College, the noted chemist and analyst, says, "Pure water is hardly second to pure air as a life giving and life protecting agent. It is the most potent servant the sanitary authorities can call to their aid."

Nicola Tesla, the celebrated electrician and inventor, in the *Century Magazine* for June, 1900, says,

> For every person who perishes from the effects of a stimulant, at least a thousand dies from the consequences of drinking impure water. This precious fluid, which daily influences new life into us, is likewise the chief vehicle through which disease and death enter out bodies. The germs of destruction it conveys are enemies all the more to be dreaded as they perform their fatal work unperceived. They seal our doom while we live and enjoy. The majority of people are so ignorant or careless in drinking water and the consequences of this are so disastrous, that a philanthropist can scarcely use his efforts better than by endeavoring to enlighten those who are thus injuring themselves.

### TYPHOID FEVER CAUSED BY IMPURE WATER

It is generally conceded that no one ever has typhoid fever or cholera unless he eats or drinks the germs that produce them. The lesson of the Spanish War should be noted. Surgeon General Geo. M. Sternberg, of the United States Army, states officially, "The total number of deaths reported in our enlarged army, including regulars and volunteers, from May 1, 1898, to April 30, 1899, is 6,406. Of these, 5,438 died of disease and 968 were killed in battle, or died of wounds, injuries or accidents."

It is well know that impure water was one of the chief causes of the great mortality. If the soldiers had been provided with an abundance of pure water, I fully believe nine-tenths of that number would have been saved. It has been stated that on the War vessels where nothing but distilled water was used, not a single death occurred from disease. The Marine Battalion, 500 to 600 strong, used distilled water from the ships while on shore duty in Cuba, and had none of the enteric fevers so common in the Fifth Army Corps.

Testimony to fill volumes could be adduced in regard to the injurious results of the use of impure water and strong as it may at first appear, I believe the statement of Tesla, previously quoted, is not overdrawn.

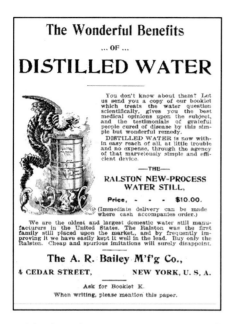
Ad for the Ralston New-Process Water Still.

During the year ending May 1, 1900, according to the last census, there were 35,379 deaths from typhoid fever in the United States, nearly all of which were caused by disease germs in water. The truths of this cannot be questioned. In the same year there were 46,907 deaths from diarrheal diseases, the great majority of which were due to disease germs and the various organic contaminations contained in water used for drinking and cooking. There are many other diseases produced partially or wholly by impure water, so that I feel I am fully justified in stating that more than one hundred thousand deaths annually are caused by taking impure water in one form or another into the system.

Let us stop a moment and consider what this means. It means two full regiments of one thousand men each marching quietly but painfully down to death each week in the year, and from a cause which is known, and wholly preventable. During the entire Spanish War our loss in battle, and deaths from wounds and accidents, amounted to less than one regiment of men, while, by the use of impure water, we are losing two whole regiments of our citizens *each week,* and still how few people ever give a thought to its prevention.

It is calculated that about ten times as many persons have typhoid fever and survive, though they never fully recover from its effects, and as many of them are seriously injured for life as there are who die from it. So it is with diarrheal, dysenteric and other water poison diseases, though the proportion of recoveries to deaths is much greater than in typhoid. From this it will be seen that more than twenty thousand people besides the two thousand who die are made sick each and every week by impure water.

Just think of it. Ponder it well. Do not forget it. Look at the 2,000 coffins stretching out in an unbroken line for nearly three miles and another line of beds of sickness extending almost thirty miles. Besides these coffins, see the crowds of sorrowing ones, mourning the loved and lost and beside the long line of the sick and suffering see the anxious friends, the nurses, and the doctors. And all this is repeated every week in the year. All this and more, is caused by disease germs and organic and mineral impurities in the water we drink and eat. It is any wonder we require the services of 130,000 physicians in the United States?

As an element of destruction, the most deadly war is a complete failure compared with the terrible results of swallowing the silent, invisible foes of human life and health which lurk in innocent looking water.

---

*The three: water, solid food and air—are all foods which help to build up and keep the tissues of the body in repair and are all absolutely necessary to sustain life.*

*Then there are the other essentials of exercise, rest and sleep, mental and moral conditions, etc.*

*The proper performance of every function of the body, digestion and assimilation of food, the circulation of the blood, the processes of secretion and excretion and the regulation of the temperature of the body, in fact, every vital action is dependent upon the quantity and quality of the water which is daily taken into the system.*

*Care should be observed not to drink so much water at a time as to burden the stomach, nor to take it so cold as to chill it.*

*During the year ending May 1, 1900, according to the last census, there were 35,379 deaths from typhoid fever in the United States, nearly all of which were caused by disease germs in water. ... In the same year there were 46,907 deaths from diarrheal diseases, the great majority of which were due to disease germs and the various organic contaminations contained in water used for drinking and cooking.*

# 1903

### RETURN TO NATURE, LIGHT AND AIR
ADOLF JUST

---

### HEALING POWER OF MUSIC
AUGUSTA VESCILIUS

---

### INTERNAL IRRIGATIONS
BENEDICT LUST

---

### HYPNOTISM IN SURGERY
BENEDICT LUST

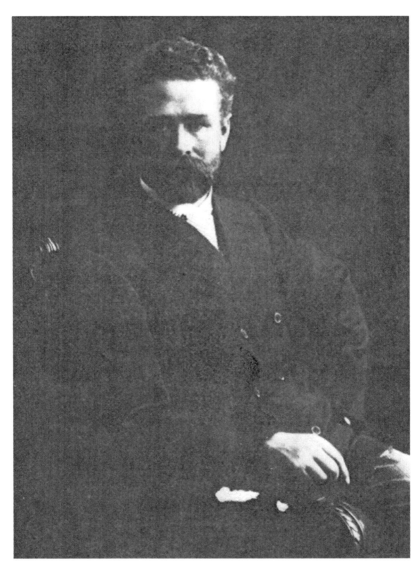

Adolf Just (1859-1936), author of the historic and pioneering book, *Return to Nature* (1896), and the architect of the "Jungborn" sanitarium.

# Return To Nature, Light And Air

## by Adolf Just, Jungborn, Stapelburg, Harz, Germany
## (Translated by Benedict Lust.)

*The Naturopath and Herald of Health, IV (3), 44-47. (1903)*

I shall speak more in detail also of the great influence which the mere earth exerts on man in all cases where he comes into direct contact with it.

If there is no opportunity to take the light- and air-bath naked, the next best thing is to take it only lightly dressed in the open or in one's room, as the case may be. The face should always be protected against the sun.

After the sun bath one must always see to the cooling of the body by means of the natural bath.*

### Light-And-Air Huts And Cottages

One great benefit to health comes from sleeping in huts and cottages situated entirely in the open, and which at all times offer free access to light and air.

We call them light-and-air huts and light-and-air cottages, but there is nothing about them in the way of appointments that would make them special hygienic apparatus and institutions.

They are huts with a roof to keep the rain from coming through, but without walls, or only lattice walls. For protection against stormy weather they are provided with curtains. For winter (for they may be used also at this season), they can be kept warm and made to keep out the snow by means of straw and partition walls penetrable by the air.

It is still better to erect more perfect cottages, with thicker walls, adapted to real dwelling purposes. But they must be sufficiently provided with windows, blinds, ventilators, etc., to permit the ingress, when open, of plenty of fresh air. "The ceiling must be provided with ventilators which may be opened when windows and doors are closed." I refer to the illustrations of the light-and-air huts at Jungborn.

Pure fresh air is required by the body, especially in the night, when it is chiefly engaged in the work of digestion. Therefore sleeping in such a hut is very important. More than is at present the case, owners of

---

*The Natural bath described in *Philosophy of Naturopathic Medicine, pages 85 – 92* was used by the early Naturopaths and provided a powerful bath for them. The Natural Bath is a vigorous bath conducted in a specialized bathtub with approximately 6-10 inches of cold water. The restoration of vitality and health is quite remarkable. —Ed.

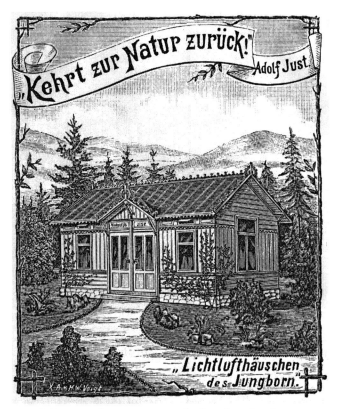

Adolf Just's Light-Air Cottage at his "Jungborn" in Germany.

gardens, parks, and woods ought to build such light-and-air huts and cottages for dwelling purposes.

The rooms of houses, even if they are in the woods, are apt to be penetrated with the odors from the cellar, the kitchen, closets, garbage heaps, etc. The air is vitiated, moreover, by the circumstance that several, often many, persons live in a house side by side, and below and above one another, and that stone walls retain foul odors a long time. They are therefore never filled with entirely pure, unvitiated air. But this is the case in light-and-air huts.

Absolutely pure air is of the greatest importance in the healing of all diseases, whether catarrh or typhoid fever, cholera, rheumatism, or gout, nervousness or consumption, cancer or scurvy, a fresh wound or a running open sore.

While speaking of the great importance of pure, unvitiated air I want to call attention to another very dangerous enemy in our present mode of living—I mean gas light. In apartments with gas fixtures, even if gas is not used, flowers never thrive; they soon begin to wilt and finally die. Shrubs and trees along promenades and in parks in the neighborhood of gas mains likewise often die. The smallest quantities of gas escaping from the stops and fixtures affect the organism most injuriously. The bad, poisonous air of the cities originates largely from the gas works. The pallor and poor health of office workers are chiefly caused by gas. In sanitariums and hospitals gas is a thing unknown. Any other kind of light (petroleum, etc.) is less injurious than gas light. The electric light is, of course, superior to all the others. It is to be regretted only that where there is no water-power for the production of electric light, recourse must be had to steam, whereby the nuisance of smoke stacks belching forth enormous masses of dense, suffocating smoke is still more increased.

Health is the foundation of all happiness, man can enjoy all earthly pleasures only in the measure of his health. Only when this shall have come to be more widely recognized will people begin to appreciate and build light-and-air cottages.

Living or sleeping in one of these beautiful cottages, surrounded by nature, will then no longer be a matter for surprise, but will be regarded as infinitely preferable to occupying dark and dingy apartments in cities, poisoned by foul odors, the breeding places of all diseases which not alone weaken and undermine the body, but are also the cause of all the defects of the mind and soul, of idiocy and insanity, of lust and selfishness, of vice and crime, of hate and envy, of contention and strife, in short, of all the ills of the earth.

One need not be afraid of freezing in one of these open light-and-air cottages, during low temperature. In the open, in the woods, one can sleep very comfortably in a light-and-air cottage during the coldest winter, if one has only a few feather beds or quilts, because the body develops more heat when breathing pure, fresh air than it does when breathing the foul and stuffy air in houses.

The light-and-air cottage protects the sleeper and his clothing during the night against rain. During fair weather it is advisable to place the bed outside the cottage and sleep entirely in the open. To this end take a straw tick or a quilt (woolen or cotton) covered with coarse linen or thick burlap for mattress, and a quilt for covering so that the whole outfit can be easily transported, and place the mattress on the ground. We shall thus soon become aware that nature rewards every step that is taken toward her, for it is still more beneficial and healthful to sleep entirely in the open than in a light-and-air hut.

In the open where we can soar unhindered to the stars, and where soft zephyrs waft about us, beautiful nights are truly enchanting, and all the infirmities of the body and soul heal quickly.

*Dann geht leise*
Then very gently

*Nach seine weise*
After his fashion

*Der liebe Herrgott durch den Wald.*
Our gracious Lord goes through the woods.

Seriously considered there is nothing ostentatious or ridiculous when a man once more puts up his bed outside of a house, entirely in the open, where hare and deer, stag and boar, and so many others of God's creatures retain and preserve their clear, bright eyes, their physical activity and strength, their perfect health, that precious talent which the Lord has entrusted to them. These do not do as the men who to-day neglect their health, yes, even trample it under foot, so that their entirely earthly existence is embittered by misery and disease and it will be difficult for them in the time to come to account for the talent entrusted to them. We shall soon see further on how sleeping on the bare ground is a most natural and healthy practice. I must observe also that light frame dwelling houses are more healthful than those built more massively.

More small houses ought to be built again, surrounded by gardens and trees, if possible. Our present large, barrack-like houses with thick stone walls in narrow-stuffy streets are obviously not conducive to health.

In cities, therefore, people ought to try to live on the outskirts.

Dwelling houses ought always to be so built and the rooms so arranged that very much light and air can at all times stream in.

So-called architectural beauty need not, therefore, be neglected. But here, too, it was well to aspire toward greater naturalness and simplicity.

*They [light-and-air huts and cottages] are huts with a roof to keep the rain from coming through, but without walls, or only lattice walls.*

*Absolutely pure air is of the greatest importance in the healing of all diseases, whether catarrh or typhoid fever, cholera, rheumatism, or gout, nervousness or consumption, cancer or scurvy, a fresh wound or a running open sore.*

*We shall thus soon become aware that nature rewards every step that is taken toward her, for it is still more beneficial and healthful to sleep entirely in the open than in a light-and-air hut.*

# Healing Power Of Music

## by Augusta Vescilius*

*The Naturopath and Herald of Health, IV (5), 152-153. (1903)*

(Extracts from Lecture delivered at the meeting of the Naturopathic Society of America.)

To one who considers music merely a pastime, a recreation or an accomplishment to be added as a finishing touch to a young lady's education, the question will naturally arise, of what vital importance can this subject be to those who are seriously seeking a solution to the problem of right living.

What are we seeking in these discussions but to gain a clearer perception of Truth, to learn how best to use the vital principle of Life in its simplest, purest, most concrete form, that we may become exponents of the gospel of harmony. Musical Therapeutics is an important department of this study of right living, as music has a distinct influence upon life and health, whether we understand it or not, and the use of music for healing, is a natural use of a natural power.

The language of music is based upon Truth. The laws governing musical Vibrations are as immutable as those governing mathematics, chemical affinities, or electricity.

Carlyle says: See deeply enough, and you see musically, the heart of Nature being everywhere music—if you can only reach it.

Music is a universal force, dynamic in its power to disturb as well as harmonize.

Malibrand was thrown into convulsions upon hearing for the first time Beethoven's symphony in C Minor. Berlioz suffered tortures when certain music was played and we know that the overpowering influence of musical vibrations set in motion by great massed choruses and orchestras, while they are an inspiration to thousands have sometimes proved fatal to a too sensitized organism.

If used without understanding, music can excite to frenzy the mentally unbalanced, perhaps the most susceptible class to its influence; and on the other hand, there is nothing that exerts a more soothing beneficial influence over the insane than well chosen music.

Key, tempo, rhythm, repetition and pause, are all important factors to be considered in the study of Musical Therapeutics.

The influence of certain keys stimulate and arouse, while others soothe and quiet.

---

*Augusta Vescilius states her address at 327 W. 56th St. New York City which was in close proximity to Benedict Lust's office at 124 E. 59th St. —Ed.

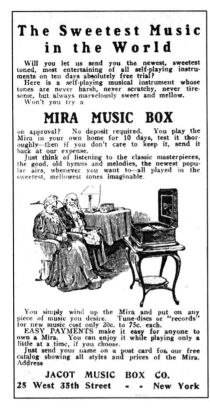
Ad for the Mira Music Box.

The major keys express affirmation, the minor keys negotiation.

The influence of the contralto and base is soothing and relaying, while the soprano and tenor with their more rapid vibration are more able to exhilarate and excite.

Experience teaches us that music when employed for general use as in wards of hospitals, to be of any value, should be harmonious, restful and attractive; all extremes of pitch and force should be avoided.

When music is selected for its therapeutic value alone, there will be no more thought of changing the character of the music to suit the day than there would be of changing the treatment.

All music based upon the true and beautiful is sacred. Then why should the jingling hymn which too often grates upon the nerves and arouses unwholesome emotions, be considered more appropriate than a beautiful composition of one of the Tone Poets that has the power to expand the soul and send a thrill of renewed life through every fibre of the body and leave a pleasing mental picture?

When preparing oneself for the practice of musical healing the musician will find that the subject calls for careful study as "every case is a new case".

There are certain qualifications necessary beside the musical gift—mental preparation that will enable one to diagnose mental conditions and their effect upon the body learn the sensitiveness to musical impressions—find the key note of the patient, the one to which they will most readily respond, and be ready to select music best suited to the requirements of the case.

To those who are attracted to this department of their profession I would say—make your calling sure by study, preparing yourself mentally and musically, and do not, by your lack of preparation, bring down ridicule upon this beautiful ministry of music.

Musical treatment has proved beneficial in such a variety of diseases that it is impossible to specify and say it is better for this or that. If all form is visible manifestations of vibration, it is possible to disintegrate or build up by the misuse or intelligent use of thought through musical sound waves.

Music creates states of mind.

The highest expression is love.

If the musician can produce a mental condition where fear, resentment, and discord are replaced by an influx of Divine Love, the result will be harmony, as every atom of physical organism will respond to the call.

Let us awake to the broader uses for music and seek to realize its deeper fuller meaning.

Too long have its wonderful resources remained a comparatively sealed book for those who have the care of the sick.

*Musical Therapeutics is an important department of this study of right living, as music has a distinct influence upon life and health, whether we understand it or not, and the use of music for healing, is a natural use of a natural power.*

*The influence of certain keys stimulate and arouse, while others soothe and quiet.*

*The major keys express affirmation, the minor keys negotiation.*

*There are certain qualifications necessary beside the musical gift mental preparation that will enable one to diagnose mental conditions and their effect upon the body learn the sensitiveness to musical impressions find the key note of the patient, the one to which they will most readily respond, and be ready to select music best suited to the requirements of the case.*

## INTERNAL IRRIGATIONS:
### THEIR USES AND PROPER METHOD OF ADMINISTRATION

### by Benedict Lust

*The Naturopath and Herald of Health, IV (11), 330-331. (1903)*

Internal irrigation has become such a powerful factor in treating the different conditions of the human body that it is necessary for people to know exactly the right way to administer this form of remedy.

Let us begin with the enema. A few years ago this was an almost unknown form of appliance and was used by doctors and nurses only in extreme cases of bowel obstruction. Today it used in every family, almost by every person. But like many another good thing the benefit that is derived from judicious and proper use of the enema can be greatly neutralized by improper and mistaken methods.

Very few persons really know the right way to give an enema. They think if they send a certain quantity of water into the intestines, that is all there is to do. But an enema given in an improper way is sure to have an evil consequence even if the immediate effect worked for is obtained.

The object of an enema is to wash out the intestines and stimulate the peristaltic action. After continued constipation an enema should never be given until a suppository has been inserted into the rectum and taken effect. This means, of course, when the constipation is the result of an accumulation of solidified feces in the rectum. These suppositories should be either of cocoa butter or glycerine and can be bought at any drug store.

After the rectum is relieved the enema should be given. The short hard rubber tube should never be used. They can be inserted only about two inches, and very little of the water entering the passage gets beyond the rectum. This causes an expansion from that section, being unable to contain the amount of fluid, and the walls of the rectum are stretched, causing, when the water is ejected, a relaxation that is frequently the cause of chronic constipation or hemorrhoids. The tube should be of soft rubber and measure from fourteen to sixteen inches long. This should be inserted about ten inches, so that it goes fairly past the rectum and enters the sigmoid flexure. This is the curve in the lower bowel next to the rectum. The rectum itself is from six to eight inches in length in the average adult, and no enema accomplishes its object unless water enters the intestine beyond that section. This sounds worse than it really is, for after the tube is well lubricated with sweet oil it enters quite smoothly. Should there be any slight obstruction, withdraw the tube an inch or two, let the water run, then turn off the water and continue to pass the tube until from ten to twelve inches are inserted.

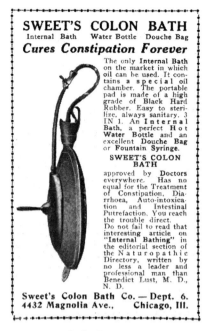
The internal bath or enema were advocated by the early Naturopaths.

The position of the patient too, is of the gravest importance. They should always be lying on the left side, with the knees drawn well up, and the shoulders well forward. Any other position for the body is incorrect and therefore liable to do harm or at least the proper amount of benefit is not obtained.

When the obstruction is actually in the upper part of the bowels, the suppositories can be omitted, and about two ounces of sweet oil be well beaten into a quart of lather made from warm water and Castille soap. Let this take good effect (it should always be retained as long as possible) then follow with two quarts of water for an enema should never be very warm, just a little more than tepid is quite sufficient, as heat causes relaxation and in such cases relaxation means weakness. Another thing, the vessel containing the water for the enema should never be hung much higher than the level of the patient's body, for the higher the vessel, the greater the force of the stream of water and these things cannot be done too gently. In cases of diarrhea give an enema always, it will wash away the irritating cause of the trouble, and save serious results if done in time.

Enemata should never be used more than once a week, unless under special directions.

There is another form of irrigation that has just as much practical value as the enema, but is not so generally used. This is washing out the stomach.

To most people this suggestion will bring a dreadful vision of the enormous stomach pump and its attendant evils. Don't be frightened; I don't like those things any better than you do. But I do say that for a foul stomach, there is nothing like a good washing out.

Start about three hours after eating; make it longer if you like but never less. Have a good quantity of warm water; you can have either one spoonful of salt to a pint, or the juice of one ordinary leman to a quart. Drink as much as you can: five or six tumblers full, more if you can.

Ad for the "J. B. L. Cascade" Internal Bath invented by Dr. Charles A. Tyrrell.

I always tell you within the line not beyond it. Drink slowly, and when you have taken enough to make you feel a decided distention of the stomach, either push your finger down your throat or tickle the back of your throat as far back as you can get. You will soon have a fine result, and as an appetite creator I don't know anything better. Do this twice, and you will rid your stomach of more foul matter than you could by taking the entire contents of a drug store.

The same method can be applied in case of a bone or foreign matter lodging in the throat. Very frequently the obstruction can be removed by something coming up the esophagus when nothing going down will affect it. An emetic will often save an operation in these cases.

Vaginal irrigations need little remark, beyond the fact that unless specially directed they should never be very hot and they should always be given with the patient lying on her back.

Intrauterine and bladder irrigations are as effectual in removing foul and irritating matter as an enema, douche, or stomach irrigation, but can never, of course, be self-administered and should always be done by an experienced operator.

Some people will argue that these things are not natural. They are, in so much as it is the only way of applying natural means to rid the system of unnatural conditions. An old lady told me once that if God had intended us to use these things, God would have put the necessary appliances in the Garden of Eden. I never heard that Adam was furnished with a tooth brush, but I think if he came back now we should find modern society more tolerant of his fig leaf costume than of his neglecting that necessary little article of the toilet.

*The object of an enema is to wash out the intestines and stimulate the peristaltic action. After continued constipation an enema should never be given until a suppository has been inserted into the rectum and taken effect.*

*The position of the patient too, is of the gravest importance. They should always be lying on the left side, with the knees drawn well up, and the shoulders well forward. Any other position for the body is incorrect and therefore liable to do harm or at least the proper amount of benefit is not obtained.*

*Enemata should never be used more than once a week, unless under special directions.*

## HYPNOTISM IN SURGERY

### by Benedict Lust

*The Naturopath and Herald of Health, IV (11), 339. (1903)*

The first case ever known in English surgery under hypnotism has been recently reported from Clapton, near London. The subject operated on was a lady of 38 years, whose leg was amputated. A local surgeon, Dr. Frank Aldrich, performed the operation. He had been studying hypnotism for nearly three years, and while experimenting conceived the idea of employing it as an anesthetic. When called to attend the lady in question, he found it necessary to amputate her limb, and her terrible dread of chloroform, he conceived, would make its use in her case unadvisable. With her consent he began to experiment on her with hypnotism, and found that when under its influence she did not seem to notice the pricking done with a needle. Each day for a week she was experimented with in this way, on each occasion being laid under the anesthetic for half an hour.

At the time of the operation she was anesthetized thirty-five minutes. When aroused she simply said, "I feel pins and needles." The doctor reported that there were absolutely no symptoms of shock, and her pulse and temperature were normal.

It is to be presumed that the report of this case will give an impetus to the study of hypnotism, even in conservative England, and that among some who will use their knowledge unscrupulously. While it may be successfully used on some, in case of minor operations, the danger to be apprehended from the free and unprincipled use of hypnotism may well be feared. Should it come to be generally employed in surgery, the only safeguard against danger will be laws to restrain its use by any except qualified medical practitioners.

# 1904

### Snow
MGR. SEBASTIAN KNEIPP

---

### Pneumathotherapy, Breathing Cure
BENEDICT LUST

---

### Return To Nature
DR. C. W. YOUNG, PH.E., D.O.

---

### Heliotherapy (Sun Cure)
### And Thermotherapy (Heat Cure)
BENEDICT LUST

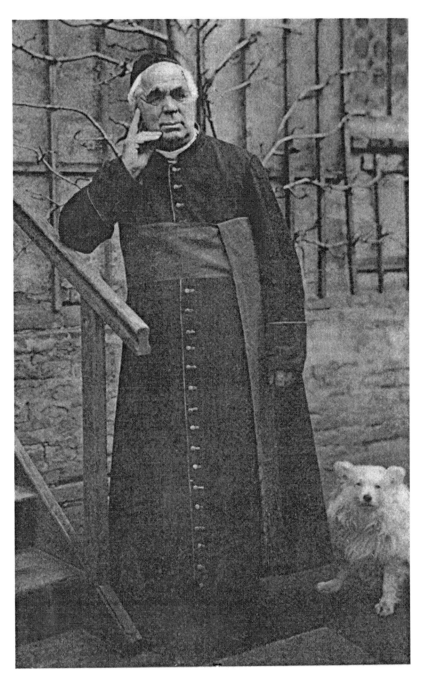

The Very Rev. Mgr. Sebastian Kneipp, 76 years old.

# SNOW

## by Mgr. Sebastian Kneipp

*The Naturopath and Herald of Health, V (2), 37-39. (1904)*

Year by year, there is a continuous change of the different seasons; we think we have the summer when autumn is before us and winter will soon follow, which, like other seasons, has its pleasant and unpleasant sides. While in summer the great God's nature stands in all its fullness and beauty, in winter we find it with a white covering of snow. Although Nature then seems to be desolate and cold and frost reign supreme, winter is not quite an unwished-for guest. Indeed, many look for it, especially the young, who find so much pleasure in romping in the snow. Look at the country children particularly, how they enjoy running around and playing in the snow. In fact, it seems as though they would not know any difference between warm and cold. Now, as also this year the winter has arrived and we soon expect to see the ground covered with snow, let us have a little talk about it, and ask of what importance snow really is to us. How can we derive any benefit from it? How could it do us harm if we do not understand to make right use of it?

Snow is not intended to be only a covering for the protection of plants, but it also does much good to mankind, and is even a means to promote health. Let us take walking bare-footed in snow. Nothing else can be more recommended to young and old than walking bare-footed in snow. But certainly further hardening, which I frequently mentioned, must also be always practiced. Children should take this exercise as much as possible, although it should not be exaggerated! For the healthy it is excellent to harden and strengthen the nerves. For the nervous as well as those who suffer from headaches, also for people that do much mental work, I do not know of anything more beneficial than walking in the snow, as this draws the blood to the feet. There are many who constantly complain of cold feet and cannot get them warm even in bed. Many such people come to me for advice. In summer I recommended to them to walk in water. In winter I advised them to walk in fresh fallen snow. Most of them, with very few exceptions, very soon obtained the desired results, and just the same as their feet were cold before they afterwards felt the most pleasant warmth. Many thought it very strange and could not understand how it was possible to get the feet warm by cold water or snow. But it is not only that, such treatment also hardens altogether and prevents many diseases, which is quite natural.

By walking bare-footed in snow, drawing of the blood to the lower extremities is accomplished, which causes uniform and natural warmth.

I want to add a few special remarks about walking bare-footed in

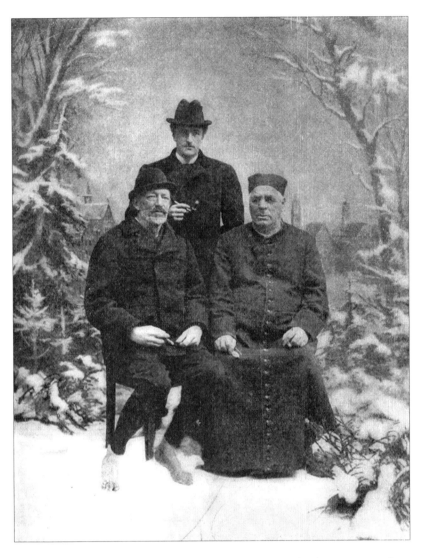

The Archduke Joseph Karl, Francis Ferdinand of Austria and Father Kneipp walking barefoot in the new fallen snow for hardening the constitution. The older Archduke was cured by Father Kneipp of Bright's disease in 1892 and presented in appreciation of his great cure a public park for 150,000 florins to the town of Wörishofen. The younger Archduke was the heir to the crown, whose murder precipitated the WWI in 1914.

snow. First, practice it only in fresh fallen snow. After the snow has been lying on the ground for some time and probably has become hard I would never advise walking in it, as it might be injurious. Second, for hardened people, it does not matter when and how frequently they indulge in it. For the weak and sick, however, the early morning hours are too raw, and they therefore will do well to set the time of their snow walks between the hours of eight in the morning and three or four in the afternoon. The length of the walk should also be regulated according to the constitution of the patient. A hardened man need not be so particular about it; but to sick and weak people I never allow more than ten to fifteen minutes for their walk. But in both cases exercise is absolutely necessary; they should not stand around and talk and finally come home with a bad cold.

While I am just writing this article someone asks me whether snow walking may be permitted during any kind of weather, and I want to say that as long as there is no raw wind no one need be afraid. But not everybody has the opportunity to go snow-walking, particularly those in the cities, where they would be stared at if they would indulge in it, and especially old people find it impossible; to those, I would recommend to have snow carried in the wash-house where they can carry out their wishes.

Many will probably find my opinion terrible or even dangerous; but after they have tried it several times they will surely come to the same conclusion I have arrived at after years of experience. There are people who never can be induced to make a trial, and who rather wear furs and wool and all kinds of rubbish, which only make the body weak and sensitive.

Wörishofen is an exception in this respect. After the patients arrive there, they at once seek the right means to harden their bodies, according to the season of the year. I hardly need to point out that in case of frozen limbs rubbing with snow is applied in order to give them natural warmth again. This rubbing with snow or snow-water has proved to be very beneficial also in other instances, as for instance, for rheumatism, cases of paralysis, etc. I remember a case several years ago of a Government official who came to me suffering terribly from articular rheumatism, and who was very near being pensioned. After he pictured to me his sad position I put him under treatment and prescribed the regular gushes. The cure was not obtained at once; on the contrary the pains increased steadily, so that he was hardly able to lie in bed; then, after the old man had given up all hope I came to him and gave him the gushes in bed, taking the coldest water obtainable, in which I put a lot of snow. This was continued whenever he felt the smallest pain, and a short time afterward he was thoroughly free from his sufferings and left me in order to take up his position again.

Snow also has excellent effect in cases of serious inflammation, such as inflammation of the lungs, pleurisy and inflammation in the abdominal parts, if used as compresses or ablutions. Only care should be taken that the patient is well covered in bed, so that the proper perspiration is attained. Compresses of ice-water, if snow-water is not obtainable, render also good service.

Those who are acquainted with the water cure, either from books or personal experience in Wörishofen, will no doubt also know the spoonful of water and the four-ply cloth for sitting which I usually recommend for constipation. The latter application gains in effect if snow-water or ice-water is used. Many who read this article will probably say that they had no idea that snow was of such great benefit and importance.

*Nothing else can be more recommended to young and old than walking bare-footed in snow.*

*For the nervous as well as those who suffer from headaches, also for people that do much mental work, I do not know of anything more beneficial than walking in the snow, as this draws the blood to the feet.*

*Many thought it very strange and could not understand how it was possible to get the feet warm by cold water or snow.*

*By walking bare-footed in snow, drawing of the blood to the lower extremities is accomplished, which causes uniform and natural warmth.*

# Pneumathotherapy, Breathing Cure*

## by Benedict Lust

*The Naturopath and Herald of Health, V (3), 52-53. (1904)*

Pneumathotherapy is the common ground of the Lung Culturists and the Atman apostles**. More than any other one phase of Naturopathy it is both physical and psychical. And more than any other it is prostituted to chicanery and charlatanism. Sumptuous Academies of Breathing offer complete courses, personal and epistolary, guaranteeing strengthened lungs, perfected digestion, quickened circulation, intensified health. One advocates abdominal respiration, another thoracic, this—the retaining of the breath, that—immediate expulsion, some—the use of Exhalers and Breathing Tubes, others—their utter repudiation.

Now the best School of Breathing is a sleeping child. You will notice that the most movement is just below the sternum, where the diaphragm is struggling to do its proper work. The convexity is greatest abdominally and least thoracically. With every full inspiration—and they are all full before clothing and stomach-distension and worry inhibit them—the diaphragm rises quite plainly, the abdomen follows perceptibly, and the chest barely moves. There is one cune [sic], one motion, one effect—no artificial distinction exists.

Thoracic breathing is peculiar to women because they bind and shrivel and mar and paralyze the abdomen, which should be the chief aid to the diaphragm. An abdominal breathing characterizes [masculinity] because they encase the throat and chest in the torture-instruments of the haberdasher and tailor. And men are stronger than women, as abdominal breathing is stronger than thoracic. Abolish collars and vests and suspenders and belts and corsets and all humanity would breathe in rhythm.

Then again are the occult respirers who devise some such formula as "Breath is Life", or "I inhale Health", or "Inspiration is Power". They appeal especially to neurotics and visionaries, whose lung-action is impeded by a stuffed stomach or a warped brain. Now Breath is Life, and Inspiration is Power, and the strong man breathes deep. But it is a living, pulsating, energizing idea that actuates him, not the spasmodic and panic-stricken repeating of a Hindoo [sic] formula. Shallow breathing and invalidism are synonymous and co-existent and any measure that remedies the one relieves the other. So that if a formula or some mystic therapeutic

---

* The original title of this article was "Health Incarnate: A Naturopathic Silhouette" which was a regular column written by Benedict Lust. —Ed.

**Atman is Sanskrit for breath or soul. Atman apostles refer to an Hindu philosophy believing in the spiritual life principle of the universe. —Ed.

Spirometers have found a place as a recognized testing device to measure pulmonary functions. The required deep inhalations can be responsible for aggravations in diseases such as asthma.

attribute of the air can develop one of the inner forces of the stunted bit of humanity, then Naturopathy bids the talisman Godspeed.

The fatal error in Lung-Culture is the confounding of measurement with capacity. Professor Doud is the most conspicuous example. His chest-expansion was the greatest in the world, and he died of consumption. The writer knows an athlete, who increases his chest-measurement six inches by simply tensing certain external muscles. Cubic capacity and circumferential girth are not necessarily proportional, and though the latter is most desirable, the former is the measure of Life or Death.

## Suggestions

1. Never hold the breath. For poise and power, a momentary pause between inhaling and exhaling is often helpful. But it should never exceed two or three seconds.

2. Never breathe through the mouth. The only exception is in certain staccato out-breathing movements for removing residual air and strengthening abdominal muscles.

3. Never strain vascular tissue. This is common with devotees of Exhalers, Spirometers and Breathing Machines.

4. Never breathe past the point of dizziness. Cerebral congestion may usually by obviated by vigorous foot exercises preceding respiration.

5. Correlate breathing-movements with body-movements. Inhale on out and up movements. Exhale on in and down.

6. Remember that posture is a vital point. Dyspeptics and neurotics carry the whole inside machinery several inches too low. And congestion, indigestion, fermentation, constipation necessarily follow. Watch a man standing on the street corner—chest in and down, abdomen out and up, and entire posture bespeaking weakness and flabbi-

ness. Chest out, abdomen in, muscles tense, and breathing will take care of itself.

7. Breathe always toward the sun or the stars. Astronomers are far-sighted, philosophical, and long-lived. And the incoming of the spirit of the air is purer and truer and deeper when the mind forgets its earthy tenement, and dwells on the grandeur of the heavens.

*The best School of Breathing is a sleeping child.*

*Never breathe through the mouth.*

*Correlate breathing-movements with body-movements.*

## RETURN TO NATURE

### by Dr. C. W. Young, Ph.E., D.O., St. Paul

*The Naturopath and Herald of Health, V (3), 66-69. (1904)*

In the great Cleveland convention of osteopathic physicians, Dr. C. M. Turner Hulett, one of the wisest and yet one of the most conservative of the members of the association, admitted that it was the Osteopath's duty to his patient to use water and heat wherever indicated. *The Journal of Osteopathy* for August, on page 266, declares editorially that all were agreed that other things can be done to assist the patient to recovery besides removal of lesions by manipulation. Dr. J. Martin Littlejohn in the *Journal of the Science of Osteopathy* says, "Water, heat, sunlight, etc., are osteopathic, because they belong to the great field of nature therapeutics, and whatever belongs to this field forms a part of Osteopathy. Osteopathy is an independent therapeutic system, and as such includes within everything natural, excluding everything foreign or alien to the body organisms."

During the last three years I have striven zealously and, as I believe, honestly, to ascertain the best natural agencies, that could be added to the marvelous discoveries of Dr. Still to accomplish health restoration in the quickest and most effective way possible. I think at last, I have run across the book of books on the subject of natural healing. The author is Adolph Just, of Germany. The title is *Return to Nature*. Price, $2.00 is published by the translator, B. Lust, 124 E. 59th St., New York. My tribute to this work is entirely voluntary, and a review was not even solicited by the publisher. I call practicing Osteopaths' attention to the book as containing more helpful suggestions along non-manipulative lines than any other book in existence. I call the lay reader's attention to it as being the most practical work on Physical Culture that has ever been published.

### EXPERIENCE OF THE AUTHOR

For years, the author had suffered the tortures of sickness. He had tried many systems of so-called "nature cures" without any very great or very permanent benefit. At last he determined to throw science and reason aside and follow instinct alone. He left the haunts of men, where disease and discord were all prevailing and went into the depths of the mountain forest and there concentrated his attention upon the voices of nature. He became entirely willing to go wherever those voices might call. He heard harmonies a hundred times more delicious and soothing than

---

*This article by C. W. Young was one of many included in a column called "Osteopathic Physical Culture". —Ed.

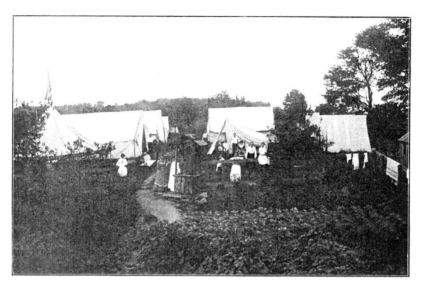

Air huts were popular with visitors to the Yungborn in Butler, New Jersey.

those produced by the most skilled of human musicians. He watched the birds and deer and other wild animals and learned how their instinct kept them in tune with nature. At last he no longer saw the misguiding hand of human artificialities. His being became attuned to the infinite harmony of nature. Every organ of his body once more vibrated with the delightful rhythm originally designed by the Creator. The jarring, discordant nerves became wonderfully changed. Instead of shrieking with pain they thrilled with joy. Life instead of being a hideous nightmare became a dream of paradise. When his health was restored, he resolved to point the way to health to the disease plagued world. He founded a sanitarium in the Hartz Mountains in Germany and called it the "Jungborn". At this place many marvelous cures have been affected.

## Character Of The Book

The book appears to me as one likely to become as useful to humanity as any that has ever been written, except the book of Divine Revelation. The language is very clear and plain. The arrangement is not as logical as some might like to have it, while others might liken it to a running brook and enjoy the lack of evenness and regularity. The author claims to have discovered the fundamental principles of the physical life of human beings. He believes he has reached bed-rock in therapeutic science. He makes astounding assertions. He claims to have discovered a method of cure that is immensely superior to all other systems of healing in existence. His claims would be preposterous if they were not true. He is human and undoubtedly there are many errors in the book, but I believe he states more fundamental truth than any other book that has ever been published on the healing art since the dawn of Creation. In his own case, so-called medical science proved to be a failure generally. He also asserts that other sciences fail to bring health and happiness. May be he is right. May be we would be better off without railroads and telephones. May be they force hundreds and thousands of people into engaging in unhealthy occupations. But I am not yet convinced that humanity would be benefited by casting aside all science. It seems to me that we may be able to return to nature sufficiently to ward off disease and reach something like physical perfection and yet enjoy the intellectual life that centers around our sciences.

### THE JUST METHOD

I presume some of my osteopathic readers will now assert with vengeance that is endorsing the Just Method, I endorse agencies for health restoration that are "grotesque" in the extreme. Let me put in a word of caution. Please do not be so foolish as to condemn any alleged healing agency until after you have investigated it thoroughly and are sure you know what you are talking about. Osteopath, let me appeal to you, do not make the ridiculous mistake our learned medical friends have made in calling Osteopathy "vile" and many other opprobious epithets before they had investigated. If you do not believe in the efficacy of the agencies advocated in *Return to Nature* used in the manner therein described, purchase a copy of the book and test the thing yourself fairly, fully and judiciously, and if it does not work, send a statement of facts to me and I will see to it that they are published. Science is advanced by accumulating facts and by demonstration and not by hurling epithets.

It is very significant that Adolph Just, the greatest of the great German naturalists, should put much emphasis on manipulation as a curative agent, indicating that perfection in the healing art cannot be attained without the use of the hand and that Dr. Still in perfecting the science of manipulation has discovered truths that will be used as long as human beings shall dwell on the earth.

### BATHS

The natural bath and light-and air-bath are described in great detail. I have often mentioned the natural bath in former numbers of the *Osteopathic World*. A condensed description appears in the June *Northern and Cosmopolitan Osteopath*. I use this bath myself, and I have found it extremely beneficial, and many of my patients are very enthusiastic over it. The light-and-air bath consists of going naked out doors or in a room with open windows. The author strongly recommends the exposure of the nude body to air as being the most efficient and most natural method of reducing fever. I tried this method in a case of quinsy in a man having strong vital powers. On the evening of the fifth day of his sickness, I was first called to treat the case. A doctor of medicine in the morning had run a lance in one of the tonsils and blood followed the lance but no pus. I found the patient in great misery. He had not been able to eat anything for two days, and his throat was so badly stopped up that he had been unable to drink any water for twenty-four hours. It was a chilly November evening. I opened three windows of the bed room as wide as possible and pulled off from the patient two heavy comforters and a sheet, and in ten minutes after I began to treat him his bowels moved. I then had him remove his heavy cotton flannel night gown and flannel undershirt, and let the cold air strike his nude skin, while I continued to give chiefly a spinal treatment. His wife asked him if he was cold. "No", he answered, very emphatically, "I am burning with fever." After twenty minutes of such treatment the fever seemed entirely reduced in a healthy way. He spit out a lot of pus, and then he was able to drink water freely. After my departure he drank a small pitcher full of lemonade and put a plaster of antiphlogistine [kaolin poultice] around his throat. He slept very nicely and thereafter made a most elegant recovery. He did not have a sign of catching cold.

## EARTH COMPRESSES

The book strongly recommends earth compresses as being superior to water for reduction of inflammations. Just would treat diphtheria by letting cold air strike the nude skin until fever is reduced, and by earth compresses around the throat. I have used antiphlogistine quite extensively, and found it very satisfactory, but maybe I can get some mud in my own back yard that will be better and cheaper than this "Denver Mud". This will be a matter of future investigation. Abdominal earth-compresses are recommended in a large variety of cases.

## FOOD AND CLOTHING

Heavy woolen and underclothing is strongly condemned. Light, porous, linen mesh is recommended. Fruits, berries and nuts are declared to be the natural diet. The author claims that our unnatural ways of living create our unnatural appetites. He condemns coffee, tea, alcohol, tobacco and meat, and he thinks cooking is harmful. He believes that we are better off on two meals a day, doing without our breakfast.

Many other hygienists have reached similar conclusions. We all will have to lay aside our prejudices and do a vast amount of honest investigation before we can be sure we have reached the correct solution to all dietetic problems.

## EARTH POWER

The most remarkable claims of *Return to Nature* are made respecting the earth power. Kneipp is given great credit for introducing the "bare-foot" cure. It is believed by some that there is an electrical connection between the body and the earth when the bare feet come in contact with the earth, and that the body is greatly benefited by this electricity. Just argues that his electrical connection is much more complete when the entire body is in direct contact with the earth. In describing his experience with his Jungborn patients he says: "But soon the patients lay down on the soft gross entirely naked, even without a shirt, and covered themselves with quilts. They soon broke out in enthusiastic exclamations over the wonderful effect of the earth upon the body during the night's rest. The opinion was often expressed that all diseases, but especially the score of serious nervous troubles of our age, would entirely lose their terrors if only sleeping and lying on the earth at night once became customary in the curing of diseases. It is indeed a fact that the effect which the forces of the earth have upon man during the night is quite incredible. Whoever has not himself tried it and convinced himself of it can have no conception of how refreshing, vitalizing and strengthening the effect of the earth is on the human organism at night during rest.

"The chief end of all healing art must be to aid and strengthen the digestion of the patient. Nothing accomplishes this end better than lying on the ground during the night, however much the natural bath and light-and air-bath may facilitate the movement of bowels.

"By sleeping on the ground, consequently, more than by anything else, the entire body is aroused from its lethargy to a new manifestation of vital energy, so that it can now effectively remove old morbid matter and masses of old feces from the intestines, and receive a sensation of new health, new life, and new unthought of vigor and strength."

I must confess the above statements amazed me as much as anything that I have ever come across, since endeavoring to learn the most effective ways for relieving pain and curing disease, though I have been greatly amazed many times since reaching the conviction that health is not to be attained by swallowing poisons. My prejudices were aroused and I declared to myself that in some way or other Just must be mistaken. I read the clinic reports in the *Return to Nature*, and the cures affected were extraordinarily marvelous, and I noticed that the most emphasized agent of cure was the earth power. Furthermore the book claimed the best results were attained in cool weather. At last instead of asserting to myself that Just was mistaken I determined to try the earth power myself.

I removed my clothing late at night, and wrapped myself in a large comforter and went out into the back yard. I then lay down with my bare back on the bare ground and the comforter over me. The wind was tinged with the chill of October in Minnesota, while the adjacent sod was hoary with frost, but I did not get cold. The ground felt cool, but it seemed to be deliciously pleasant from the start. I lay there for half an hour and I could distinctly feel a soothing, normalizing effect taking place in all the abdominal viscera. The next day I felt the arousing from lethargy and new manifestation of vital energy so vividly described in Just's wonderful book. I caught no cold whatever.

The time is coming when the hospitals will be emptied of their multitudes of sufferers, and when aching brows and pain-racked bodies will be almost unknown. It is the time when humanity shall return to nature and to natural methods of healing. (*The Osteopathic World,* Minneapolis)

---

*Please do not be so foolish as to condemn any alleged healing agency until after you have investigated it thoroughly and are sure you know what you are talking about.*

*The book strongly recommends earth compresses as being superior to water for reduction of inflammations.*

*It is believed by some that there is an electrical connection between the body and the earth when the bare feet come in contact with the earth, and that the body is greatly benefited by this electricity.*

*By sleeping on the ground, consequently, more than by anything else, the entire body is aroused from its lethargy to a new manifestation of vital energy, so that it can now effectively remove old morbid matter and masses of old feces from the intestines, and receive a sensation of new health, new life, and new unthought of vigor and strength.*

*I read the clinic reports in the Return to Nature, and the cures affected were extraordinarily marvelous, and I noticed that the most emphasized agent of cure was the earth power.*

# Heliotherapy (Sun Cure) And Thermotherapy (Heat Cure)*

## by Benedict Lust
*The Naturopath and Herald of Health, V (4), 87-90. (1904)*

With the exception of the sun-bath and hot applications, these treatments are reserved for sanatorium use. Rheumatism, neuralgia and kindred ailments yield most readily to dry heat—the baking process or the electric light bath or the sun-bath. Most nervous and digestive disorders are relieved by proper application of heat. The sun-bath, as described by Adolph Just, in his work, *Return to Nature*, and as used in his sanatorium, "Jungborn", is somewhat as follows: One lies on the ground, preferably in the woods, without clothing. If the sun be uncomfortably warm, novices may protect themselves by a covering of porous cloth, or still better, fresh leaves and branches. Sunburn, while not dangerous or injurious, is decidedly unpleasant, and may be best obviated by rubbing the body with moist earth before exposure. If scorching should occur, the surest remedy is cold water and wet compresses (moist earth serves satisfactorily); avoid altogether oils, salves and like alleged allayers [pain relievers].

In the hot sun the bath must be modified, perhaps alternating between sun and shade. Direct contact with the earth is essential; mattresses, hammocks, roofs and other go-betweens vitiate the treatment. In case propriety demands covering, a single thickness should suffice, whether in the open air or in one's room: the face and head should always be protected, moistened grape-leaves being excellent. The natural bath (elsewhere described in *Return to Nature*) should always follow the sun-bath, or the next best substitute be provided.**

The duration of exposure varies from a few minutes to perhaps an hour or longer, and if a delightful sense of warmth and life and power does not thrill palpably from the sun-bath, it has been taken wrongly and the bather is to blame, not the bath.

### Phototherapy (Light Cure) And Aerotherapy (Air Cure)

The beneficence of light is no longer doubted by the most benighted pre-hygienic practitioner, and needs no eulogy here. A most striking example of its recent development is the Finson Institute at Copenhagen: similar establishments exist also at Paris and Berlin. Prismatic baths, of

---

*This article by Benedict Lust was Part XVI of a series called, "Health Incarnate, A Naturopathic Silhouette". —*Ed.*

** The Natural Bath is found in *Philosophy of Naturopathic Medicine*, pp. 85–92. —*Ed.*

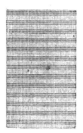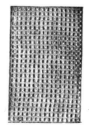
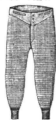
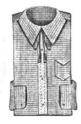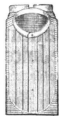
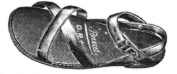
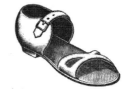
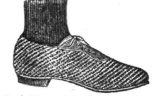
Benedict Lust began the first health product store in NYC and expanded to the "Yungborn", in Butler, New Jersey selling natural attire.

sun and electric light, are used in conjunction with cold water for the relief of bacillary, nervous and other diseases. Red, gold, blue, white and purple rays are practically the sole method of treatment. And cancer in its most virulent form yields to the germicidal potencies of the sun-god.

The effect of certain colors on the nervous system has long been known, e.g., a person confined in a room virulently purple becomes shortly a raving maniac. But the Germans, as usual, have first reduced theory to practice and science. And Phototherapy will soon be recognized among the indispensable measures of Naturopathy. The Finson Institute is described in detail in the *Kneipp-Blätter* of August, 1901.

Aerotherapy is as yet a stranger among the legion of "pathies", and deserves elaborate introduction. Benjamin Franklin understood it and took an air-bath daily. But the early apprehending of great truths by great men does not involve their general acceptance and application.

The Indian is never sick; the American is proverbially so. And there are reasons for it. The Indian papoose is born with a tendency toward health. His birth was but an episode of a few hours in the vigorous free, happy life of his mother; his early months are passed on a board, his childhood is free from prohibitions not to play in the dirt, or go barefoot, or do things the normal child-animal delights in; his youth is spent in the forest, with Nature, and among the animals.

And he grows up a straight, strong, symmetrical son of Nature.

The American is cursed before birth. Instead of exercising and bathing and breathing and rejoicing, the expectant mother stitches and nibbles and sighs and dreads; and the puny, fretful, nervous babe is the incarnation of her abortive attitude. From the feverish pillow and fretting blankets he is tossed into the heinous baby-carriage and jolted into spasms or spinal curvature. The play-spirit is crushed, the study-spirit is defied, the natural child-longings are pressed into mathematical moulds and set rules, and the little old man grows up a nervous, dyspeptic, cantankerously one-sided specimen of a civilization-pervert.

Now the Indian has no flannels or houses or carriages to box up his body from the earth and air and dew and rain and light. And nervous dyspepsia is out of his ken [understanding]. The American takes particular pains to barricade himself from light and air. Not satisfied with building a gloomy, stuffy, foul office and a dark, narrow, fetid flat, he fiendishly devises close-woven underwear and airtight hats and blood-curdling gloves and catarrhal mufflers and effeminate furs. He has observed with family tradition and religious punctiliousness the day in November for the first scratching of the flannels and the day in May for their gleeful discarding. He believes heat and warmth synonymous, so he shivers his bloodless frame over his poison-spouting register, buries himself frantically in his great ulster, and rushes, congealing, to the overheated car that bears him to his steaming office.

On the way he passes Naturopathy, without overcoat, mufflers, gloves or flannels, warm as toast, walking briskly, reveling in the pure air of the early morning and smiling compassionately at the hot-house product of super-civilization. The underwear question is too intricate to discuss here, but the following brief arraignment of wool next the skin may suffice:

1. It clings tight to the skin, thus vitiating transpiration.
2. It conducts heat readily, thus promoting loss of bodily warmth.
3. It fails to adapt itself to temperature conditions, thus inviting extraneous cold.
4. It readily becomes saturated with perspiration, thus chilling the body.
5. It absorbs and holds impurities, thus retarding pore-excretion.
6. It irritates the skin, thus inducing discomfort and nervousness.
7. It invites rheumatism, malaria and like diseases.
8. It is conducive to "colds"; its constant wearing means overheating, its removal means overcooling.
9. It is often the shearing of sickly animals, and is wholly subversive of cleanliness, rather than productive.
10. It is repulsive to a normal person, and proves thereby its unnaturalness.

Now *atmospheric air* is the Naturopathic undergarment. It is non-conducting, non-irritating, non-saturable, refreshing, comfortable, clean. Wool is distinctly anti-atmospheric; linen and all loose-wove textures have always a lining of air. Aeropathy, therefore, and Naturopathy advocates as the best: linen, net, China-grass and maco (Egyptian cotton). Kneipp's linen tricot, Kneipp's linen, Walser's China-grass, Mez' net, Walser's Rippenkrepp, Mahr's correll maco, linen mesh, Ramie all these meet the requirements most satisfactorily.

Perhaps next to the "flannels" fallacy, in point of importance, comes the footwear travesty. Cold or sweating feet, corns, and like pedal distresses are the legitimate result of ill-fitting or ill-made shoes. Fashion decrees that footwear be uncomfortable, unanatomical and unhygienic. We Americans care little for the first specification, less for the second and nothing for the third. And not until the advent of the chiropodist's bill do we begin to suspect the fallibility of our shoemaker. The differences are many between the ordinary shoe and the aeropathic. The former binds the foot, retarding circulation; it absorbs moisture, hindering perspiration; it is unyielding, causing corns, bunions and abrasions of all kinds: it is uncomfortable, causing chafing, discomfort and nervousness. The latter is loose, adaptable, porous, comforting. And it wears. Soled with the solidest German leather, it is just nicely fitting itself to the foot by the time the department store bargain shoe is a forgotten wreck.

The Naturopathic shoe suggests a long winter evening: a coal-fire, a rocker and Ik Marvel or his kin. Pure linen socks are a valuable re-enforcement to the Natural Sandal and Low Shoe, but are not indispensable.

The corset question is not strictly aeropathic, but may be noted in passing. So-called "female weakness" is the outcome of a woman's corset, or a man's passion, or both, of the former in the case of a virgin; of the latter, or of both, in the case of a wife. Dr. Rosch's fearless essay on "The Origin of Most Chronic Diseases" defines very plainly the crimes of husbandhood. (Published in pamphlet form by *The Naturopath*; price 25 cents postpaid.)

As for the corset, explanation, ratiocination [logical reasoning], argumentation, any and all pleas to the brain, the body, or the heart, have failed for centuries to win women from bondage. And we do not purpose any extended dissertation. Among other things the corset does, are the following:

1.  It paralyzes intestinal action, inducing chronic constipation.

2.  It renders the abdomen flabby, inert and unresisting a hot-bed for all diseases.

3.  It prevents movement of the diaphragm and necessitates chest-breathing.

4.  It tends to substitute fat for muscle, changing the lithe, dainty symmetry of maidenhood to the clumsy, porcine corpulency of matronhood.

5.  It vitiates the contour, life and beauty of the breast, producing induration, atrophy and worse perversions.

6.  It retards digestion and assimilation, and is the direct cause of the worst forms of dyspepsia.

7.  It gripes the glorious tokens of womanhood into a helpless heterogeneous heap, whence spring an infinity of uterine and ovarian abuses.

8.  It is a preventative or abortive of motherhood.

9.  Its whole function is the dwarfing and shriveling and perverting of pure womanhood, in health, beauty, influence, ideals. And its existence is a hideous witness to the bowing of women before the false standard of men.

The Grecian bust girdle, the Venus physical culture waist, and other admirable substitutes are fast superseding the corset with women who know.

Thermotherapy and Aerotherapy may be briefly summed up in the following suggestions:

1. Never wear flannel next the skin. If purse or preference contraindicates the getting of the best, use a gauze undershirt beneath a thin woolen.

2. Never let the feet or other parts of the body remain cold. Hair insoles—Porous [Adolf] Just socks—exercise—massage—even hot applications—but keep warm.

3. Learn to discard mufflers, gloves and furs whenever possible. A rational course in Naturopathy will soon make effeminating garments odious to you.

4. Never close your bed-room window. Always a few inches at the top, usually a few at the bottom, and the rapid swinging of the door before retiring, to facilitate ventilation.

5. Take an air-bath for a few minutes at bed-time. This may or may not include exercise-period, and should be gradually increased to a half-hour or longer.

6. Use few bed-covers. The feet should be well protected, but a course of hardening by the Kneipp method will obviate the need for artificial warmth.

7. Use discretion and moderation. In Aeropathy and in Hydropathy, Dietotherapy and other branches of Naturopathy, the lesser extreme is always preferable to the greater.

---

*In the hot sun the bath must be modified, perhaps alternating between sun and shade.*

*The natural bath (elsewhere described in Return to Nature) should always follow the sun-bath.*

*The American is cursed before birth. Instead of exercising and bathing and breathing and rejoicing, the expectant mother stitches and nibbles and sighs and dreads; and the puny, fretful, nervous babe is the incarnation of her abortive attitude.*

*Never let the feet or other parts of the body remain cold.*

*Never close your bed-room window.*

### How Shall We Live
#### Benedict Lust

---

### Chiropractic
#### Bartlett Joshua Palmer, D.C.

Benedict Lust's Naturopathic School of Regeneration was located beside his Kneipp Health Store at 111 E. 59th St. in New York City.

# How Shall We Live?

## by Benedict Lust

*The Naturopath and Herald of Health, VI (1), 3-5. (1905)*

Health is the best rudder on the voyage of life.

Natural! This short word means the shunning of all the sins considered in the last chapter, the unlimited use of our mental capacities and a strict obedience to our nature.

It is to be regretted that we so easily misconceive Nature's will, for the cyclone of our present super-civilization has blown us to faraway side paths where we find ourselves scarcely able to hear the voice of our great teacher. Then let us hasten to return, let us diligently read the book of nature and we shall come to the following conclusions, which will teach us "The art of living a long life, free from care".

*An abundance of Light and Air is the first condition of Life.*

Sunlight especially is a leading factor for the prevention and healing of disease.

"The Doctor is not required where the sun shines." Sunbaths, as they are called, have shown marvelous results. Is not the sun alone the mainspring of all life and motion in nature?

Let us not shut it out, neither from our rooms, by curtains and shades, nor in the open air by parasols and other devices.

While the sun gives us our life, the air, or rather fresh air preserves it. We make it serve us during the day by frequently ventilating our rooms, if our daily task keeps us within and during the night by leaving the windows open. As long as we do not take the care to constantly breathe good air, all our hopes for the recovery of real health remain a delusion and a snare.

## Care Of The Body Is Nature's Law

We can obey this law:

1. By a systematic care of our skin, consisting of Sun and Air Baths and in summer of a Natural Bath daily, in winter 2 or 3 times a week.

2. By a frequent cleansing of the mouth and teeth.

3. By a proper care of our hair, by using fresh pure water, as most hair tonics, pomatums and essences are known to cause irritation and must necessarily have a bad effect on the scalp and the whole nervous system.

4. By the frequent change of our underwear.

### Simplicity In Dress Is The Third Requirement Of Nature

The less, the better; the best guide is the comfortable condition of the body. But away with all excess of undershirts and protectors, drawers, shawls, fur collars, and fur coats, for our skin must have contact with the outer air and it takes severe revenge for any infringement on its rights. Man is a creature intended for living in air and as such would be really better off by going through life in the costume of Adam. Let us take the following examples of such "undress" to heart, that it may open our eyes to the uselessness and the danger of all needless ballast in the form of clothing.

On the shores of Oakland Bay, there lives a German Captain, Edward A. von Schmidt, a very tall man of splendid physique, a veritable giant. This powerful specimen of humanity, tanned and ruddy, has been going naked for 20 years (except for a belt and a pair of cotton bathing trunks) during this time he has defied all the climates of the world, being "feared" as far away as the South Sea. On being asked why he did not wear clothes in this climate, like other people, he answered:

> Well, to make it short, on account of my health. I am the descendant of a family in which consumption is frequent; when I was yet a boy, people would predict that the weakness of my lungs would cause my death. And when I went to sea, my friends believed I would never return. Now, when in the tropics I always wore very little clothing and the less I wore, the better I felt, and whenever I commenced wearing additional clothing, I would not feel as comfortable.

> A year thereafter I brought a vessel through the straits of Magellan, and there I noticed that the natives of Fireland went naked. I saw old men hale and hearty, and mother who were nursing their children, all going naked. They were quick in their movements and full of strength.

> Then I said to myself: I have found the secret of health. From that time on I go dressed, like the powerful natives of that wintry land, just as you see me now. I also dress my children in accordance with these principles and have never spent a penny on my family for the services of a physician or for medicine.

### Our Nourishment Must Be In Accordance With Nature

Everything that is harmful to our body that tends to destroy it, to weaken it, to stir up passions and therefore everything that is directly harmful is contrary to nature. The words: "man is what he eats" contain some truth, as we must admit when we observe that our "refined" diet, with all its irritants, harmful beverages, alcohol and tobacco is conducive like nothing else to poison our body, weaken our energy and to stir up passions.

Let us then reform our diet, let us cease our indulgence in deleterious pleasures, if we do not wish them to become tyrants over our free will, and to be ourselves the martyrs of adopted weaknesses and desires. The basis of all diet reform is:

1. The greatest possible diminution of our meat diet.
2. The diminished use of spices.
3. A more liberal use of vegetables of all kinds.
4. An abundant daily supply of fruits and nuts of all kinds, according to the season.

These are Hygeia's most important commandments. In obeying them we shall gain health of body and purity of soul. They put alcohol and all pertaining thereto under the ban, because we are no longer in need of stimulants. They close to us the saloon doors, but open to us the delights of happy contentment with the beauty of simple customs and a quiet home life, as well as the joy of feeling morally satisfied with ourselves. Before everything else, let us exchange the disadvantages arising from the use of expensive meats for the benefits derived from the enjoyment of cheaper fruit and nuts—for fruit and nuts alone is the original and natural food of man. An abundant daily fruit and nut diet has in truth regenerative qualities; it gives new impulses to flagging vitality; it has a favorable effect on the brain, quickens and facilitates the production of blood, prevents piles and their complications, promotes the activity of the kidneys, is a preventive against disturbances of the digestive organs, aids the secretion of bile, and, lastly, induces regular, quiet sleep. (People with weak stomachs ought to accustom themselves *by slow degrees* to a daily fruit diet.)

Let us now add to these observations the final conditions of a life in accordance with nature's laws.

## MODERATION, LABOR AND REST

Moderation in eating and drinking is a further means for attaining enduring health, and bodily as well as mental efficiency. It is not the luxurious meal of the aristocrat and the epicure that guarantees capacity and energy, but the modest diet of the honest laborer, where simplicity serves the plate and moderation the bread.

Labor is balm for the blood, that is: bodily labor. Those to whom it has not been given to perform, may seek a substitute (and *must* seek it) by work in field and garden, or by frequent walks through meadow and woods, over hill and dale. Nature holds in her lap an inexhaustible supply of rich blessings for all of us. Unnatural sedentary habits always bear the stamp of deterioration and weakness, and we therefore honor the attempts to obtain an 8 hour day for those performing sedentary work indoors.

Rest tastes well after our task is done. But this rest is not to be sought in smoke filled saloons, badly or not at all ventilated, odorous with liquor and beer, breeding places of intemperance and debauchery, but in a little circle of dear friends, with whom we may share the comforts of cheerful home or the blessings of God's all-loving nature.

We shall close here, for we have now given a plan for leading a natural life, worthy of the name of man. It remains for you, dear reader, not only to know what such life means, but to *lead* it.

In wisely living in accordance with these preliminary conditions of a natural life—strength to conquer evil desires and passions, hygienic self-government over your body—in this consists true worldly wisdom. It will prove an unconquerable bulwark against sickness and disease, against physician, surgeon and apothecary, patent medicine sharks and medical quacks; against morphine, mercury, Pasteur's and Behring's serums, Koch's Tuberculine and other hellish inventions.

Living according to nature is the threat of Ariadne, which safely guides deluded humanity from out the maze of social misery, and back to a happy life, free from care.

Therefore: Awaken, dear people! Recognize the cancer of our times, and the cause of all misery! See the degeneration and debility of mankind! The vast host of the sick and crippled! Count the innumerable institutions which contain your orphans, your widows, your sick, your poor, your blind and your insane!

Consider the highest average duration of life in our generation (50-55 years!). And then bear in mind that it was nature's intention to give man a lifetime of 150 years!

Think also of the depths of degeneration into which the deteriorated Spanish and French (Anglo-Saxons included) races have already begun to fall, that you may at last understand the causes of bloom and of decay; of the rise and fall of the lost Empires of antiquity!

It is still time for retracing our way, therefore, turn back, dear friends, return to nature! Stop on the mazy path of unnatural living! Throw off the delusions of vaccination and medicine! Put an end to false pretense and false civilization! Control vices and passions! Let us light the torch of a new, true worldly wisdom, that its rays of promise may penetrate into the deepest depths of the world's misery and rekindle the flame of long lost happiness on earth!

True wordly wisdom as nature teaches it! Therein is contained the

Jethro Kloss and Otto Carqué had an immense influence on the growing Natuopathic profession.

exalted enjoyment of physical strength and health, the bond for success and for all pure joys of life, the joyous consciousness of the inner harmony of the mind and soul! Return to Nature! It means the rebuilding of humanity, the regaining of lost prosperity, the renaissance of all wellbeing, of all happiness, of pure enjoyment of life and of all joy within us.

Godspeed, my people! Ascend the height where freedom lives, true freedom, happiness, and lasting peace! Godspeed!

---

*While the sun gives us our life, the air, or rather fresh air preserves it.*

*Moderation in eating and drinking is a further means for attaining enduring health, and bodily as well as mental efficiency.*

*Unnatural sedentary habits always bear the stamp of deterioration and weakness, and we therefore honor the attempts to obtain an 8 hour day for those performing sedentary work indoors.*

*In wisely living in accordance with these preliminary conditions of a natural life—strength to conquer evil desires and passions, hygienic self-government over your body—in this consists true worldly wisdom.*

## CHIROPRACTIC

**by Bartlett Joshua Palmer, D.C.**

Secretary, The Palmer School and Infirmary of Chiropractic, Davenport, Iowa

*The Naturopath and Herald of Health, VI (10), 284-289. (1905)*

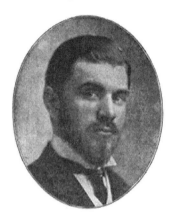

B. J. Palmer, D.C.
His father D. D. Palmer
invented Chiropractic.

When Ontario, Canada, was a wilderness, covered with its primeval forests, when Toronto had but one house, the grandparents of the writer of the present sketch were among the first settlers, a short distance east of Canada's beautiful city. Their pioneer experience was similar to that of others. There, the future discoverer of Chiropractic was born March 7, 1845, nestled in a primitive cradle made of hemlock bark, which the sun had warped into shape, suggesting the ready-made infant couch. There he listened to his mother's sweet lullaby and received his first impressions toward making this world the better for his having lived in it.

His early life was similar to that of other boys, except that he was inclined to think for himself and never accepted an idea as true, because everybody said so. He was radical in thought and work.

At the age of twenty he came to Iowa. For twenty years he was engaged in raising fruit, honey and the grocery business. Surrounding circumstances compelled him to think of those afflicted with disease. His constant thought and questions to physicians were, "What and where are the causes of symptoms called disease? What is wrong with the patient that causes distress?" Medical answers that they would "give such and such drugs to relieve" were not satisfactory.

Dr. D. D. Palmer wanted to know *what* was wrong, believing that if he knew *where* and *how* the wrong was he might be able to remedy it. He reasoned that the body was a human machine that every act done and all feelings were but the sensations of the nerves; that if those nerves were natural there would be no such symptoms as disease. He eventually learned that most of the wrongs could be corrected by the hands, so he called his new mode of healing Chiropractic, which means hand-fixing.

Millions of people have been dissected, both dead and alive, by the medics with the vain hope of finding the cause of disease.

They have utterly failed. Each new moon looks down ascant [sic] on a new theory and a different remedy for the symptoms. They never have thought of fixing the cause.

While Dr. Palmer has made many friends, a few practitioners, from a spirit of envy and ignoble rivalry, are his enemies.

He has not escaped the usual disagreeable experiences of all originators. He has envious opposition from dishonest competitors, who claim to have taken a Chiropractic course. For this reason this school gives a diploma to each student who proves himself competent to practice this science.

There never was a time when the mind of man has been so restless in regard to therapeutics. Thousands of suffering people are waiting and anxiously looking for some other way outside of operations and poisons. There is an unrest; every conceivable thing seen and unseen is being tried. The evolution of the human mind is progressing at a remarkable rate of speed; we are learning to think. Our thoughts are rapidly and daily changing. The beliefs, theories and the entire educational foundations of our childhood are often overturned in a day. We are so accustomed to this rapid change of thought that we are only surprised that each practicing physician has not in and of himself learned to do what we are doing. That which is considered unprofessional today is liable to become the orthodox of tomorrow. The idea of our present liberalists will be venerated by future generations.

In the mighty sweep of human progress all sciences except one have been wonderfully advanced. The science of healing the sick and afflicted—misnamed medicine—has been enshrouded with mystery and ignorance, pretention and despair. Physicians study the effects of medicine on disease; they are ignorant as to the cause. A medical man describes disease by naming the effects.

That which should be the science of healing the sick and afflicted has been enshrouded with myth and mystery. The physicians of the future will adjust the cause of disease instead of treating the symptoms.

Different schools follow their own blind theories. The bacteriologist clings to his theory of microbes; the savages and spiritualists to the control of evil spirits; the many forms of faith, prayer and mind cures to evil thinking. Thus they wrangle over pills, principles and prayers, while their patients get well or die.

The regulars, irregulars, faddists and fakirs all claim equal success with equal evidence. All have similar successes and failures. Each despises the other's mode of practice.

Of late, science has discovered the simple fact that the human body is a fine, sensitive piece of machinery run throughout all its parts by nerves. That disease is a condition in which nature is trying to carry on its work of repair and growth with the machinery out of gear—a human machine out of order.

Chiropractic is the only mode of healing which exactly locates the cause of disease and teaches how to correct it. It is not faith cure, Christian Science, medicine, magnetic, electric, osteopathy, hypnotism, massage nor anything else but Chiropractic. It stands in a new field of thought; its foundation is a correct knowledge of anatomy and physiology.

Instead of benumbing and deadening the sensory nerves with poison, give them freedom to act and to feel naturally; instead of pain, give them ease and comfort.

In 1886, Dr. D.D. Palmer began healing as a business. He desired to know why such a person had asthma, rheumatism or other afflictions. He wished to know what difference there was in two persons that caused the one to have certain symptoms called disease; that his neighbor living under the same condition did not have. Physicians answered by saying that they would give such and such remedies. He did not want to know what remedies they would give; but desired to learn what difference there was in the man of health and the one who was diseased. He wanted to learn the cause of disease; why one was afflicted and the other not.

In his practice of the first ten years, under the name of magnetic, he treated nerves, followed and relieved them of inflammation. He made many good cures, as many are doing today under a similar method. His constant thoughts were that there was a difference in the person affected and the one not so. He was fully aware that he was treating effects. What was the cause of those ailments was what he desired to learn. He had progressed far enough to learn in what region the cause of any described symptoms were.

There must be a turning point, it was so with Chiropractic. But it took years to discover and develop that which was named Chiropractic, which means hand-fixing. A Chiropractor is one who adjusts or repairs with his hands.

Ninety-five percent of all deranged nerve functions are made so by subluxations of vertebrae which pinch nerves in some one of the 51 joint articulations of the spinal column.* Therefore, to relieve the pressure upon those nerves means to restore normal action, hence normal functions, perfect health.

The laws upon which this science is founded are so old as the vertebrata of the animal kingdom, but have been overlooked because of inherent superstition misdirecting the unenlightened mind of investigators.

The cause of disease has been, and is yet, mysterious to the great mass

---

*The author of this article states 51 joint articulations and later in his article states 52 joint articulations. —Ed.

of humanity. Chiropractic has solved the mystery. The old idea, that the cause of disease is outside of man, still prevails in most of the schools of healing and the cure consists in finding something outside, which, by being introduced into the body of the sufferer, will drive the disease out. Therapeutic methods give remedies to treat the effects. The chiropractic idea is that the cause of disease is in the person afflicted and the cure consists in correcting the wrong that is producing it.

Chiropractic finds the cause in pinched nerves of the person ailing, and releases that pressure by adjusting some of the 52 articulations of the vertebral column. In doing this there is no rubbing, slapping, knife, drugs, artificial heat, electricity, magnetism, hypnotism, stretching or mental treatment, in fact nothing but the adjustment of the displaced vertebra. This is not done with any surgical appliances nor any apparatus whatever, but simply by the use of the hand on a table. The adjustment is almost instantaneous. The movements are unique and chiropractic in every respect; no other system has anything similar. Chiropractic is the only system that exactly locates the case of disease and cures by hand adjusting.

A large share of diseases is caused by nerves being impinged in the foramina, which is occluded by the displacement of the vertebrae. These vertebrae are replaced by the hands; using the processes as handles.

To illustrate, he had decided that all diseases of the throat, such as goitre, croup, diphtheria, bronchitis, quinsy, and tonsillitis had their origin in the region of the stomach. Now, under the science of Chiropractic, he had ascertained that the nerves of innervation to the stomach emerge from the left side of the spinal column and the nerves which produce the above diseases by being disarranged, proceed from the right side. The nerves of the stomach may be impinged only, but usually when there is a displacement of the vertebra that pinches nerves on one side, they also impinge nerves on the opposite side.

On September 18, 1895, Harvey Lillard called upon Dr. Palmer. The doctor asked him how long he had been deaf. He answered, "Seventeen years." He was so deaf he could not hear the rumbling of a wagon. Mr. Lillard informed the doctor that at the time he became deaf he was in a cramped position and felt something give in his back. Upon examination there was found a displaced vertebra, a spinous process that was not in line. Dr. Palmer informed Mr. Lillard that he thought he could be cured of deafness by fixing his back.

He consented to have it fixed; we now say adjusted.

Two adjustments were given Harvey Lillard in the dorsal vertebra, which replaced a displaced vertebra, freeing nerves that had been paralyzed by pressure. This explains why so many persons "have been deaf ever since they had the measles". The measles were the acute stage and the deafness was the chronic effect from the same cause.

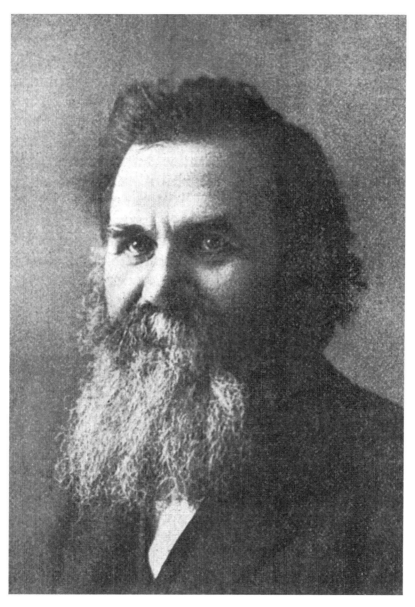

Daniel David Palmer, D.C., inventor of Chiropractic.

Mr. Lillard can hear today as well as other men. He resides at 1031 Scott Street, Davenport, Iowa.

The science of Chiropractic is being developed. It had to have a beginning. Osteopathy had a beginning. Dr. A. T. Still says in his book, "I began to give reasons for my faith in April, 1855." Thirty-seven years after, we find him teaching a class of less than a score of students. When he named the science, developed by him, Osteopathy, we are not informed. The principles of Osteopathy had to be collected, even if they were already known. To sum it up, Dr. A. T. Still made a science of certain principles and movements; it was he who gave Osteopathy a start for such he has now the credit.

Chiropractic had its beginning in September, 1895. We did not wait 37 years before teaching it. We, however, often wish that we had not placed it on the market until it was ten years of age. If we had done this, it would have saved much discussion and confusion in regard to who discovered the principles and movements of Chiropractic. It is of such a nature, that we could have retained it within ourselves, as long as we desired.

We have seen fit to date the beginning with the first adjustment given by Dr. D. D. Palmer, the discoverer and developer of this science. He was not the first person to replace vertebra by any means. For fear that someone might so construe his writings, *The Chiropractor*, number seven, gave 29 authors who believed in and set more or less vertebral joints, many of them before the discoverer of Chiropractic was born.

D. D. Palmer simplified the replacing of vertebrae. He discovered a simple method of using the processes as handles. Instead of finding a few rare cases of slipped vertebrae, that had been wrenched from their natural position, he found them very common. Indeed, it was the rule instead of the exception.

Others who had preceded him allowed that vertebral displacement might occur; that such might cause diseased conditions. D. D. Palmer said in print and person that 90 to 95 per cent of all diseases were caused by displacement of the spine. It was he who first described how and why luxations were the cause of disease.

He has created a science of vertebral adjustment. True, there were others, perhaps thousands, who had replaced joints of the backbone, but none had knowingly used the spinous and transverse processes as handles.

To say that D. D. Palmer discovered the principles and varied movements of Chiropractic at a fixed hour, of a certain day, of such a year, would not be correct. He has been many years developing that which has culminated into a science. Many principles which go to make up that which he named Chiropractic were studied by him during the previous ten years of 1895.

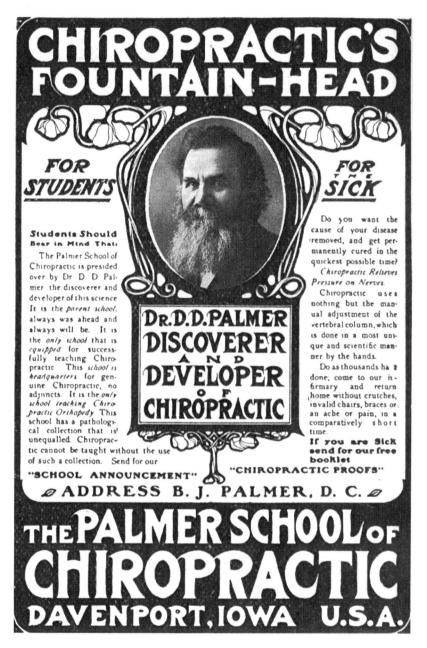

This ad and many other Chiropractic ads appeared in *The Naturopath* in the early days.

We look upon the giant locomotive as a thing of strength and beauty, and are charmed with its herculean power of locomotion as it can be hurled over the rails at the rate of 100 miles per hour, carrying its freight-age of human life. Yet after all, the secret of its momentous force lies in a simple principle—drive wheels to which it is connected. Chiropractic, like the locomotive, is another thing of beauty, for it demonstrates the strength of a simple principle in unique Chiropractic adjustment.

Giant strides have been achieved by inventive genius, but it would seem that little has been done in adjusting the cause of disease, until within the last few years. Why not advance in this field equal to that of others?

Allow me to call your attention to the advantages to be derived from a Chiropractic education:

1st, It is rational because it is anatomically correct for the removal of pressure, opens up the spinal foramina, thus the nerves respond to the normal functions and the patient is freed from disease.

2nd, It is practical, because it strikes directly at the root of the trouble, and therefore removes the cause.

3rd, It prepared one to fight life's battles, because he can immediately demonstrate its efficacy to cure, and in turn make for himself a substantial livelihood.

4th, The Chiropractor can give sciatic rheumatism to the most skeptical patient in an instant by a lateral lumbar adjustment, and just that surely is it the proper means of cure in arthritis, caries, osteomalacosis, scoliosis, torticollis, spastica, periosteomedullitis and all other ills.

5th, A Chiropractic adjustment is quickly given, thus enabling one to adjust hundreds of patients daily, multiplying his usefulness for the relief of suffering humanity.

The illustration so often repeated by Dr. Palmer, impresses one with the truth and virtue of Chiropractic. Let us for a moment fancy a beautiful dwelling with an opening in the roof whereby the water trickles in from every raincloud, and it is very devastating to its elaborately carved furniture and rich Brussel carpet. This foolish man applies varnishes and secures new furniture and carpet, only to find that the next storm causes the same sad havoc. Why does he not secure the service of a carpenter to fix the leak in the roof?

Again, let us imagine a wise man whose wife is suffering from an attack of typhoid fever. He at once secures the service of a competent Chiropractor, one who dexterously removes the pressure on the nerves which cause this dreadful disease. And behold, after two adjustments, she is well again. Think of the common sense of removing the cause instead of doping one's self with useless remedies which only relieve for a short time and are powerless in adjusting the subluxated vertebrae, which is not only the cause of typhoid fever, but the whole category of disease.

I commend Chiropractic to you and to the world, and if you will keep in mind the illustration of the rich man's dwelling, you will no longer continue to treat effects but will wisely remove the cause by fixing what is wrong. In the face of the world's suffering, I can fearlessly assert that the crying need of the hour can be met by Chiropractors for he does know how to permanently remove the cause of disease.

> There's a worth in Chiropractic,
> That is even more than gold.
> It is like the first love story—
> Better experienced than told.
>
> One lies in easy position;
> The next he hears is a click,
> He feels the pain has vanished
> And relief has come that quick.
>
> The world needs Chiropractors—
> Needs them on every hand,
> For to those in pain and anguish,
> This is a weary land.
>
> Then let us strive to be masters
> In the science that we employ;
> To make the whole world better
> And more full of peace and joy.

*Instead of benumbing and deadening the sensory nerves with poison, give them freedom to act and to feel naturally; instead of pain, give them ease and comfort.*

*Chiropractic finds the cause in pinched nerves of the person ailing, and releases that pressure by adjusting some of the 52 articulations of the vertebral column. In doing this there is no rubbing, slapping, knife, drugs, artificial heat, electricity, magnetism, hypnotism, stretching or mental treatment, in fact nothing but the adjustment of the displaced vertebra.*

*He [D. D. Palmer] has created a science of vertebral adjustment. True, there were others, perhaps thousands, who had replaced joints of the backbone, but none had knowingly used the spinous and transverse processes as handles.*

# 1906

Nature Cure Publishing Co. was one of Benedict Lust's enterprises specializing in health books.

# THE VALUE OF EARTH AS A REMEDY

by Dr. Adolph Just

*The Naturopath and Herald of Health, VII (1), 23-25. (1906)*

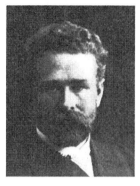

Adolph Just.

The following notice appeared some time ago in all newspapers,

A few days ago in the village of Recale, near Caserta, a young girl of twenty years, when mowing hay, was bitten by a snake. Her foot and leg were greatly swollen in a few minutes and the poor girl suffered the most acute pains. Her father put her on a truck and wheeled her to Caserta. Upon arriving there the right foot and the right arm of the unfortunate girl were horribly swollen. The physicians declared her case to be beyond help. The girl lost consciousness and the father wheeled her back, more dead than alive. He then tried a remedy that, a century before, had once saved the life of a young girl who, too, had been bitten by a snake. He dug a hole in the earth, stripped the girl of her clothes, put her naked into the hole and covered her again with earth up to the head. The mayor of the village ordered the man to take the girl out of that hole; but the whole village sided with the father of the girl, and a fight would, certainly, have taken place, if the mayor had insisted. After twenty-four hours the girl was dug out again, and was sound and well.

This incident was published by the *Corriere di Napoli*, according to the affidavit of the Prefect of Caserta.

Many times I have been told by people who had traveled in foreign countries that they had been surprised to read in my book, *Return to Nature*, of the earth applications which they found to be in such common use among the natives of many lands in different parts of the world.

Who revealed to these natives the healing powers of earth? The voice of Nature—their own instinct.

From this incident in that Italian village we learn that in Europe also people have used earth in cases of blood poisoning. We also know that when, for instance, a person is stung by a bee, old women will instinctively take earth, wet it with their saliva and put it on the painful part. Animals also, especially horses, have had leg troubles cured by applications of earth.

But nowadays we are far more enlightened, and better educated; we do not care any longer for nature, nor do we understand her language.

If we really care for our health and bodily well-being, we have again to listen to the language of Nature and try to understand it. Then we also will use earth as a remedy and it will often prove far more effective than all Priessnitz's water cures, and will probably in the end become a universal panacea for many troubles.

It is not always necessary to put the body in or on the earth; but we may put the earth on the body. Its power for strengthening and healing is wonderful; it often surpasses everything that has been done in the way of healing or curing.

The earth is replete with life; she unceasingly pours forth a tremendous force on the man who touches her. This is shown by the legend of Anateus; and that is the reason why doing barefoot is so refreshing. The animals in the forest remove all leaves, grass and snow before they lie down, in order to come in close contact with the earth; every forester will certify to this. Animals also bathe in the mire.

We ought to rest on the ground as often as possible. Wonderful good can be derived from sleeping on the earth, in warm nights, or even on an earth-couch, made up in the bedroom.

Earth or clay applied to suffering parts of the body draws out all morbid and foreign matter. Herein lies its wonderful value if applied in any malady, no matter its name, be it gout or consumption, or abscesses, or female troubles; in a word, it is a cure-all for almost every evil of the body.

As the damp earth produces such wonderful effects on the abdomen by drawing out heat and strengthening of the digestive organs, its application is of great importance in such diseases as nervousness, insomnia, melancholia, fever and so forth.

The results attained through earth applications, pointed out in my book, are quite remarkable. I will mention only a few.

Mr. F. suddenly became blind on one eye. All remedies were of no avail. He applied damp earth and after a few days the eye improved, and after four or six weeks the visual faculty was restored. This reminds us of the way Jesus Christ healed a blind man. He spat on the earth, and thus made a piece of mud, which he put on the blind eye and the man was healed.

Mr. P. had chronic articular rheumatism; his leg was to be amputated. In this emergency my book fell into his hands, and he put packs of clay on his leg; within a few weeks it was healed and Mr. P. was the happiest man in the world.

The Rev. Dr. S. told me that in his congregation was a man whose leg was to be amputated; "I prescribed packs of clay and within six weeks the man was cured."

Mr. M. made a compress of clay for the back of his head, and during one night he was cured of a chronic toothache.

A Mr. N. had suffered for years from toothache; no dentist could cure him. After a few days his toothache was thoroughly cured by applying earth; and pains have never returned.

Mrs. G. had often cramps and fits; she was cured by earth compresses.

One man, who had for years suffered of rheumatism, was cured by sleeping for a fortnight on the bare earth.

For months Mr. Z. had been suffering from retention of urine, which brought him almost to the verge of death; he applied earth to the abdomen and the sexual organs; and after a few days the secretion of urine became normal and the man was out of danger.

Mr. V. S. had stomach complaints; he was continually vomiting and could not retain any food at all. As soon as damp clay had been put on his abdomen, the vomiting stopped and after a week he was able to retain food. In this way he had been saved from death, and bye and bye, his health was restored. Leprous eruption, scurvy and hydrophobia have also been cured by this natural method.

By its intense cooking effect, damp earth proves its wonderful curative power in inflammations, fevers and so forth.

Packs of earth strengthen and cure the limbs or any part of the body; while lying on the earth cures excitements and feverish conditions. Since I have made earth applications a regular part of my medical treatment, I have seen many cases which prove the great healing power of the earth, which may appear doubtful to those who have not witnessed these cases; but whoever listens to the voice of Nature, understands her simple laws and is not in the least astonished at these phenomena.

Man is made of dust and must return to dust. Earth is his real element.

The over refined and utterly enervated man can attain a certain physical and psychical brightness, elasticity and composure of soul only by adhering to earth. For this reason I recommend all nervous people to the Earth-Power.

The applications of earth can never do any harm, if they are not made in a stupid way.

When men no longer understood the voices of Nature, they, cut off from their original starting point, fell victims to fear and cold, to bacilli and other scientific theories by which they were led astray, and no more understood the causes and circumstances which underlie all facts; consequently, they have made mistakes on mistakes.

I can only draw attention to the value of the earth and her curative powers.

Anyone who wishes to inform himself on this subject will find an excellent text-book in my *Return to Nature*.

Of course, success does not always appear at once; not always even within a few hours or a few days. Sometimes it is necessary for us to exercise patience.

Nature has also other good remedies, as light, air, water, diet, mental influences, and so forth; these applied in the right way, as has been done by myself in many a case, increase the effects of the earth cure. Much is always accomplished by proper diet. Other natural remedies by which we may conquer diseases by the use of earth are also outlined in *Return to Nature*. Most people who read this book have been attracted by what I have written about the earth power; even physicians have accepted it knowing the value attributed to it be primitive people.

It is the inmost desire of my heart to put this simple remedy into the hands of the plain people.

*But nowadays we are far more enlightened, and better educated; we do not care any longer for nature, nor do we understand her language.*

*It is not always necessary to put the body in or on the earth; but we may put the earth on the body.*

*Earth or clay applied to suffering parts of the body draws out all morbid and foreign matter.*

*Since I have made earth applications a regular part of my medical treatment, I have seen many cases which prove the great healing power of the earth, which may appear doubtful to those who have not witnessed these cases; but whoever listens to the voice of Nature, understands her simple laws and is not in the least astonished at these phenomena.*

*When men no longer understood the voices of Nature, they, cut off from their original starting point, fell victims to fear and cold, to bacilli and other scientific theories by which they were led astray, and no more understood the causes and circumstances which underlie all facts; consequently, they have made mistakes on mistakes.*

# THE KUHNE CURE

## by Hans Knoch

Sanitarium at Woltersdorfer Schleuse on the Erkner River

*The Naturopath and Herald of Health, VII (2), 53-58. (1906)*

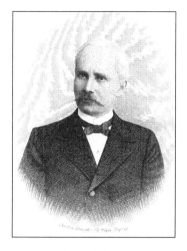

Louis Kuhne.

There seldom was a physician whose methods had as many enemies and who was so much slandered as the late Nature physician, Louis Kuhne, who was active at Leipsic from 1883 to 1900. Nevertheless, the assertion is true that there were not many other physicians and healers that could show such astonishing results in curing all kinds of diseases, as this man and his disciples. His method became known all over the world within less than ten years; from all countries patients came to Leipsic to be treated by him.

The observation that in case of disease the shape of the body is changed, and that when recovery follows the original shape is restored, brought him to the conclusion that diseases are caused by deposits of certain substances which disturb the harmony of the organism and which are foreign bodies to it. Another reason for his conclusions was that during a disease, and especially during treatment by Nature cure, there followed strong sensually noticeable excretions by the intestines, kidneys and skin. So he came to his known sentence: "Disease is the presence of morbid matter or foreign bodies in the organism. Thus there is only one cause of disease and also only one disease which comes up in different forms, according to what organ is affected." He was the first one to emphasize the unity of all diseases.

The loading of the body with foreign matter he ascribes to different causes. On one hand disease is caused by heredity, as sick parents have sick children. On the other hand large quantities of foreign substances are stored up in our body by breathing spoiled and used up air, but wrong and unhealthy nourishment, which, besides nutritious parts, contains also poisonous substances, and by eating and drinking much more than is needed to replace the used up cells and to produce and to preserve one's energy. These foreign bodies and excessive nourishment, he continues, cannot be completely assimilated in accordance with the general mode of living at present, and cannot be removed by the excretory organs, which are already overworked. The result is their storing up in the body and consequently functional disturbances. According to his view, the foreign bodies are stored up first in the abdomen and from there reach the extremities and the head by way of blood circulation. He asserts that the removal of these substances must take the opposite course; and therefore he tried to remove them, first, from the abdomen, so that the foreign substances from the other organs could return to the abdomen and thus be nearer to the excreting organs. So it came about that in his method the treatment of the abdomen was the most important; and as there is only one cause of disease, so there is also only one remedy to treat all diseases, namely, applications which stimulate and increase the activity of the excretory organs of the abdomen (intestines and kidneys). This brought him to these two applications: The board sitz-bath (or rubbing sitz-bath), and the trunk rubbing bath.* While the former was his own invention, he took the latter from the general Nature cure and improved it in many ways. To stimulate the activity of the skin, he soon took up also the steam-bath in which he applied the useful system of reed-banks. He relied mostly on the application of board sitz-baths, and practically obtained the greatest successes with these alone.

Kuhne's opinion is that these two baths produce a particular cooking of the inside of the body, in which high heat is developed during disease; and these baths cause the foreign bodies to be conducted to the kidneys and to the intestines. At the same time they act upon the important nerve-trunks, which end in the genitals and raise the power of the nerves in general. The influence upon peristalsis (activity of the intestines) by board sitz-baths is so great that constipation of long standing is frequently removed by a few such baths. Whoever, like myself, has used this board sitz-bath on himself and on others, knows that with no other application can one obtain so normal a stool as the one that Kuhne described: plentiful, consistent stool, solid, yet not hard, well and uniformly surrounded by mucus, so that no pieces break off and remain in the body.

Here is a description of Kuhne's procedures:

### BOARD SITZ-BATH OR RUBBING SITZ-BATH

Necessary utensils:

A sitz bath tub** or a water-tub or a small bath-tub which contains 25-30 liters of water (8-9 gallons);

A small wooden foot-stool, which fits into the tub or pail, or a small board which can be put over it;

A rag or rubbing-cloth of soft sack-cloth or of coarse linen.

---

*Kuhne's treatments were also known as friction hip baths. —Ed.

**Men can also use a large pail, if needed, which they must put in such a position as to be able to sit in front of it. Afterwards, the bath can be made as described above.

# Sitting Bath Cubs

## OF ZINC,

(will never grow rusty)

| No. 1. | No. 2. |
|---|---|
| $3.50 ($4.25). | $4.25 ($5.00) |
| No. 3. | No. 4. |
| $5.00 ($6.00). | $7.50 ($8 50) |

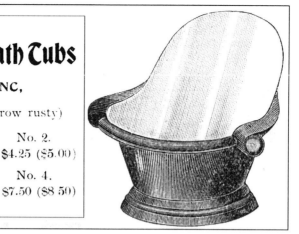

Application: The foot-stool is put into the sitz bath-tub, the tub is filled with water of the temperature as prescribed, up to the upper border of the foot-stool and the patient is sitting completely in the dry. The prepuce is drawn over the glans penis (which hangs down, so that the gland is covered by the prepuce), and the prepuce is kept between the thumb and the index finger or between this and the middle finger of the left hand, so that the gland is fully covered and cannot be touched; the prepuce is drawn down into the water and the outer edge of the prepuce is washed under the water with a rubbing-cloth. It is to be recommended to do the washing in one direction, either from above downward or from right to left or in the opposite direction, and so that the whole circle of the prepuce is touched.

Women wash by moistening only the external genitals with the rubbing-cloth. Under this washing, not a strong rubbing back and forth is understood, but a mild touching upon the labia majora, not minora, from above downwards. It does no harm if the buttocks become wet. During the monthly period these baths should not be taken; if lasting more than four days, treatment should begin carefully on the fifth day, but the baths should be taken warmer and shorter and only after a few days are to be taken just as cold and as long again as originally ordered.

The board baths are best taken with the body naked and in a warm room. Where this is impossible, one has to cover himself with a woolen cover or airy clothing, so that the body can perspire freely (which is very important). If well-water is used, let it first stand for half an hour in the room. The body must be warm when one wants to take a bath: besides, one has to look out for quick and thorough warming up again after the bath by a walk, physical exercise, or, if this is impossible, by good covering in bed.

### Trunk-Rubbing Bath

Necessary utensils: A sitz bath-tub or a sponge bath-tub, or a not too small water-tub, and a rubbing-cloth of sack-cloth or of coarse linen.

Application: The tub is filled with water of the ordered temperature and only so far as to reach the navel of the patient, who is sitting in it comfortably, leaning backwards. Then the abdomen is rubbed in its soft parts with a coarse linen cloth and in the middle line from the navel downwards, as well as back and forth over the back from the region of the kidneys downwards. During the bath the water is cooled down to the required temperature by adding colder water.

One must take the bath in a warm room and be himself warmed up first. The feet, which remain outside of the bath, are wrapped in a woolen cover.

To avoid disturbance of circulation in the legs, which may result from their lying on the edge of the tub, put a foot-stool under the feet.

After this bath one must try to warm himself thoroughly by walking, etc., and then only nourishment is to be taken.

The effect of these board sitz-baths is generally best when they are taken quite cold, about 10° to 12° C. (50° to 54° F.). But many patients cannot stand so low a temperature, even with their hands, and are forced to take warmer baths, sometimes even 20° C. (68° F.), very seldom warmer. Number of baths, one to three daily. Duration of baths, ten to sixty minutes.

The trunk rubbing-baths are best begun at about 34° C. (90° F.) and gradually cooled down 4° to 12° C. (39° to 54° F.), according to the requirement of the case. Duration of the bath: three to twenty minutes; number: one to three daily.

There is no general rule in regard to number, temperature and duration of the baths, as in the Kuhne cure there must be considered the condition of the patient's body, as well as the temperature of the body, the power of reaction, the kind of disease, etc. Many failures which were reported may have been caused by bathing without taking into consideration the above mentioned facts. Whoever wants to have the Kuhne cure should always consult an expert. This cure is to be used in all acute and chronic diseases in which it can be performed.

When Kuhne combined his bath procedures with steam-baths and used them for years, he recognized the one-sidedness of his system in many cases and took in many of the other curative factors, as sun-baths, air-baths, mud compresses and partial packs.

One of the most important advantages of the Kuhne cure is, besides its great effect, its simplicity which enables everyone, even the poorest to apply it.

Kuhne was one of the few Nature cure physicians who required his patients to keep first of all a vegetarian diet. He went further than the others, as he asked his patients to use exclusively vegetables and fruits, sometimes even raw and unripe. He considered the use of meat, meat broth, spices, salt, alcoholic and narcotic drinks, etc., the chief source of tainting the body and, therefore, he ordered first to avoid all these substances.

Finally, it should be mentioned that Kuhne put up a new form of diagnosis, to which he was led by observing the change in shape of the body during disease. He called this form of diagnosis science of physiognomy, which is not correct, according to my opinion, as the question is about the forms of the whole body in disease. Kuhne became so experienced in his diagnosis that frequently his patients were amazed at the correctness of his judgment.

### THE ATMOSPHERIC CURE BY RIKLI

Vincent Priessnitz had already recognized the importance of air and of light, and used both these important elements quite freely.* What this talented empiric judged of the air is shown in his well-known expression before the district judge, when the use of sponge-baths was to be prohibited: "And even if you prohibit the use of water, I shall treat the people with air, and they will become healthy." But those men were not so enlightened on this subject as Priessnitz. Water should accomplish everything. The expression, "Water does it, of course," governed the spirits up to the moment when the Swiss "Arnold Rikli" brought into general use the words that were honored by all: "Water does it, of course; higher (better is air, and highest (best) is light!"

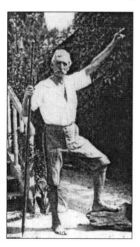

Arnold Rikli.

Arnold Rikli, the founder of the first sanitarium for atmospheric cures in Veldes is at the same time the founder of the light and air cure in general. For thirty-two years he was alone in this sphere and was not only laughed at by physicians but even misunderstood by Nature cure physicians, until finally his work, *The Atmospheric Cure* received due attention.

Arnold Rikli was born in February, 1823, at Wangen on the Aar, in Switzerland. His education was managed by his father, who was a genuine Swiss, and who owned a dyeing-establishment. When his friends

---

*The importance of light and the sun bath was understood by Naturopaths long before our current recognition of Vitamin D deficiencies. —*Ed.*

advised him to engage a tutor and thus throw the care of his children off his shoulders, he said: "Money and property, everyone is trying to keep away from strangers as well as possible. How can I let my children, who are dearer to me than all the treasures in this world, become systematically spoiled?" Among his brothers and sisters little Arnold was distinguished by his sharp talent of observation and judgment, common sense and youthful haughtiness. He was especially attracted by the river near his father's residence. His greatest pleasure was to play ashore or to swim in its silvery white waters, and there could not be a higher punishment than to keep him away from the river for a day. At the school of that place, which was quite a good one in those times, Arnold Rikli received his elementary education. Brought up by his parents in virtue and honesty and always near Nature, he learned its wonderful effect on the physical and mental development of men; unknowingly he was led and directed by it. The clear, fresh water, the warming sun rays and the pure mountain air were his nurses from whom he received the first hygienic rules, power and courage for his later activity and later struggles.

Thus his first years of boyhood passed by, and he grew up to become 14 years old. Now, he bid good-bye to his father's home and entered the polytechnic school at Ludwigsburg, where he graduated successfully in 1839. After his graduation, he returned to his father's house and gave himself up to manufacturing, according to his father's wishes, though against his own ideals. Yet he was too good a son to go against the will of his father, for whom he had unlimited respect. He studied chemistry at leisure, together with his older brother, Rudolph. Their father's laboratory gave them opportunity enough to complete their theoretical knowledge with corresponding practical experiments.

At this time the young Arnold suddenly got an idea that the judiciously regulated influence of air and light on the human body must have a healing and strengthening effect similar to that on plants. The result fully confirmed the correctness of his view. During the summer months he tried many experiments with light, water and air, which were very successful.

In 1843, he graduated from the military school at Berne, as a volunteer and was sent by his father to other places to find out similar factories, and their new regulations. Rikli remained also a whole winter in the neighborhood of Triest, where he first saw Dr. Munde's *Hydropath*, and his work on *Cornaro*, the temperance preacher. He gave up manufacturing and began to study both the above mentioned works. To try all the hints and remedies, he went through all the hydropathic cures himself. Well, he followed temperance so far that he became very pale, thin and weakened. With special partiality, he was studying Professor Meissner's *Theory of Circulation of Warmth*, which later on gave him very good hints on equalization of warmth in the human body and also on judicious ventilation in living rooms and stables.

On his return home, he soon afterwards married, at the age of 22, a Miss Mary Landerer of Basel, by which marriage three sons were born. At the same time many water cure sanitaria were opened in Germany and in Switzerland, which interested Rikli most and which were repeatedly visited by his brothers, relative to their cures.

In April 1845, Rikli went along as a special officer during the short campaign against the volunteer corps of Canton Luzern. At that time he caught a severe cold which resulted in diarrhoea and kept him in bed for a long while. A military surgeon and a private physician stood near the dying bed of the patient (according to their opinion), without advice. Yet fate decided differently. Rikli chose to undertake a hydropathic cure and the result was a complete cure in three days.

In 1846, Rikli and his family, with his two older brothers, moved to Seebach on Milstatt in Oberkärnten, to establish a factory similar to his father's.

The business flourished and soon there was working at the new factory about three hundred persons. It is understood that there was no want of diseases of all kinds, and Rikli took into his hands the cure and care of the sick, while he left to his brothers the management of the factory and gave himself up almost entirely to medicine. The neighborhood took his success to notice, and he soon received patients from the best families. He went so far that he was treating free of charge and even paying some workmen to have them stand the cure and to enable him to observe the course of their diseases and the final result of his method. By this time he invented the first bed steam apparatus, which, after many improvements, was sold in large quantities all over the world.

In May 1852, Rikli fell ill with pleurisy. Being already then against doctors and their systematic poisoning, he did not call in any physician, but gave his attendants the necessary instructions, and cured himself hydropathically in a very short period from the violence of this acute disease. Completely cured, he was advised by a friend to go to Valdes in Oberkrain for recuperation. The pure balsamic air, the wonderful beauty of nature and the excellent and very healthy climate of this especially beautiful place did him much good, and he decided to transfer his share in the factory to his brothers and to build a Nature cure sanitarium at Veldes and to settle there as a Nature physician. Finally, in April, 1855, he was enabled to accomplish this. Then began hard fights with the prejudice of the lower classes against everything new and unusual, as well as with the power of the medical faculty, who were afraid for their existence and incomes. Yet Rikli kept up with his strong arms the banner or progress and science high above the heads of the masses. The latter could bespatter it but not trample on it!

Unexpected objections and obstacles were in the way of introducing the vegetable diet, the sun-baths and especially the beautiful light-and-air baths. The patients were suspicious of the unusual orders which were against the old custom, and they partly opposed them. In public papers as well as in all classes of the population he and his system were laughed at. But finally the truth conquered. Arnold Rikli has received recognition and admiration even from his opponents and opened the way for the triumph of the light-and-air baths. The many newly erected light-and-air baths, the air-hut treatment in large institutions, the ventilated assembly halls in the popular lung cure places are the best proofs to the general appreciation of the atmospheric cure. The sanitarium at Veldes is of course thriving. The 80 year old man stands at the head of this institution, full of physical and mental vigor. Every year, many sick persons, more foreigners than Austrians, wander there and return to their homes completely satisfied, with kind wishes and congratulations on their lips for the old veteran of Nature cure.

*"Disease is the presence of morbid matter or foreign bodies in the organism. Thus there is only one cause of disease and also only one disease which comes up in different forms, according to what organ is affected." He [Kuhne] was the first one to emphasize the unity of all diseases.*

*So it came about that in his method the treatment of the abdomen was the most important; and as there is only one cause of disease, so there is also only one remedy to treat all diseases, namely, applications which stimulate and increase the activity of the excretory organs of the abdomen (intestines and kidneys).*

*Arnold Rikli" brought into general use the words that were honored by all: "Water does it, of course; higher (better is air, and highest (best) is light!" ... In May 1852, Rikli fell ill with pleurisy. Being already then against doctors and their systematic poisoning ... he cured himself hydropathically in a very short period from the violence of this acute disease.*

*The many newly erected light-and-air baths, the air-hut treatment in large institutions, the ventilated assembly halls in the popular lung cure places are the best proofs to the general appreciation of the atmospheric cure.*

## Try The Laugh Cure

**by Edward Earle Purinton**

*The Naturopath and Herald of Health, VII (7), 270-274. (1906)*

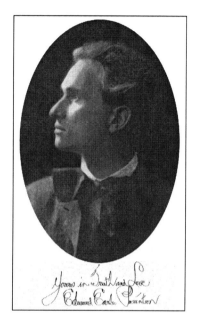

If I ever needed a doctor I'd call Mark Twain. Because he's the only one that takes his own medicine. Indeed that's the test of any man's truth—does he *take* it or *talk* it?

*Life is the only one antidote to learning and the only cure for loquacity.*

The American public is sick. Sick of graft, of corruption, of political, medical and theological spoilage, of upper tedium and lower milliondom, of medieval pedanticism, of swelling promise and scant performance, of a thousand and one things that all betoken the single universal malady of civilization: *Insincerity.*

And the American public has called Mark Twain. Praise be for that. It doesn't much matter what a man's symptoms are if he only has the right doctor. Time was when we had Chauncey Depew for our national counselor and family doctor; that was when we didn't know how sick we were. Now we're bewailing our sundry symptoms—but we've called Mark Twain. And this latter is the healthiest sign in the history of the case.

Doctor Depew was an old-school practitioner; he gave placebos—and grinned as he pocketed the fee. Doctor Twain is a Naturist; he finds the cause—and smiles because he knows the cure. Doctor Depew laughed *at* us; Doctor Twain laughs *with* us. And it took the wholesome contagion of the second to show up the sickly grin of the first. Laughing at a man is likely to give him a pain—laughing with him is sure to take it away. Make fun of a sick man and he's your enemy; make fun for him and he's your friend.

Mark Twain is everybody's friend because he makes fun for everybody. He is our benefactor moreover; and doubly so, because we don't know it—the wisest way to help a man is to let him think he's helping

## LOOK PLEASANT, PLEASE

Wipe that frown off your face. Laugh. A sour stomach and a sour face always go together. Don't get in the Down and Out Club. Cut Mr. Gloomy Gus off your list of acquaintances. He isn't a fit associate for you. This is the message in

# THE
# LAUGH CURE

by E. E. Purinton. This little pamphlet is written in this popular author's happiest vein. Like all Mr. Purinton's writings, it contains also a lot of sound practical advice. If you feel "blue" or disposed to look at the world through dark spectacles, get this pamphlet and laugh your troubles away. Price 15 cents.

Published by

BENEDICT LUST, N. D.

BUTLER, NEW JERSEY

E. E. Purinton wrote long articles and often for Benedict Lust's publications.

you. We generously buy a ticket for some charity entertainment where Mark is to speak; and we're the charity. For a man's laugh is the gauge of his sincerity; to enhance one is to augment the other. Wherefore is every humorist a healer—a soul-healer.

Long faces make broad graveyards. And they do it quick.

Nobody ever died laughing. People die doing everything else—but not that. Even Hundred Year Clubs die if they haven't learned how to laugh. The normal life is half-love, half-laughter and nobody ever got sick who kept the balance between the two. Fears inside and frowns outside are the established hall-marks of simon-pure invalidism. There is no fatality but fear. And the lad or lass, who laughs enough sends fear into the everlasting limbos on the double-quick.

The newspapers have been telling us of a shrewd Paris doctor, a specialist in psycho-nervo-hypnotic-machinations, who maintains a large institution devoted solely to the Laugh-Cure. By means of highly erudite and fetchingly ornate cajolery he lures to his Dispensary of Corrective Cachinnation hosts of the hysterical rich and lazy; whereupon he seats them solemnly in a circle, gives the momentous signal and orders them to laugh religiously for a full half-hour. Then he makes some mumbo-jumbo passes, looks preternaturally wise, collects a most ambitious fee, dismisses the class till next day and retires to his sleeve for his turn to laugh. They laugh at each other, he laughs at them, we laugh at him and Heaven knows who laughs at us. A goodly store of merriment forsooth.

I wish every Nature-Curist and "New Thoughter" in America could take instruction from that French doctor. Because of all the grumpy, dumpy, gloomy, gruesome graveyard avenues on earth, the average Advanced Thought sanitarium is it. A few of the saner metaphysicians try to make you laugh because it's your duty! But outside of this howling farce, scarce indeed is the sound of good, old-fashioned, wholesome, hearty laughter. Out on the sickly imitation—the gasping gurgle or eerie chortle of soul-less cackle or spasmodic gush! Give us neither the simpering grin or the coarse guffaw. A man can't change the fibre of his nature—he can and should change the fidelity of his nature. And it's the unfaithful whose smile is a simper.

Every sanitarium needs on its staff a sleuth photographer likely to snap the patients at any moment they aren't watching. Maybe they wouldn't "look pleasant" then! I actually believe they'd stop talking symptoms if they knew their friends might behold how uncanny and altogether frightful they appear during the process. There ought to be a fine in every health resort for any symptom caught skulking around in the atmosphere. With a strip of adhesive plaster handy for the mouth that let it escape. Swapping symptoms may be a lovely pastime, but it's an all-fired poor trade. Because whichever one you get is worse for the giving—and the ghost of your own comes back. Say nothing but what is bright, beautiful, beneficent. Remembering too that silence always tells more than words.

Laughter is the universal solvent of human woes. In every woman's smile you can see the tears just coming or just going; for a woman knows by intuition when to laugh. A man never knows unless some woman taught him. And the reason most women grow hysterical is that men have robbed them of the power to laugh. There is heart in a woman's laugh—there is only head in a man's. Women lack less the "sense of humor" than the cruelty of wit. Take the sting from a man's wit and you have the secret of a woman's humor. But whether it be a woman's smile or a man's chuckle, the essence of longevity is still there. Laugh long, live long.

### What A Healthy Laugh Does

### 1.   Jiggers The Diaphragm And Unkinks The Solar Plexus

The first muscle to get lazy in a sick man is the diaphragm. And death always starts in the solar plexus; whence the profuseness of "Breathing Exercises" and the prolixity of "Affirmations". But all the respiring and affirming on earth can't equal the rejuvenating effect of a good laugh on the lungs and emotional centre. Ever notice how much easier you breathe after a season of mirth? Without trying, too—and that's the beautiful part of it. The greatest good always comes unconsciously. And the very *strain* of attempting to breathe naturally often defeats its own purpose. As for "Affirmations", what they most affirm is the negation of the man that makes them. Imagine Morgan, Edison, or Hearst retiring supinely to a cushioned corner at a specified hour each day to murmur in tremulous parrot-fashion, "I—am—success" alas! The men who succeed get up and hustle; the children who live go forth and play; the women who love serve and sacrifice—and smile. Next to Love is laughter fullest of soul-thrills.

### 2.   Mollifies Surly Stomach And Corrects Recalcitrant Liver

The man who takes *Puck* after dinner doesn't take pills. Nor eat at a vegetarian restaurant—where laughter is the second daily sin, beef broth being the first. The man who laughs over a plate of pork is a lot saner than the one that shivers over a bowl of bran mash. This everlasting fussing about what we shouldn't eat is enough to sicken a well man. You insult your stomach every time you question its ability to handle the food it selects. It knew its business from A to Z before Battle Creek was a post office in a dry goods-store. Throw dietetic dissertations into the fire and study the wondrous wisdom of your own instincts. Sit up straight and enjoy your food. Remembering every laugh is an alarm-clock to a sleepy liver.

### 3.   Elevates Internal Organs To Their Normal Position

The "Down-and-Out Club" so exquisitely pictured by our friend, Cartoonist Powers, is the right name for the Has-Beens; a man once down is soon out. Everything drops when a fellow's sick. He is down in the mouth, down at the heel, down on everybody. Simultaneously the bottom falls out of his thermometer and his purse. His stomach sags, his chest caves in, his lungs collapse and his heart feels like lead. I don't blame him I've been there. But now I can look back and laugh at it all. The whole performance seems ridiculous. Because I have spent some while cultivating a laugh that shakes every bit of the inside machinery back where it belongs, I have ceased needing pills and props. You can do the same—won't you try? Things grow the way they face. And if we faced the sky with a smile instead of the earth with a frown, we'd always feel as perfect as the flowers.

### 4.  LOOSENS ARTERIAL DEPOSIT AND PREVENTS OLD AGE

I know an old man of seventy with the complexion of a child. And he has the merriest laugh in the neighborhood. Perhaps just a coincidence, but I think not. The dancing eyes and racing blood of youth are most evident in a child's unaffected, unashamed, undiminished, shout of laughter. Folks who laugh till they're red in the face may not be strictly elegant, but they'll be more consoling than the tombstones destined presently to draw conclusions on their critics. Laughing is essentially a limbering process— it beats any "setting-up" drill ever invented. Because it not only rejuvenates the unbending, it reforms the childlike. A feeling of dignity is more than egg-shells to walk on, yet most old people tread that precarious path for years, such as walk with a cane walked first with dignity. Get down on all fours and play menagerie with the little tots, if you want to preserve your youth. "Play bear" and you won't act bear.

### 5.  RELAXES THE NERVES AND RESTORES SPONTANEITY

Laughing is the lost art of America. Study the faces you see in the stores, street-cars and railroad stations—even at the play or in church the same joyless, hopeless, useless tension draws the features, pales the cheeks, furrows the brow, haunts the eyes and drives all semblance of a smile form the stern-set lips. What's the use? Does it pay? Give me rather a Swiss peasant who can view with a smile his thatched roof that the sky peeps through or a Swedish immigrant maid with all her worldly belongings on her back and her heavenly heritage in her heart, knowing only enough English for her native laugh to slip out between the words. That's all words are good for anyway—to serve as partitions between the smiles and tears of silence.

### 6.  CHANGES VIBRATIONS FROM NEGATIVE TO POSITIVE

This point is of special note. Microbes always choose an inert body for their lodging place. Local congestion is but a symptom of general stagnation. Sick folk are proverbially the prey of the first marauder that come along—whether a germ, a pessimist, or a medical shark. And the first thing an invalid needs is *initiative.* Some positive force from within himself must be aroused to [*] come to the baleful influences without. And the quickest way to scatter the rubbish that's accumulated on his soul is to get him laughing. At least while he's seeing a joke he isn't looking for bacilli, spooks, and hobgoblins. Which latter respected citizens come only when they're called.

### 7. GIVES MICROBES THE AGUE AND SENDS SPOOKS INTO A DECLINE

I can fairly see both cohorts uncanny turning in a mad rush and flee-ing for their lives before the general alarm of a hearty laugh. I sort of imagine microbes are mundane ministers to spooks—they prey on sick bodies while spooks prey on sick souls. And the human species is so inor-dinately helpless in the presence of both bands of prowlers that they're apt to grow unduly vain. Some people are actually proud of their sick, spook-pestered souls; as theorizers, reformers, clergymen, poets and spiritualists. The man who isn't happy is somehow twisted in his doctrine or shrunk in his life. Let him learn how beautifully the Laugh-Cure will stretch him back to the normal with no hiding place left anywhere for crepuscular intruders, whether physical or psychic.

### 8. TAKES YOUR MIND OFF YOUR SYMPTOMS AND HELPS YOU SEE STRAIGHT

A clear laugh, like a ray of sunlight, shows just where cobwebs are. With the furtive whereabouts of the psychic spider that spun them. Most people's mental habitation is thickly festooned with the subtle strands of alien thought. And they're so busy unmeshing themselves they forget to look where their soul-window used to be; indeed somebody has very like-ly stolen up in the night and nailed a shutter on the outside—somebody by the name of *either* Bigot or Freethinker, *either* Prude or Freelover, *either* Doctor or Antidoctor. Now a single breath of sincere laughter blows the cobwebs down, another sweeps the dust from the window and a third makes you want air enough to smash the shutter into bits too small for even a memory to hang to. Blessed be the freedom of mirth.

### 9. ACTS AS AN ALL-ROUND BRACER

The only one with no bad after-effects. Nothing is so potent as the laugh-habit for discouraging discouragement. Physical tonics always leave a man's will weaker than before. But laughter is mixed in the laboratory of the soul. And the formula is guaranteed. Moreover you can "treat"

---

*A word appearing in the original document was missing due to damage. —*Ed.*

as often as you will, making neither yourself poorer nor others worse. Indeed the slaves of society, with a pitiful irony but beautiful intuition, call their liquid overtures "smiles", a wan substitute, verily.

## 10. Cleanses Your Aura To Its Original Hue

Wisdom always looks so sepulchral I never dared come close enough to ask advice. Folly smiles so entrancingly I just naturally sidle up to her for a comforting kiss on the cheek. Wherein is Folly the wiser than Wisdom. I was just thinking of Theosophy; how gorgeously it tells about auras—and how hideously it paints its own! Stupid truly to forget the act of joy in studying the effect. Every time you frown, fear, hesitate, or err, you put a coat of ugly brown over the radiant blue, pink or yellow of your soul at birth. Every time you laugh you dislodge some of this encrustment, disclosing your true self more nearly in reality. And the oftener you laugh, the prettier you will look, the finer you will feel, the better folks will like you. Babies are so attractive because so sincere—with that society women knew this most magical of all beauty secrets.

## 11. Improves Your Business Chances

The man Fortune smiles on is sure to smile back. And if you smile anyhow, the world is more than likely to court you as Fortune's favorite. Often you can fool Fortune by the same ruse; she's a forgetful, heartless, fickle jade at best, and with a little coaxing instead of sulking she'll elope with you as quick as with the other fellow she started to smile on. Ashamed though we be we must acknowledge that a bold, brave, showy front goes vastly further in the business world than a profusion of the rarest violets blooming in the back yard. The man who makes it his business to smile is the man whose business enables him to smile. You can never scowl away competition, adversity or failure; you can smile it away. And by the same token popularity comes.

## 12. Unites Fool And Philosopher

They're really one in the fully developed nature, where all opposites meet and merge into unity. But they don't know it usually until they've laughed away their differences to delight in their similarities. Men diverge infinitely in their doctrines, their studies, their personal pursuits of health, wealth and happiness. But their amusements are much the same. And social clubs do quite as much as unsocial churches to promote the feeling of universal brotherhood. Did you ever think the only place a man dare laugh hilariously is in a saloon? Someday the W. C. T. U. busybodies will awake to the fact that the Corner Café has its hold not in the physical dissipation it affords, but in the *psychic, mental* and *emotional relief.* Then they'll begin smiling to the wine-bibber instead of frowning at him. Every sinner, every sufferer, every partaker of mortality is starving for the smiles of an understanding soul. You never really love a man until you can laugh with him.

### 13. MAKES FOR SANENESS, SWEETNESS, AND LIGHT

The Infinite is one vast reservoir of joy, whence healing currents flow constantly to the finite being ready to receive. The rose smiles sweetly to the sun, the lark carols rapturously to its mate, the stream swoons delirious to meet the tossing sea, the winds sound their wind joy and the hills echo it back. Ecstasy is the Love of Nature and the life of God. And the human overflow is laughter. Let us give our bodies back to Nature, till once more we can revel in the simple sense-delights of childhood. Let us give our souls back to God, till the promise of the image be fulfilled and the halo of supreme bliss be our enduement forever. Birth is the smile of Nature. Death is the smile of God; let life be the smile of Man!

---

*Laughter is the universal solvent of human woes.*

*If we faced the sky with a smile instead of the earth with a frown, we'd always feel as perfect as the flowers.*

*[Laughter] CLEANSES YOUR AURA TO ITS ORIGINAL HUE.*

*Jiggers The Diaphragm And Unkinks The Solar Plexus*

*The first muscle to get lazy in a sick man is the diaphragm.*

*Every time you frown, fear, hesitate, or err, you put a coat of ugly brown over the radiant blue, pink or yellow of your soul at birth. Every time you laugh you dislodge some of this encrustment, disclosing your true self more nearly in reality.*

# 1907

## THE SPRING CURE
### BENEDICT LUST

Louisa and Benedict Lust's Butler Jungborn was a model for Naturopaths, offering the therapies of Kneipp, Just, Kuhne, Rikli and others.

# The Spring Cure

## by Benedict Lust

*The Naturopath and Herald of Health, VIII (5), 139-140. (1907)*

### Spring Best Time for Treating Disease—Quick and Permanent Cures Obtained—Convalescents Rapidly Improve—Yungborn, Only Sanitarium in America Making Specialty of Spring Cure.

Most of the readers of the *Naturopath* are no doubt acquainted with the inspiring poem of the late J. J. Ingalls, entitled "Opportunity", and wherein words to this effect occur, "I pass and knock but once at every door. Those who are ready, open up! If not, I pass along to come no more!"

To every sick man and woman, to every sufferer from some long-standing disease there comes a golden opportunity, charged with hope and promise for them. This opportunity is the hour of great natural changes, the hour when everything in Nature is quickened by the mysterious creative force that operates in and through all created things, the wonderful hour of rebirth! If any season of the year bears a message of good cheer and hopefulness to the sick and suffering it is the season of Spring. At this time of the year we witness a quickening of life, especially among the plants. The dormant sap quickens, shoots up through the dead stems and in a short while we see this new life manifested in millions of bright-colored blossoms. In the human organism a like process takes place. The vital spirits are quickened, the dormant cells stirred into activity and, where the body is sick, efforts are made by the organism to cast out its poisons. Sometimes the body succeeds without any external assistance. But usually the vital spirits of a sick person are at a low ebb and while the patient may earnestly wish to become well and while the system may make efforts along the line of self-cleansing, vitality is lacking and the patient drags along in the same miserable way as before. Even where treatment is suggested a sick person usually has not the will power or energy to take it up or else he seeks some easy method like taking pills or medicine, instead of adopting a radical cure. Those who have been laid up all Winter seek to delay treatment until the summer months under the deluded idea that the hot summer days are the best for treating sickness. By such unwise delays complications often arise which may have most serious results. In all things given us to do, we should act promptly! The highest duty of man is to maintain himself in a healthy condition and if sick, to promptly get himself back to health. The vital time for the sick to do this is now!

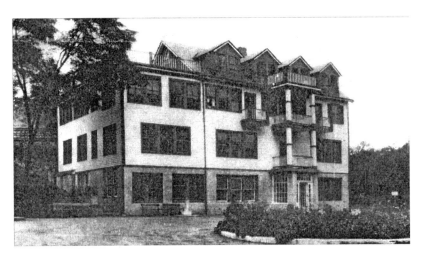

The Headquarters at the Jungborn in Butler, New Jersey.

Springtime is the time to assist the organism in getting back to its normal, healthy, condition. So-called modern diseases, such as neurasthenia, stomach and bowel disorders, impoverished blood, disturbances of the organs of assimilation, lung troubles and the various diseases of women, yield readily to treatment at this time of year. Spring fever, "that tired feeling", and other spring ailments that have been brought on by lack of exercise, stuffed rooms and a wrong diet during the winter months, are also amenable to quick treatment and cure at this time.

The question arises, where should one go for treatment? All of the health resorts and sanitariums throughout the country close in the Fall and do not open until the summer season is well under way. This is undeniably true and, we might add, also fortunate since the average health resort is no more fitted up to take care of patients during the Fall, Winter and Spring than is an ordinary country boarding house. In Europe places like the establishments at Carlsbad, Homburg, Wiesbaden, Nauheim, etc., have made provisions to take in patients all through the year, but in this country no such sanitarium existed until the Yungborn opened its doors for all-the-year-round patients. The Yungborn Sanitarium is admirably situated for this purpose. Located in the delightful Grace Valley, in the heart of the Ramapo Mountains, and half hid by the growth of heavy pine woods on all sides, it is protected from the north winds and enjoys a mild, pleasant climate for the greater part of the year. Special cottages have been constructed for cooler days and known as Northern Log Houses. These houses are solid, charming private place of abode, constructed according to Dr. Lust's ideas. They contain two finely furnished rooms and a pretty balcony and inside are pleasant and warm even on the coolest days.

All modern curative methods known to Naturopathy are employed at

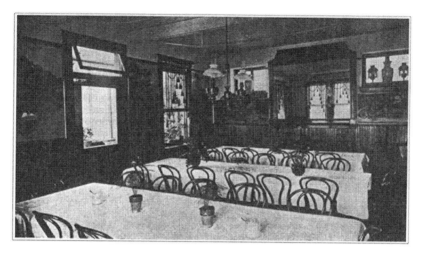

Dining Room of "Yungborn" Health Home at Butler, New Jersey.

the Yungborn and patients have the advantage of mountain climbing and walks for hours in the beautiful private parks belonging to the sanitarium, etc.

The table board at the Yungborn is admitted to be the best of any in the country. Separate tables are provided for vegetarians and a course of individual diet is prescribed for all those needing dietetic treatment. Fruit is abundant at the table. To the various kinds of nuts which must be deemed principal ingredients of human food and to the fine fruits and berries that are raised and gathered on the property, there is always found a bountiful supply of imported foreign fruit, such as oranges, figs, dates, mangoes, bananas, etc. The richest milk, cream and butter, cottage cheese, buttermilk, and fresh eggs, all home products, are served daily as well as fresh vegetables in season.

The cost for exclusive room, board, lighting, heating and individual treatment, which includes the light, sun and air baths, clay and earth treatments, masso-therapy, Kneipp applications, etc., including personal advice, is $2.50 per day, $16 per week, $60 per month. For convalescents and visitors who do not take the treatment and who desire board and room only the cost is $2 per day, $12 per week, $40 per month.

Two Naturopath doctors and one "regular" physician are in constant attendance and an extra Ladies' Department is maintained, presided over by a lady physician (gynecologist) and a staff of experienced lady attendants.

Butler, New Jersey is reached easily in an hour from the Pennsylvania R.R. depot, Jersey City. Well-equipped trains leave the depot about every two hours.

A richly illustrated prospectus of the sanitarium, showing glimpses of the beautiful scenery surrounding the place and describing the treatment, will be sent free on application. We kindly ask you to send in the names and addresses of invalid friends and we will mail them prospectus postpaid.

---

*Usually, the vital spirits of a sick person are at a low ebb and while the patient may earnestly wish to become well and while the system may make efforts along the line of self-cleansing, vitality is lacking and the patient drags along in the same miserable way as before.*

*Springtime is the time to assist the organism in getting back to its normal, healthy, condition.*

*The Yungborn Sanitarium is admirably situated for this purpose. Located in the delightful Grace Valley, in the heart of the Ramapo Mountains, and half hid by the growth of heavy pine woods on all sides, it is protected from the north winds and enjoys a mild, pleasant climate for the greater part of the year.*

# 1908

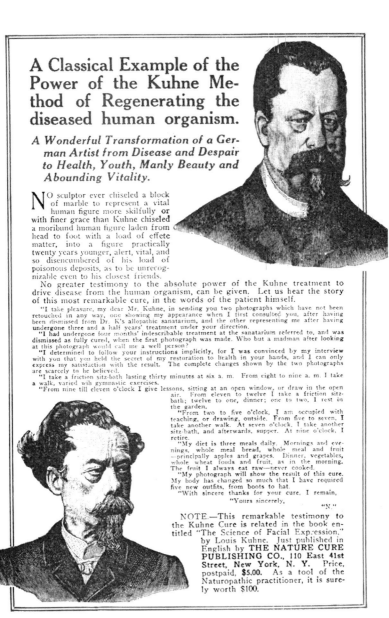
Louis Kuhne wrote two foundational books for the early Naturopath: *The New Science of Healing* (1891) and *The Science of Facial Expression* (1895).

# THE SCIENCE OF NATURE-CURE

Lecture Delivered By The Editor Before The German Nature-Cure Society In New York

## by Benedict Lust

*The Naturopath and Herald of Health, IX (1), 1-3. (1908)*

It is not the first time that I have the honor to appear before you and to lecture about "The Science of Nature–Cure". We all know that this country has been called that of inventions, but none of these is so grand, so far-reaching as "The Science of Nature-Cure".

The essence of most inventions is profit and advantage, but Nature-Cure aims at the physical, and consequently, at the spiritual and intellectual well-being of man; a healthy, strong constitution is the foundation of happiness; a man healthy in body and soul is able to face any emergency; energy and will-power will always be at the command of any well-balanced man or woman. As the science of Nature–Cure is new to many I have to demonstrate it.

Ladies and gentlemen: you may be familiar with the fact that the views about sickness and diseases have lately changed. If we compare the diseases of our times with those of the middle ages and those of the old Germans, everybody will admit that with every year new diseases come up. The more we go back to the primitive conditions of humanity, the healthier and stronger were the people. When still at school I asked my teacher what is the reason "that the old Germans were so healthy and strong?" And he answered, "Hardening."

The keynote of Nature–Cure is: "Without hardening no strong health". The old Persians, Romans and Greeks harden their bodies, even by the command of the government; nature alone was their guide, not physicians. Some will state that those people had neither the culture nor the institutions as we have them now. But that is a poor way of living, where not only a few but all suffer; where people instead of hardening their bodies, effeminate and weaken them. The old Germans when passing the Alps which they did in the winter, naked, only a bear skin thrown over their shoulders, slid on their shields down the Alps; in this way entering sunny Italy. Nowadays man, when taking a bath, does not only go into a warm room, but even in to a warm bathtub, thereby annihilating the power of resistance in his body. If such a man is then exposed to rough weather he wonders why he catches cold; when this cold is intensified by a cough, and he will consult a physician. The latter gives it a name, calls it inflammation of the throat and the patient must scrupulously follows all directions. He takes three times a day chlorine with distilled water; gargles and even swallows some drugs every two hours. To this very day such processes are supposed to be excellent. That by such drugs and poisonous matter

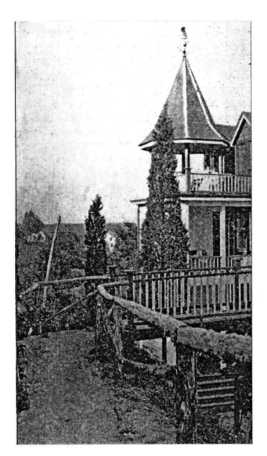

Yungborn's new building and observation tower.

mucus membranes, the inner organs, the nerves, even the whole skeleton will be affected, people believe to be perfectly right, but bare foot walking and water applications they think vulgar and common. I admit that medicine can soothe pain, but it can never affect a thorough, a permanent cure. How does Nature–Cure proceed?

Every man has a certain, mysterious power within him which regulates his health and strength and which may be called *natural power*. If the physician understands this power, understand its suggestions, he will bring about a marvelous successful cure. An intelligent physician will not apply poisons, but elements taken from nature, as water, air, light, rest, exercise, diet and so forth. No physician can bring about a cure minus these remedies.

Water is applied in three different forms, either warm, or cold, or as steam. The Nature–Cure is based on the old, great, irrefutable, external laws: heat expands or dissolves; cold draws together, makes strong and hard. There is only one law: Follow Nature. Every man needs air to breathe; the purer the air, the healthier the man; the better he feels, the purer his blood. In order to remain in good health, the body has to inhale as much fresh and healthy air as possible. What a healthy man must have in order to remain in good health, a sick man ought to have in order to come back to health. The same holds good to light, air and rest. Of very good effect are the sun baths which, especially, further assimilation. A cripple can, of course, not take any exercise, but he has to be massaged, has to submit to passive exercises and to rest. That the science of Nature-Cure rests on a good basis is proven by the fact that our masters, Kneipp, Schroth, Kuhne and others have well plowed the soil into which they planted their seed; for many physicians have changed their minds and from science have come to nature. How much people are in sympathy with this method we learn from the fact that everywhere associations of Nature-Cure are formed. The more physicians depart from nature, the more laymen will have the recourse to the natural remedies.

Persons, not yet familiar with the powers of Nature, imagine, if a Naturopathist treats them and cures them in no time, their ailments were but slight, but if a physician takes a very long time, causes the patient a great deal of expense and pain, and the latter recovers, notwithstanding the poisonous drugs he had to swallow, is quite another case. People ought to understand that a physician can never cure but only support the natural powers of the patient. The natural power is backed by natural means. Our country overflowing with prejudice and mistakes lacks in natural thinking and knowledge. We partisans of the natural cure live up to our principles: "Follow Nature", while the principle of the physicians is: "Poison the system with drugs; take its consequences." Many people think Nature-Cure too simple to enlist anybody's confidence. But our methods are far more many-sided and varied than those of the physicians. Many physicians who have exhausted the store–house of the pharmacopeia apply then diet, water, electricity, indicating thereby that they themselves were not fully convinced of the efficacy of their pills and powders. In this way not only the physicians but also the patients will become convinced of the value of this method. But this is not sufficient; people have to study the subject, have to acquaint themselves with this literature, have to listen to the lectures of the Naturopathists and should become members of the associations of Naturopathists. Whoever is in doubt how to treat the case, ought to read about it consult an expert and in this way broaden his knowledge.

Nature's remedies are far more powerful than those of medical science. Violent head or stomach pains will be quicker and more thoroughly cured by Nature than by medicine. Whoever has really been relieved his pain by drugs, has incurred some other evil, though this is still hidden; but if the pains are stilled by water or massage, the body will be thoroughly regenerated. Four thousand years ago people still lived up to Nature; then, no physician would have succeeded in building up a practice; but since humanity degenerated, she has tried to cure diseases by drugs.

Most people are averse to poisons, but their indifference to everything except money-making, blunts their plain commonsense. This indifference is nowhere more appalling than in everything concerning health; people are too lazy to study or to listen to lectures, otherwise they would not entrust their most sacred property to the first one coming. Just this indifference is a great obstacle; but all good things take time. Hundreds of physicians have already endorsed the science of nature's cure; that is, in part, because many of them still continue to give medicine. These have not yet fully realized the wonderful effects attained by baths and other natural applications. Nature-cure is still supposed to be identical with physical culture. By this natural method the body will be hardened, the physical power be strengthened and not only be able to resist disease but also to throw out poison hidden in the body. And there is one great mistake all people, physicians included, make, that they believe medicine cures, while, in fact, it is the natural power in the body that cures. The reason why Naturopathy is still a child, a young plant, is that people believe too much in medicine and are too indifferent. Finally, I beg to impress upon each and all the request: "Help me to propagate the science of Nature-Cure; lend your hand to the erection of this great structure."

---

*The keynote of Nature–Cure is: "Without hardening no strong health".*

*What a healthy man must have in order to remain in good health, a sick man ought to have in order to come back to health.*

*There is one great mistake all people, physicians included, make, that they believe medicine cures, while, in fact, it is the natural power in the body that cures.*

*There is only one law: Follow Nature. Every man needs air to breathe; the purer the air, the healthier the man; the better he feels, the purer his blood.*

---

# PREVENTION IS BETTER THAN CURE

## by Benedict Lust, N.D.

*The Naturopath and Herald of Health, IX (3), 82. (1908)*

The most noble object of the Nature Cure is to prevent all diseases. If diseases and all the evils of the body are to be prevented each individual must first of all begin to live a more natural life. Almost everybody is guilty of transgression against Nature; and these transgressions are far more frequent in the families of the rich than in those of the poor. Not until humanity has returned to Nature and has begun to obey her laws can the general condition be improved. A life in harmony with Nature is the first step and the first requirement for coming up to those conditions. This wisdom includes the following points:

1.  Nutrition which excludes everything that is unwholesome; the kind of food we take is of the greatest importance. This statement can only appear to be unimportant to those who are themselves unimportant. A wholesome diet from the vegetable kingdom is the following:

    a.  All kinds of grains, such as wheat, rye, barley, oats, Indian corn, rice, buckwheat, millet, and so forth, and the products manufactured from them, as oatmeal, macaroni, groats, flour and bread minus leaven.

    b.  All kinds of fruits and berries, either raw or cooked, and nuts; grain and fruits are the very staff of life.

    c.  All legumes (peas, beans, lentils) are an excellent food, especially for those who do hard work. They contain more albumen than any kind of meat.

    d.  All vegetables and salads, including mushrooms and potatoes.

    e.  Milk, butter, mild cheese, eggs, pure oils and honey.

    f.  Wholesome drinks, such as pure water as Nature yields it, though fruit juices may be added.

    The warm drinks we recommend are coffee prepared of barley, wheat, rye, acorns, and so forth; malt-coffee, nutritive salts, cocoa, tea of young strawberry, and blackberry leaves, and so forth.

    Kneipp's and other vegetarian cookery books ought to be used in the preparation of good and wholesome food.

2.  The careful culture of the body and care bestowed on sanitary environments are of first necessity.

    a.  Continually admit fresh air into your dwelling by proper ventilation; sleep with open windows, though in the cold weather the

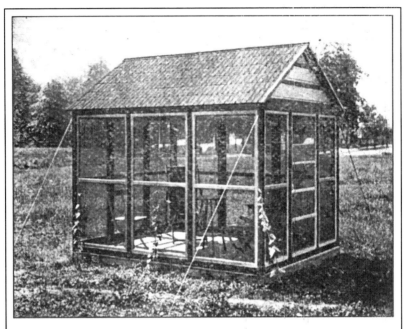
The precursor to the modern tent, screen houses were ideal for those seeking the air cure.

shades may be pulled down. Breathe through the nose and not through the mouth.

b. Take much exercise in the open air; also practice gymnastics; in winter before the open window in summer out of doors.

c. Take sufficient rest and sleep, from six to eight hours within twenty-four hours. Always retire and rise early.

d. Be scrupulously clean about your body and your treatment of it (baths, washes, rinsing of mouth and nose).

e. Wear light, comfortable and porous clothes; corsets and tight pressing clothes are injurious to health.

f. Your dwelling should be light, sunny and airy.

g. Family life must be pure, sexual excesses must be avoided.

On the other hand, because living contrary to Nature is harmful, the following things must be avoided.

a. All meat of killed animals, even broth and such products as sausages.

b. All alcoholic drinks, beer, wine, brandy.

c. The use of tobacco in all its forms.

d. All narcotics and stimulants, such as coffee, tea, spices, pickles and such things; vice, idleness and overwork of the body as well as of the mind, unclean and unhealthy rooms.

e. Also all drugs, vaccination, injections with morphine, serum or lymph.

If these lines should benefit people who think rightly and seek the health of body and soul the writer will be thoroughly satisfied.

*The most noble object of the Nature Cure is to prevent all diseases. If diseases and all the evils of the body are to be prevented each individual must first of all begin to live a more natural life. Almost everybody is guilty of transgression against Nature.*

# THE EARLY MORNING WALK

## by S. T. Erieg

*The Naturopath and Herald of Health, IX (6), 179. (1908)*

There is a division of opinion as to the advisability of a walk before breakfast. Without doubt there are those whose vociferation would be antagonistic to anything so wholesome, but this is not the fault of the early morning walk, but of their own inability. Some persons have by their own way of living unfitted themselves so that an effort becomes a task. To such the early morning walk may not appeal; it is one of the sane things that is not contained in their mode of living.

One of the obstacles against the early morning walk is lack of time. Yet I have known very busy persons who could find time for this healthful recreation, while others less busy pleaded lack of time. It is generally idle persons who never have time for anything and have the greatest number of excuses to offer for their misdeeds. When it pertains to spiritual or bodily welfare, no hindrances should be tolerated; nothing should be so great or so loved that cannot be thrown aside.

Walking is good at any time, but the early morning walk is a luxury in itself. This is the time when half the world is asleep, while the other half is awake and about, especially is this true in the spring and summer months, when animals and birds are out at the break of day. The air at early morning is different than at any other time of the day; it is more invigorating, more life-producing; it permeates the body with health and the brain with clearness. This is the time when all the lower creatures are out and enjoying life. The feathery songsters are at their best; they seem to be bubbling over with happiness, and sing as they do at no other time of the day. What a great privilege it is to walk in the green fields and woods as the sun is making its appearance in the east, and inhale the pure air and enjoy nature. If there is one thing for which we should thank God above some other things, it is for pure air, although we are sometimes confronted with the inconvenience of leaving the smoke and soot of the city behind, and journeying for the unadulterated air from the immediate vicinity of our domiciles.

It may be thought that the walk from home to work is sufficient as a morning outing, but how is this walk usually carried out? Usually by lying in bed to the limit of time, swallow the breakfast whole and in a very uncongenial state of mind rush off to the place of work. This is no exercise. Exercise should be congenial; it should be indulged in with both body and mind, the mind should assist in the exercise. Effort accompanied with enjoyment leads to excellency. The more we enjoy our work the greater progress we will make and the greater the degree of perfection in our chosen work. The same holds good with reference to our bodies.

The Naturopathic School of Regeneration had a second New York City location at 135 E. 58th Street in 1902.

Walking is an excellent means of exercise; it is an all-around exercise. It preserves the physical strength and is a means of acquiring health. It is a beautiful exercise and an educational exercise. It leads through beautiful places, through sunny lanes and cool woods, up the side of lofty moun-tains and in beautiful ravines and by the side of beautiful streams. Many places can be visited and many lessons learned and knowledge acquired only by this means of exercise.

While walking will not develop the entire body, yet it can be said truth-fully that no one means of exercise can develop the entire body. There are various exercises combined which will develop the entire body sym-metrically. But when all is said and done, there is no exercise that affords so much pleasure and holds so much in store as the means of walking. It is an exercise that you can always look back upon with pleasure, and as it were, paint mental pictures of scenes along its path.

*One of the obstacles against the early morning walk is lack of time. Yet I have known very busy persons who could find time for this healthful recreation, while others less busy plead-ed lack of time.*

*Walking is good at any time, but the early morning walk is a luxury in itself.*

## HOMEOPATHY AND ITS RELATION TO NATUROPATHY

**by Dr. Rudolf Weil, Berlin**
Translation made by *The Naturopath*
*The Naturopath and Herald of Health, IX (10), 297-299. (1908)*

Before going into the question it is necessary to explain briefly to the reader some of the points of Homeopathy. Among physicians and laymen there exists a very great ignorance of the nature of Homeopathy. In their college days, doctors hear no more perhaps than an occasional cheap witticism on the part of some professor at the expense of Homeopathy. The sons of Asclepius usually receives this with a loud, stupid laugh and the incident is closed. The graduated physician has perhaps in the course of an afternoon's nap idly glanced over the pages of some book on this subject and then with an expression of disgust, at its simplicity, thrown it into a corner. That, in most cases, represents the study of a science that, to be properly understood and applied, requires years of theoretical and practical work. Laymen consider homeopathic medicines either as strong poison or no medicines at all. Their family physician charmingly assures them that he would eat the entire contents of a homeopathic drug store for breakfast.

We have not the space here to discuss the question pro and con. However, let it suffice to say that thousands of learned doctors are devotees of this study; that the literature of this science is magnificent; that multitudes of sufferers find relief in Homeopathy after all other methods of curing have been tried; and, finally, that if all other systems of healing were as efficient as they are claimed to be by their adherents, it would be unnecessary for any sick man to seek relief in Homeopathy. In laying down the principles of Homeopathy, Dr. Dahlen, a recognized celebrity, says,

Three pillars support the structure of our science:

1. *Similia similibus curantur* as the main point of all.
2. The tests of medicines on healthy persons as the assumption of No. 1.
3. The science of dosing as result of No. 1.

The law, that like is cured by like, is no child of the brain of Dr. Samuel Hahnemann, the founder of Homeopathy. Traces are found in the literature of hundreds of years ago, sometimes distinct, sometimes almost obliterated. To consider these references individually would be to exceed the boundaries of this paper. Scarcely one of the leading ideas beginning with Hippocrates would be found missing from this collection.

An important argument in favor of Homeopathy is the test of the many different medicines on a healthy person.    From this we first learn the nature and extent of their effect on the human organs.    In this manner the appearances of poisoning and their different manifestations are brought to our notice.    We must study the effects of the different medicines from the most innocent to the most deadly, thereby obtaining a regulated instrument for our own purposes, the efficacy of which we could in no other manner learn.    For if a certain remedy influences a certain part of a healthy organism; it will have the same effect on a diseased one.

Dr. Hugo Schultz and Dr. Arndt, professors of the Greifswalder University, had the courage to openly advocate this main principle of Homeopathy.    The former performed valuable tests of this kind with his scholars about which the greater number of physicians maintains silence.    Allopathy employs larger and frequently injurious doses of medicine, entirely ignoring and neglecting the finer means, to the study of which Dr. Schultz especially devoted himself.

Professor Arndt has firmly established the fundamental biological law in connection with Professor Pflüger's law of convulsions by electric currents on the living organism which reads:

1.    Weak sensations arouse life activity;
2.    Middle strong sensations strengthen vitality;
3.    Strong sensations suspend activity;
4.    Very strong sensations destroy life.

Diseased organs are in a state of great irritation.    Provocations that would otherwise pass unnoticed almost loosen reflections of variable intensity.    According to this law the smallest doses of medicine must exercise some effect more or less distinct on the affected organ.    Thus is declared the working of homeopathic medicines which leave the sound organ unaffected.

Homeopathy is accused of influencing the progress of sickness very little or not at all.    Everyone not a partisan must admit that Allopathy often influences the diseased organ in a rough manner and inflicts direct injury.    As a result cases of poisoning by medicine, even nowadays, are very common and to which the public, believing them to be unavoidable, quietly submits.    Poisoning by mercury, salicylic acid, digitalis, etc., are matters of daily occurrence.    The amount of harm caused by the use of too much medicine, according to experienced physicians, is almost inconceivable.    Two excellent books by the eminent Professors Lewin and Robert will greatly enlighten anyone who may care to hear more of this subject.

That Homeopathy, even if applied by a layman, is often urged in its disfavor, but in fact it is something very much to its credit.    How much more efficient ought it to be in the hands of a physician?

It speaks well for this science that the practical American has built as

Ad for homeopathic tissue remedies.

many homeopathic hospitals as allopathic; that Homeopathy is taught at the universities; the number of followers of each school is about equal. Mindful of the proverb, "Time is money", the American will entrust his body only to the safest form of treatment. The waiting rooms of homeopathic doctors would not be as well visited if sick people obtained sufficient relief at the hands of the other physicians.

The various peculiar ideas of Dr. Hahnemann, the founder of Homeopathy, which are frequently used as an argument against it, have been laid aside by the modern Homeopathy. Homeopathy has not stood still. It has been industriously developed and perfected. The work and researches of the former school have not been ignored, even if another course in its therapeutics is being pursued. Nor should it be claimed that Homeopathy affords a perfect and comprehensive cure for all diseases of the body. It can be asserted, however, that among all existing methods of healing, Homeopathy occupies a foremost position. The really learned doctor should know everything that will assist him in restoring the diseased body to health. He can render his patient the greatest assistance by the individual and combined application of all therapeutic methods and means. Nothing hinders the art of healing more than narrow-mindedness and stubborn loyalty to a certain principle. No single method can accomplish everything. Each method applied individually or combined with others can attain the greatest success possible to human learning and intelligence.

The adherents of nature cures are quite as opposed to the use of medicine as are the devotees of Allopathy to Homeopathy. And for what reason? Shall we discard fire, gunpowder or water because, in inexperienced hands, they have caused much damage? No one will deny that Nature contains herbs and substances that have great healing powers. Why ought not the physician employ these means in the proper cases? Only fanatics firmly devoted to some principle can hold such views.

Our second question can be answered very briefly. Homeopathic treatment is entirely in harmony with the water, light and air cure. No one can deny that water, light and air properly applied will improve the health of a sick man. By treating the diseased body both internally and externally we can obtain better results than by confining ourselves to one method. Homeopathic methods, which can never harm since they exclude the danger of poisoning, cooperate successfully with water, light and air cures. Large doses of medicine, on the other hand, in forcing the healing efforts of nature, produce more harm than benefit.

The knowledge of possible ill results of medicals [medicines] induced the doctors of the University of Vienna in the last century to treat their patients, whenever possible, without the use of medicine.

It shall not be denied that water, light, heat, diet, etc., alone are capable of curing, but after long experience I believe that Homeopathy combined with the natural healing agents will produce the best and speediest results.

---

*An important argument in favor of Homeopathy is the test of the many different medicines on a healthy person.*

*It speaks well for this science that the practical American has built as many homeopathic hospitals as allopathic.*

*Homeopathic treatment is entirely in harmony with the water, light and air cure.*

*Nothing hinders the art of healing more than narrow-mindedness and stubborn loyalty to a certain principle. No single method can accomplish everything.*

# 1909

## THE SANITARY POWER OF THE CLIMATE OF HIGH ALTITUDES
DR. THEO. J. JAQUEMIN

## THE RELATIONSHIP OF THE INORGANIC SALTS IN THE VEGETABLE AND MINERAL KINGDOMS
LUDWIG H. STADEN

## THE HEALING POWER OF CLAY
ROBERT BIERI, N.D.

Henry Lindlahr used this ad and it last appeared in Benedict Lust's publication, the August issue, 1920.

In the following month, the September issue, Lust borrowed Lindlahr's ad above and posted his version. In 1920, $5,000 to $10,000 would be in today's currency equivalent to $60,000 to $120,000.

# THE SANITARY POWER OF THE CLIMATE OF HIGH ALTITUDES

## by Dr. Theo. J. Jaquemin

*The Naturopath and Herald of Health, XIV (7), 416-420. (1909)*

Healthy people feel better in a cold climate; while weak, old and young people feel more comfortable in a warm climate, because their blood has not sufficient warmth to equalize the assimilation. Medium degrees of heat are more agreeable to sick people, because they give rest to their mucous membranes, especially to the respiratory organs, which have less power of resistance. In any case it is of prime necessity that a climatic health-resort be always protected against severe cold and dry winds, as these produce fatal effects among patients inclined to consumption.

Hot and dry air increases the perspiration and is more pleasant than air that is hot and damp. The latter brings on a profusion of perspiration, impedes the functions of the kidneys, causes a lack of appetite and impedes assimilation.

Dry air is stimulating for the skin and mucous membrane, while dampness tends to produce rheumatic diseases. Climatic health resorts ought never to have one degree of dampness over 60 degrees to 70 degrees (16° to 21° C.) on the hydrometer.

When warm air comes in contact with cold air clouds, fogs, rain and snow are formed; all these are detrimental to the patient. For this reason all clear, cloudy, rainy or foggy days have always been carefully registered at health resorts.

Rain clears the air; and it will always be noticed that after a rain-shower patients feel better. Snow like-wise has a cleaning effect; when falling down it carries with it the organic dust in the air, and while it lies, all dust remains on the soil. Of fog we have only evil to report. It makes breathing difficult; exaggerates all ailments; depresses the mind, and frequently produces fatal results in pulmonary diseases. Days free from fog, most frequent on high altitudes are therefore, of the greatest importance.

Whatever the differences of climate and of the meteorological factors at the various health resorts may be, one thing is demanded of all: air free from dust and smoke. We have all experienced disagreeable, oppressive sensations when we have inhaled foul or dirty air. We also know the delight of inhaling fresh, country air when we go to the country after a day's work in the dusty city.

What we call "dust" is the combination of the most carried matter of inorganic, organic living, and organic dead atoms. The city air is especially loaded with dust; even the country air is not free from it. Where there is but a slight current of air the inorganic dust falls to the bottom, but the organic dust, especially, all the small atoms, such as: bacilli, microbes, bacteria, spirilla will be raised by the slightest current of air.

In ordinary diffused daylight one cannot see dust, but any ray of sunlight shows us that the dust hanging in the air as something tangible. Nobody would care to open their mouths in this focus of electric rays of light and inhale that mass of dust. Nevertheless, we all inhale, every minute, millions of dust particles without being aware of it.

This inhaling of dust is highly injurious: it irritates the mucous membrane, enters the tissue of the lungs, and propagates contagious diseases. The thinnest, invisible dust is the most dangerous. Let us, at the same time state that a really healthy subject is able to resist injurious influences. But not so the sick man, whose cells are weakened to such a degree that the injurious noxiousness results in a serious deterioration of the general condition. This constitutes one of the very first reasons for sending the patient out into fresh, healthy air; there his condition will soon improve, because his nature has now to conquer only the disease, and consequently, his hope is greater.

Conditions of the soil also have an important influence on climate. Where the soil is too dry, there is too much dust; but wherever it is too damp, we have the best foundation for producing indifferent as well as pathogenic bacteria; the influence of the soil is especially observed in its vegetation and in the quality and purity of the drinking water.

At no health resort should the hardships of life ever be mentioned. Everybody ought to be free from care and live in the open air night and day. The performance of gymnastic exercises should be regarded as a matter of duty.

These factors and curatives differ according to the latitude and altitude of the health resort, to its location, whether in the middle or on the border of the country; so that we may classify these various climates, as forest, sea, plain or highland-climate; the latter is most favorable for therapeutics.

The most important agencies are the tempered atmospheric pressure, the greater purity of air, the dryness of the soil, the increased caloric and chemical intensity of the sun-rays, the cooler temperature and the scarcity of oppressive foggy days. For many places one has besides altitude:

1.  The local grandeur of Nature, the limitless vista and its beneficial influence on the mind.

2.  The rich contents of oxygen in the air, as well as disinfecting etheric oils if fir forests are in the neighborhood.

3.  The necessity of climbing a little when walking, thus strengthening the whole muscular tissue, and stimulating the lungs to deep breathing.

Everybody who has made a study of these conditions, even those who from the pressure of air infer the physiological effects of the health resorts on high altitudes, admit that strength, appearance of good health, respiration, power of resistance, appetite and digestion greatly increased. Whether these results are obtained by the pressure of air cannot be ascertained; they would seem rather to be caused by much walking and climbing. If we bear in mind that plain country life has a magical influence on the worn-out subject this effort will naturally be increased on high altitudes where the cooler atmosphere, the grandeur and beauty of Nature stimulate the appetite.

The respiration, the circulation of the blood and the beating of the heart increase in high altitudes, though on these of medium height a quick equation of these functions takes place. Besides, the dryness of air on high altitudes, the excretion of carbonic acids and the exhalation of steam from the skin and lungs increase. But I must impress upon my readers the fact that climbing enlarges and deepens the respiration, increases the activity of the lungs and strengthens the circulation of the blood. Everybody will notice that mountaineers have a larger thorax chest, not because of hunger but because of steady climbing and because of the energetic, slow, deep breathing imperatively connected with climbing. Consequently, the strength and large development of their respiratory organs accounts for the like strength of the muscles of their thighs. Tourists, too, who have lived for some time on mountainous heights, usually return with a larger chest and deeper respiration. Finally, I must say that the greater purity and coolness of the air have a more beneficial influence on the general health than the mere situation of the most beautifully place located place in the country.

The climate of high altitudes is highly recommended for consumption, especially in winter. Sufferers from phthisis are greatly benefitted by living for some time on such altitudes. Though all theories do not agree as to the physiological effects of this or that health resort, that fact is well established that strong sunlight, dust-free, fresh air, cold washes and douches and plain, non-stimulating diet far surpass the antiquated methods of teas, drugs and dark rooms. Because of all these considerations the physicians will often find it hard to select the right place. He can only be guided by certain rules. First he should never send a poor patient to a distant health resort. He should bear in mind that health resorts are never meant for persons without means.

One physician remarks on this subject,

If one were to send a poor man into the very best climate, the desolation of his situation, the burden of care, the hunger, the poor lodging, and the insufficient food of his home will follow him everywhere. And, harassed by these mental pictures, he would feel uncomfortable even in an earthly Paradise. In fact, far away from his home, the cure would really injure him, and intensify the melancholy of his disposition; while staying at home in his wonted surroundings with his friends and family would help to facilitate his recovery.

Anybody who has not sufficient means to pay for the accommodation of a health resort, or who can only obtain these means through great sacrifices, should try to recover his health at home. There are many illustrations of the foolishness of sending poor patients to distant health resorts. Sometimes a poor widow has to sell almost all she has in order to get back the dead body of her husband (who was sent away by a physician) in order to bury him at home. Or, a hard-working man, denying himself and his children all manner of comfort, spends the last cent on his sick wife at some remote health resort; only after a few weeks to stand with his family by her coffin. These are considerations which should be borne in mind by people in like circumstances. Such sufferers ought to remain at home and avail themselves of all these remedies Natures affords at far less expense. Patients, too, who have not time to devote to the recovery of health, should remain where they are.

We trust that in the United States, the great leader in philanthropic enterprises, there will soon spring up Sanitaria in every state, where the poor may be restored to health. As the poor have to consider their purse, so any rich people have to consider the weakness of their characters. These should also be treated at home; for, within the last decades many health resorts have come to contain dens of gambling and other vices. What extravagances and excesses are not committed at these places by the devotees of Bachus and Venus? Many guests, because of the weakness of their characters, are more injured than benefitted in these places. Common sense tells us that all forms of excitement, love, hatred, gambling, intemperance and so forth in every country and in every clime produce the same injurious effects. The recovery of health is never a miracle; it is only attained by assiduously submitting to the laws of Nature, which are altogether contrary to a life of luxury. Only, under the most weighty considerations is any physician justified in sending a patient to any remote place for recovery, but never, if the home climate is good enough to bring about an average condition of health. If, however, the patient himself is convinced that only a stay in the South or on the mountains, or at the seashore will restore him to health, and if he has sufficient means and a relative to accompany him, let him go for months, or even years, if necessary, to recuperate.

As a general axiom we may assume that health resorts must be exempt in summer from any enervating weather, and in winter must not be extremely cold, and must be sufficiently pleasant to keep the guests outdoors. Health resorts on high altitudes are excellent for most patients; notwithstanding the cold, there are many sunny days, no fogs, few changes in the temperature and many days may be spent out of doors.

To speak more definitely, let us consider the health resorts in Switzerland. They are situated from 4,750 to 6,250 feet above sea-level. Though the fundamental peculiarities of the respective climates are everywhere almost the same; they have a distinctly characteristic gradation; and even so far, that this gradation goes hand in hand with the altitude as well as with the locality. On high altitudes the sky is of a deeper azure blue; the sunlight and heat are intensified; and though the snow period is long, the temperature is pretty low.

The increase of the intensity of all climatic factors is especially noted if one goes from Leysin (Canton Wardt) (4,750 feet above sea level) to Wiesen (4,770 ft.), Claradel (5,459 ft.), Samaden (5,670 ft.), St. Moritz-Kulm (6,090 ft.) and Ober-Arosa (6,028 ft.). All these are in Canton Graubuenden.

The fundamental qualities of these climates culminate in the following factors:

- Dimunition of the pressure of air;
- Constantly cold winter days without sudden changes in the temperature;
- A long snow period;
- Dry, pure air; dead calm;
- A cloudless sky;
- Exceptionally little fog;
- Magnificent sunlight, and powerful, splendid sun heat.

Such conditions produce marvelous effects on the human body, whether in good or poor health; of special benefit are they to consumptives. Not only do the appetite and the muscular nervous power greatly improve, but the blood, the life-given stream, undergoes great changes. The number of blood corpuscles and the haematoglobulins [sic], the pigments of the blood, are improved both in quality and quantity; consequently, the absorptive capacity for oxygen is greatly intensified. The circulation of the blood and the lymph becomes more energetic; the expansion of the lungs is more pronounced, and so their contents of blood diminishes, and finally, the cold, dry air will by and by absorb the rich bronchial and pulmonary secretions.

After these detailed demonstrations the reader will understand that the climate in high altitudes is a heroically effective potency. This fact admitted; the question again arises, how is the right place for the patient selected? Because what is one man's meat is another man's poison. High nervous temperaments, neurasthenia, a number of pathological conditions, heart-failures, disposition to hemoptysis, emphysema of the lungs and asthma, do not admit of a cure of high altitudes, the efforts of which are on a level with those of an average country-seat.

Here we have to individualize and to find out if we have to deal with the so-called pneumonia forms, or cases where constant fever symptoms prevail. To this category belong all those patients in whom the destruction of tissues has reached such a point that need of breath is very great, and the absorption of oxygen is limited to a minimum that their lives just hang by a thread; for such patients lower lying resorts must be selected.

It would be a mistake to suppose that people with cavities in their lungs should be excluded from the treatment on high altitudes; as we know by experience that such cavities often enough entirely heal. Galloping consumption, laryngitis, intestinal consumption and chronic renal diseases are so intractable that the patients are almost beyond recovery.

How can we turn to good account the modern curative methods of the climates on high altitudes? There are rules which have to be followed if one would not risk one's life and purse as well. The time for treatment on high altitudes should be as long as possible, though one may go from one place to another if their healing virtues are much the same. As long as improvement is noticed, the treatment may be continued. A pause of six weeks may be made during the period of the melting snow and the atmospheric perturbations of the vernal equinox.

The cure should always begin late in summer or early in the fall, so that the patient may become so acclimated as to be able to stay during the winter. Patients, who cannot stand the high climates mentioned above, may go to Goerbersdorf in Silesia (1,827 ft. high), Reinboldsgreen in Saxony (2,259 ft. high); Falkenstein, in the Taunus (1,640 ft.), or Canigon in southern France (2,297 ft.). At all these places the leading physicians follow Dr. Brehmen's principles, fresh air, as much exposure as possible to the daylight and profiting by the sunlight wherever you find it.

Pulmonary diseases with pronounced lesions should be sent to the highest altitudes; and in the fall and winter to lower ones which, though in a less degree, have the peculiarities of the high altitudes. That such patients must be isolated goes without saying.

During the long evenings in winter, living at these resorts becomes very monotonous; it would be a relief to find such places where treatment and entertainments might be combined. For instance, Innsbruck, in the Tyrol, would answer this purpose.

Lying at an altitude of 1,912 feet in the Inn Valley, this city has a population of about 36,000 inhabitants. Surrounded by mountains, it is well protected against the winds from the north; there are the Calk Alps with their peaks and points; from which the sun rays are thrown back as from a gigantic reflector; to the south rises majestically the 8,900 feet high pyramid of the Serlos, while the valley of the Inn, in progressive sinuosity, extends to the foot of the historic romantic Iselberg, which is scarcely twenty minutes' walk from the city gate. Besides the soft zephyrs of Italy make a southern vegetation possible in a country surrounded by snow-capped mountains. In the West the Martinwand and the Hohenberg fence in the Inn Valley which extends in the east to Hall and then runs out into a narrow valley.

The city of the Inn has many points of interest. It has beautiful, wide streets, public works, shady avenues and artistically arranged promenades. The soil is excellent; after the heaviest storm the soil dries up within two hours. The drinking water coming from the mountains has a pure, invigorating taste. Epidemics are unknown. The temperature is never extremely cold. Dr. Pertner, professor of the high school at Innsbruck, gives us the following schedule of the average temperature during the years from 1896 to 1900:

October............ 7.7 ° Celsius
November......... 2.5° Celsius
December......... 0.4 ° Celsius
January............. 3.9 ° Celsius
February........... 0.2 ° Celsius
March............. 3.3 ° Celsius

We have then in the month of October, November and March an average temperature of 30 to 45 degrees Fahrenheit; while the months of December, January and February show a fluctuation between 39 degrees and 25 degrees Fahrenheit. The monthly rainfall reaches 1 ½ inches. The amount of moisture in the air is on an average 76.2. The pressure of air is of the Innsbruck climate is, more or less, uniform; it is between 712 and 709 mm. mercury in extremes, and, therefore, it is of priceless value to the equipoise of the organism. Winds are very rare; consequently, the perturbations at the vernal equinoxes are of some importance. Only a few rainy days introduce the equinoxes; then, from the 10th of October to December there are the loveliest fall days. The mild winter begins in December, and the soil is covered with solid snow which affords the best opportunity for the healthy sport of sleigh riding.

*Rain clears the air; and it will always be noticed that after a rain-shower patients feel better. Snow like-wise has a cleaning effect; when falling down it carries with it the organic dust in the air, and while it lies, all dust remains on the soil.*

*Conditions of the soil also have an important influence on climate. Where the soil is too dry, there is too much dust; but wherever it is too damp, we have the best foundation for producing indifferent as well as pathogenic bacteria; the influence of the soil is especially observed in its vegetation and in the quality and purity of the drinking water.*

## THE RELATIONSHIP OF THE INORGANIC SALTS IN THE VEGETABLE AND MINERAL KINGDOMS

by Ludwig H. Staden

*The Naturopath and Herald of Health, XIV (10), 618-619. (1909)*

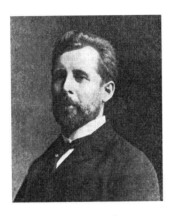

Ludwig H. Staden.

That which gives the herbal essences, or commonly called herbal teas, such high curative value is not only the presence of the inorganic cell salts in the herb, but especially that unknown life force, inherent to organic matter in a high degree, though this same life energy exists also in inorganic matter, but in a lower degree. It is the same wonderful power which has been the cause of crystallization of the mineral, has developed in the plant and become the road of sentient life, leading in the animal and human being to lower and higher consciousness.

The mineral kingdom underlies the same fundamental laws as the vegetable or animal kingdoms, all the organic life is there, though in a latent condition, not perceivable by our senses, therefore the life force which the Eastern scientist calls the "prana" is attached to it in a lower degree than in the vegetable kingdom, and this is the reason why man and animals take their food principally from the vegetable kingdom. Properly spoken, there does not exist any inorganic matter.

There is a similar relation with atoms and molecules. An atom, science says, is the minutest matter which cannot be divided. But matter, be it ever so minute, yet can be divided in infinity, because divisibility is the characteristic nature of matter, consequently an atom does not exist really, it is nothing more or less than a molecule.

However, we have to make a difference between an atom and a molecule, as well as between organic and inorganic matter, as we cannot prove physically the organic condition of inorganic matter. Western science has not yet penetrated in nature as far as that.

The question whether inorganic matter can be assimilated to any advantage of our system from the mineral kingdom must be answered in the affirmative; that means, it refers only to the twelve inorganic cell salts (Dr. Schuessler's), which are real constituents of the human body, and then they must be taken in infinitesimal small portions. It stands to reason that we cannot look for food in the ordinary way from the mineral kingdom,

# The Schuessler
## Tissue Food Remedies

### Calcarea Fluor.

Glandular swellings, hemorrhoids, varicose veins, prolapsus of womb. ...  **$1.25**

### Calcarea Phos.

Anemia, bone diseases, teething disorders, cholera infantum. .......  **$1.25**

### Calcarea Sulph.

Ulcers, suppurating skin diseases, chronic catarrhal conditions, advanced stage of lung diseases. ..........  **$1.25**

### Ferrum Phos.

Fevers, inflammations; early stage of all congestive diseases. ............  **$1.25**

### Kali Mur.

Second stage of inflammatory diseases, croup, coughs, diphtheria, glandular swellings, gastric disorders, constipation, sluggish liver. ............  **$1.25**

### Kali Phos.

Mental disorders. Nervous diseases, neurasthenic conditions generally, neuralgia, sciatica, insomnia. .............  **$1.25**

### Kali Sulph.

Late stage of inflammatory and catarrhal diseases. Bronchitis, pneumonia, scarlet fever, etc. .....................  **$1.25**

### Magnesia Phos.

Neuralgia, convulsions, spasmodic conditions, nervous headaches, sciatica, dysmenorrhœa; whooping cough. ...  **$1.25**

### Natrum Mur.

Skin diseases, with thin, watery discharges. Influenza, hay fever, coryza. Leucorrhœa. Diabetes mellitus. ..  **$1.25**

### Natrum Phos.

Gastric and intestinal disorders with sour or acid symptoms. ..........  **$1.25**

### Natrum Sulph.

Intermittent fever, bilious attacks, jaundice, diarrhœa, Skin diseases with yellowish scales. .................  **$1.25**

### Silicea.

Chronic, deep-seated ulcerations and suppurations. Chronic glandular swellings, tumors, carbuncles, etc. Phthisis pulmonalis. ....................  **$1.25**

**Prices of the Schuessler Tissue Remedies**

Bioplasma a general reconstructive for Vitality and Regeneration, a combination of the 12 Schuessler Tissue foods, **$2.25**, postpaid.

**DR. BENEDICT LUST**
**110 East 41st Street, New York**

Scheussler Tissue Salts continue to be used.

even the table salt, so much pretended as a necessary food article, is absolutely unnecessary, for the man who lives on the only natural diet—fruits, raw vegetables and nuts—for the simple reason, because fruits, etc., contain sufficient sodium chloride, as well as all the other organic salts.

The question arises: are the inorganic salts better and more profitably assimilable from the vegetable or from the mineral kingdom, especially in case of disease, or is there no difference at all in the assimilation from the two kingdoms?

There is without doubt some difference, although an inorganic salt remains an inorganic salt, whether we find it in the mineral, vegetable or animal kingdom.

Naturally man does not look for food from the mineral kingdom; consequently, if the inorganic salts constitute such an immense importance in building up and maintaining the physical body, nature has surely well provided for that man should become sufficiently supplied with all the needful inorganic constituents through the vegetable kingdom, provided he eats fruits, etc., abundantly in all varieties. If this is not the case, we have to take an extra supply of inorganic salts either from herbal decoctions or directly from the mineral kingdom.

Now we have said that some unknown vital force or life energy is inherent to organic matter in a much higher degree than to inorganic matter, and this should decide the question whether we prefer to compensate the deficiency of inorganic salts from the vegetable or mineral kingdom. However, in case of disease, I consider it best to use both ways. The herb cure harmonizes very well with the biochemic system of medicine.

Whether the inorganic salts, once assimilated by the vegetable kingdom, suffer a transmutation in form of a vitalizing process may remain an open question. My opinion is that the vitalizing process lies in the whole plant itself, and this is the point where arises the difference in the assimilation from the two kingdoms. If it is the inorganic salt the body requires solely, it may be taken from either kingdom, respectively, it is more convenient to take it from the mineral kingdom.

To discuss this question any further is perhaps not the most important task; it is sufficient to become convinced that the inorganic salts are of the highest importance for our physical welfare. The late Dr. H. Lahmann, in his book, *The dysaemia of the blood as the cause of all disease*, shows that he perfectly agrees with this theory, and the celebrated chemist and Dr. Hensel, likewise Lahmann, indeed refers entirely to the vegetable kingdom, and Dr. Hensel, though more of Dr. Schuessler's conviction, yet recommends the farmer to fertilize the soil with powdered stone manure, in order to produce the fruits of the fields richer in organic salts.

Coming now to the conclusion and remembering that the same life force is the quintessence of organic and inorganic matter, higher in degree in the vegetable, lower in the mineral, we comprehend why we will look in general for the supply of inorganic salts from the vegetable and in special from the mineral kingdom.

Dr. Schuessler's biochemic system is an astounding fact, almost beyond criticism, through its wonderful simplicity, and Naturopathy should, under all circumstances, accept this system in its great domain of healing.

---

*The question whether inorganic matter can be assimilated to any advantage of our system from the mineral kingdom must be answered in the affirmative; that means, it refers only to the twelve inorganic cell salts (Dr. Schuessler's), which are real constituents of the human body, and then they must be taken in infinitesimal small portions.*

*The question arises; are the inorganic salts better and more profitably assimilable from the vegetable or from the mineral kingdom, especially in case of disease, or is there no difference at all in the assimilation from the two kingdoms?*

*Coming now to the conclusion and remembering that the same life force is the quintessence of organic and inorganic matter, higher in degree in the vegetable, lower in the mineral, we comprehend why we will look in general for the supply of inorganic salts from the vegetable and in special from the mineral kingdom.*

## THE HEALING POWER OF CLAY

by Robert Bieri, N.D.

*The Naturopath and Herald of Health, XIV (10), 620-622. (1909)*

Nothing more interesting could be found in the way of historical research than what comes under the scope of this article. Was it custom among the ancient races to use clay or virgin earth as a remedy against bodily affliction, or has the statement to that effect been the speculative work of modern therapeutists to give bias to their respective systems? The question has long been the center of speculation; not until 8 or 10 years ago was it settled, when the noble Adolph Just sounded the first bugle call for the true *Return to Nature* movement. Then the false theories subsided. But he was not the inventor or discoverer of this wonderful remedy. Ages have passed since man and beast became aware of that positive restorative element oozing from the earth. The natives made use of it in many ways, describing its wonderful efficacy in records, some of which are preserved in the Babylonian section of the British Museum and elsewhere; these can be read to-day on stones, tablets, temples, obelisks, memorial documents and in war reports, all carved in stone. The still more ancient races living in the valley of the Ganges and north of the Himalayan Mountains treated their wounded soldiers with earth bandages, having little else apart from that resource.

To-day innumerable savage tribes and nations are still using moist earth for their open wounds and all skin diseases. African missionaries and Oriental students have repeatedly told me the mode of treating the sick and wounded with this universal remedy, never having failed to witness among them the quick, astonishing cures thus achieved. Dr. Michaud, a recent African explorer and ethnologist, whom I had the pleasure of meeting in London on his way to Paris, told me how the superstitious tribes living west of Zanzibar were being doctored by their quacks. Bad spirits, so they believe, had taken away or killed the good spirits in the earth and only the clay of the witch doctor could possibly save them from the highly poisonous bites of native snakes and scorpions, or from the terrible wounds inflicted by poisoned arrows, spears and assegais [iron-tipped spear]. The Balis have a most elaborate system of curing, not only wounds, but all diseases and tropical epidemics. This is a tribe of mighty warriors, living in Odogomakumack, far back in the interior of the English Gold Coast and German Cameroon (East Africa), first discovered by Ramseyer and closely studied by Dr. Michaud. Their fantastic conception of religion, superstition, or mythology, is closely involved with the scheme of the great physician, "Mother Earth".

Among the classic literature we find much space devoted to the claim that earth possessed great healing and magnetic qualities. Early Greek mythology furnishes among other narratives the well-known story of Antaeus.

When the giant Hercules was in the service of Eurysthens, he was ordered to fetch the golden apples of the Hesperides. But these were guarded by the giant Antaeus, son of Geca, the Earth Goddess. Hercules, who never to that time had been defeated, opened combat with his powerful opponent. During that immortal struggle Hercules observed that Antaeus always was refreshed and strengthened when he stood upon the earth, but became weak and powerless as soon as he was separated from the earth by being lifted into the air. Therefore, Hercules uprooted Antaeus bodily, thus he could easily strangle him and bring the golden apples back to his master.

The magnetic qualities of the earth need not be enlarged upon, since we are not familiar with the natural phenomenon, such as the compass and its needle, the thunderstorm, and other signs of this wonderful life force. Our own largely perverted impressions of a correct life lead us faithfully, even yet, to the feeling of what we should do and how we should live in accord with Nature's laws to regain perfect happiness. It does not take us long to see for ourselves that the earth has a most refreshing, invigorating and salutary influence as soon as you come into direct touch with it.

As an illustration, I will quote to you a few lines from the works of Adolf Just, who came to his conclusions through close observations at his sanatorium in Germany. He writes: "Animals and man are still as much subject to the laws of Nature as plants, and they still draw their strength and vitality from the earth.

Knowing this, I attached still greater importance to going barefooted on the earth, and became more than ever convinced of its great curative effect. But I asked myself if this influence of the earth could not be utilized on behalf of man in a still greater degree. For the first thing, I no longer had my patients sleep in high bedsteads, but on strawticks or quilts, on the ground in the open air, or in light and air cottages. They were thereby brought closer to the earth during sleep. This was at once felt as a gain; sleeping became pleasanter and much more invigorating. But soon my patients lay down on the soft grass entirely naked and covered themselves with quilts. Soon I heard their enthusiastic exclamations over the wonderful effects of the earth upon their body during the night's rest.

The author is of the opinion that most diseases, but especially the number of serious nervous troubles of our age, would entirely lose their terrors if only sleeping and lying on the earth once more became habitual in the curing of disease.

By sleeping on the ground, more than by anything else, the entire body is aroused from its lethargy to a new manifestation of vital energy, so that it can now effectively remove old morbid matter from the assimilating organs and receive a sensation of new health, life, and unsuspected vigor. (Illustration from the animal kingdom.)

We have seen from the foregoing remarks that the earth as a whole possesses great healing qualities, but you justly ask, has that anything to do with the subject in question?

The question is warranted, since we were going to speak about clay as a therapeutic agent. But remember that the forces manifested in the ground are exactly the same when earth is moistened and applied in the form of clay compresses, packs, etc. Of course, there is the presence of water in the clay bandage, which is of a special value, as we soon shall see. Clay derives its vital power from the ever progressing law of generation, and has as its basis the forming of new life cells, which, in the ordinary course of nature, are used to bring forth new concentrated organism, as manifested in plants, trees and vegetables. When earth has no chance to perform this reconstruction for us, then we are prompted by natural instincts to make use of that stored-up vital energy for many of the ailments that have befallen the human race. Animals, once more, have demonstrated the right way for us to adopt. If an elephant, for instance, has been wounded, he at once moistens the earth with his saliva, stirs it into a soft mass, and covers his wound with it.

I am of the opinion from the short observation made at the "Yungborn" Health Home, Butler, New Jersey, that clay, as prepared there, is an incomparable remedy for all wounds, inflammations, fevers, skin diseases, boils, open sores, accidents of cutting, stabbing, burning, shooting, etc., for ulcers, impoverishment of the hair follicles, eruptions of all kind, stings and bites of animals, including hydrophobia or bites of mad dogs, blood-poisoning; for all dermatological troubles such as cancer, lupus, tetter, dandruff, syphilitic skin troubles, leprosy and elephantiasis.

Here at our establishment we employ the clay in its most simple and natural form, and I am prepared to testify that the mud bath taken in a prone position has still greater advantage than the clay compress locally applied. Of course, people to-day will think an earth bandage much too simple. Their restless mind tries to concoct salves by means of great scientific research, and with the aid of complicated apparatuses and costly drugs; although a simple bandage of earth will heal the wounds exceedingly well without any risk, while salves are often most dangerous.

We shall not choose clay or earth for a pack or bandage from a place where impurities have been disposed of, or where we have reason to believe that the clay is contaminated. Blood-poisoning may result when earth is taken that has been over-cultivated with manure or chemical compounds.

When it is not possible to apply the clay pack as prescribed at the

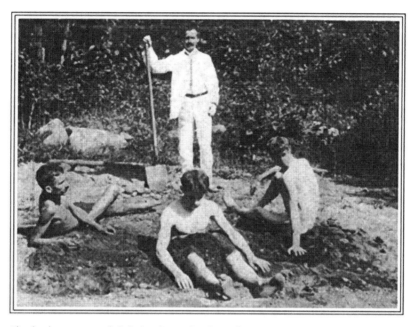

Clay baths were used daily by the Butler, "Yungborn", visitors. Benedict Lust leans on a shovel in the background.

Yungborn, then another method may be resorted to, and this is the earth compress. The moist earth is simply spread over the affected spot, on the abdomen, the chest, the eye, the foot, the hand, the sexual part, on the region of the larynx, thorax, the aorta, the heart, kidneys, liver, pancreas, spine, etc. It is then first overlaid with a linen cloth, somewhat larger than the spot covered by the earth. Then another cloth of cotton or wool is placed over the linen, and the whole wound about with bandages, so as to remain in place. The physiological action is in all process of healing the same; and notwithstanding that clay has not found a ready acceptance among the medical profession, we may be sure it will continue to be a most important factor in the history of natural therapeutics.

In the Kneipp Cure a very fine salve is used, made from clay. Excellent results have been obtained therefrom.

The action of clay is first of all absorbent, acting as a sponge, capable of extracting uric acid accumulation from any part of our body, and all other poisonous matter which has caused us acute or chronic diseases. Then, again, a good clay compress will greatly assist nature in dissolving an army of bacteria, warring against us in our arteries, veins, hearts, lungs, etc. It can therefore be relied upon in acute diseases, such as typhoid fever, scarlet fever, malaria, yellow fever, whooping cough, measles and influenza. Clay will act as a fine heat and cold regulator if mixed with cold water. Internal fever, as shown by a quickened pulse, a hot skin surface, pains and burning sensation in our interior organism, as well as in cases of nervous disorders, melancholy, etc., will soon lose its hold on the patient if put to flight by a clay compress. Clay applied in cases where it has to battle against positive living enemies, such as bacilli, bacteria, microbes, carcasses, liniocacas [sic], streptococcus, tubercles, and the like, will gain the victory through its stimulating and expelling qualities. Again, clay will soothe, it will help to give back to us through a cleansing process of the lungs a normal balance and poise for our physical and mental well-being. Would it not be worthwhile to consider these few suggestions and be benefited to the uttermost by familiarity with this heaven-sent earth force?

*From the short observation made at the "Yungborn" Health Home, Butler, New Jersey, that clay, as prepared there, is an incomparable remedy for all wounds, inflammations, fevers, skin diseases, boils, open sores, accidents of cutting, stabbing, burning, shooting, etc., for ulcers, impoverishment of the hair follicles, eruptions of all kind, stings and bites of animals, including hydrophobia or bites of mad dogs, blood-poisoning; for all dermatological troubles such as cancer, lupus, tetter, dandruff, syphilitic skin troubles, leprosy and elephantiasis.*

*Of course, people to-day will think an earth bandage much too simple. Their restless mind tries to concoct salves by means of great scientific research, and with the aid of complicated apparatuses and costly drugs; although a simple bandage of earth will heal the wounds exceedingly well without any risk, while salves are often most dangerous.*

*The action of clay is first of all absorbent, acting as a sponge, capable of extracting uric acid accumulation from any part of our body, and all other poisonous matter which has caused us acute or chronic diseases.*

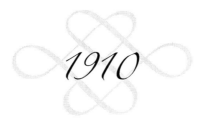

# 1910

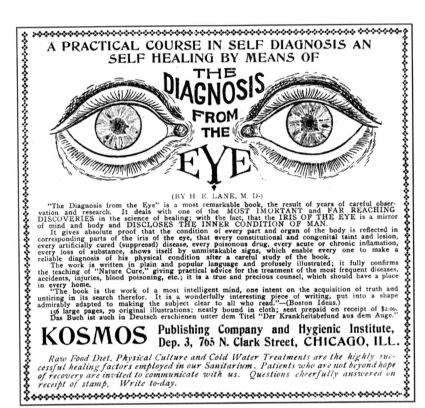
Kosmos Sanitarium, owned by Dr. H. Lane who wrote a much valued book, *The Diagnosis of the Eye*, taught many Naturopaths including Henry Lindlahr.

# The Scurf Rim*

## by Henry Lindlahr, M.D.

*The Naturopath and Herald of Health, XV (5), 263-266. (1910)*

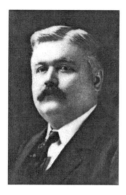

Henry Lindlahr, M.D.

The name Scurf Rim was applied by German diagnosticians to the dark ring often visible in the outer iris of the eye, because it usually appears and is always intensified, after suppression of milk crust, scurf, sycotic and other eczematous eruptions on the head and bodies of infants and children.

The outer rim of the iris, where the iris color joins the white of the eyeball, corresponds in the body to the cutaneous surface or skin. If the skin is normal, healthy and active, the rim of the iris shows no abnormal discoloration. If, however, the skin is weak, enervated, relaxed and anemic there appears in the rim of the iris a dark ring.

Sometimes this dark ring is complete all around the iris, sometimes it appears only in certain portions or segments of it.

Suppression of skin eruptions, mercurial inunctions, hot bathing, steam baths, heavy, dense clothing and anything else which weakens skin action tend to intensify the scurf rim.

Heredity, as we have learned in former articles, is indicated in the iris of infants by a general darkening of color. Sometimes, however, in the offspring of scrofulous, psoric or mercurial parents the scurf rim also is, shortly after birth, more of less distinctly visible.

Nature endeavors to purify the tender, plastic body of its hereditary taints and miasms, not only through the natural channels of elimination, but also the various forms of acute infantile diseases, such as diarrhoeas, skin eruptions, colds, catarrhs, febrile diseases, etc.

One of Nature's favorite means of purifying the infant organism seems to be skin eruptions on head or body. If these are suppressed by salves, drugs, drying powders, oils, creams, soaps, etc., warm bathing, warm, dense clothing and coddling, the scurf rim appears, or, if already present, becomes more prominent, indicating that the skin action has been weakened and paralyzed by such unnatural treatment.

It would probably be going too far to attribute the scurf rim always

---

*The original title of this article was "Diagnosis From The Iris Of The Eye" which was a series written by Henry Lindlahr published in his own journal, *The Nature-Cure* and later re-published in *The Naturopath and Herald of Health*. —Ed.

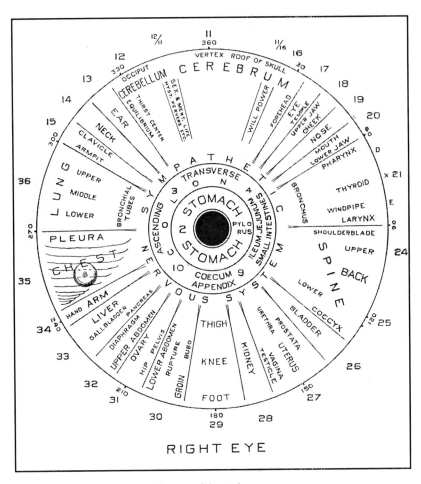

The iris of the right eye.

to suppression. As before intimated, the dark rim may be the sign of a naturally weak and inactive skin not virile enough to produce eruptions. Such an individual, however, has but few chances to survive in the battle for life, and usually succumbs to the first serious disease crisis.

On the other hand it is very interesting to observe how even in later life the scurf rim diminishes and gradually disappears when under the influence of open air, sun and light baths, cold water treatment, massage, osteopathy, etc., the cutaneous system becomes alive and active, and when the latter, by means of skin eruptions, furuncles, carbuncles, etc., throws off the latent chronic taints.

The scurf rim is therefore a reliable indicator of the normal or abnormal condition of the skin. This becomes of eminent importance in diag-

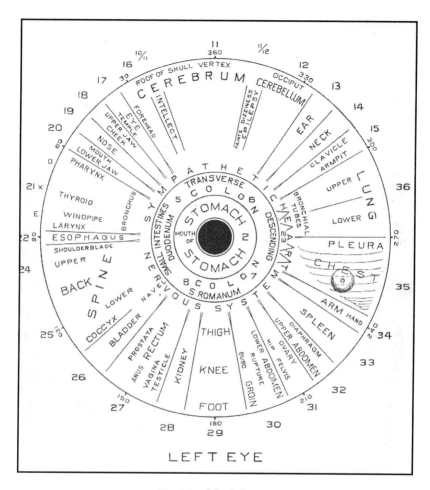

The iris of the left eye.

nosis and prognosis when we consider that the skin is the largest and most effective organ of elimination. If by burns, scalds or by other causes one-third of the cutaneous surface has become inactive or is destroyed, the elimination of systemic poisons is interfered with to such an extent that auto-intoxication or self-poisoning takes place and death is the inevitable result.

The skin besides containing the superficial organs of touch has two very important functions, viz., heat radiation and excretion. Our temperature constantly stands near 99 degrees F. [37° C.], no matter whether we are at the equator or in the polar regions; whether we swelter in the heat of summer or shiver in the cold of winter. Deviations of a few degrees either way from the normal heat are symptoms of severe illness. The body is able to maintain this equality of temperature only by the instrumentality of the lungs and especially of the skin. If the skin is tense and occluded, then inner blood pressure and temperature rise too high. If the skin is too weak and relaxed, then the loss by radiation is too great and as a consequence inner blood pressure and temperature sink too low. If heat radiation is interfered with, as in high fevers, uric acid poisoning, enervation of the skin, etc., then result in the interior organs a tendency to congestion, high blood pressure, catarrhal, feverish and inflammatory conditions.

The healthy skin excretes large amounts of carbonic acid, urea, xanthine, creatinine, and numerous other systemic poisons. It does therefore an immense amount of vicarious work for lungs and kidneys. If the action of the skin is inhibited by sudden chilling, uric acid precipitation, or by other paralyzing, enervating or occluding influences, the inner organs of elimination, in addition to their own, have to do the work of the skin, and become congested and overworked, and catarrhal conditions are the result.

We can now understand why the Scurf Rim, in a measure, stands for what we call the scrofulous constitution because it betokens an inactive, weakened skin system, suppression of hereditary taints, weakened circulation, cold extremities, pale, clammy skin and therefore a tendency to chronic catarrhal conditions, all of which prepare the way and form the congenial soil for tuberculosis in later life.

### The Third Lung

For these reasons we often say that we cure tuberculosis by the regeneration and cultivation of the "third lung", that is, the skin. This at once brings out in full relief the immense importance in the cure of lung diseases of the nude, open air, sun and light baths, cold water treatment, massage, osteopathy, of porous or no underwear, light clothing, nude sleeping, out of door sleeping, etc.

Heavy, dense clothing alone is sufficient to enervate and suppress the natural eliminative activity of the skin because it prevents free ventilation and keeps the body bathed day and night in its own poisonous exhalations, and this causes and aggravates a multitude of catarrhal ailments and uric acid diseases.

Often we hear remarks like the following, "I cannot understand why my face is full of blotches, pimples and eruptions when my body is perfectly pure and clean."

There is no mystery in this very common phenomenon. The face in such cases has to do the work for the rest of the cutaneous surface because coming in contact with light, air, rain and cold, the face has the only healthy piece of skin on the body capable of active elimination.

If these blemished ones would expose their bodies as freely as their hands and face to the health giving, stimulating influences of air, light and water, elimination would become normal and general all over the body, and their complexion would soon clear up and become as pure and beautiful as that of a child. This we constantly prove to be a fact in our work. Nature Cure is therefore the best and most rational of all cosmetics.

As explained in the previous chapter on density, dark discolorations, signs and spots stand for lack of blood, sluggish circulation, chronic catarrhal conditions and destruction of tissues in the corresponding parts and organs of the body; therefore the dark scurf rim is the sign of an enervated, vitiated skin, of poor surface circulation and of very defective elimination.*

### Uric Acid And Skin Action

The question may be asked, how is it that persons without a scurf rim often suffer from defective skin action?

In our article on Natural Dietetics we shall bring out the fact that elimination through the skin may also be diminished and checked by precipitation of uric acid in the surface capillaries, the result of which in extreme cases would be complete cessation of elimination through the skin and uraemic poisoning.

Weakening or suppression of the surface circulation by uric acid deposits in the capillaries (collaemia) may occur in people with otherwise good skin action as a result of faulty diet or disease of the kidneys. The degree of uric acid precipitation in the surface blood vessels may be accurately determined in the following manner by the reflux test:

> Press a fingertip on the skin. If the white patch thus produced fills up with blood immediately, say in 3 or 4 half seconds [1.5 or 2 seconds], then the circulation is active and normal; if, however, the reflux of blood into the white patch occupies from 4 to 20 half seconds [2 to 10 seconds] then the circulation is impeded by uric acid precipitates and the degree of occlusion can be estimated by the length of reflux.

### How To Efface The Scurf Rim

Massing of the scurf rim in certain segments of the outer iris is always a sign of weakness or morbid encumbrances in the corresponding part of the body. If the scurf rim is very marked in the lower half of the iris and if the upper part, especially in the region of the brain, shows the whitish signs and clouds or inflammatory conditions, so is this an indication that the circulation in the cutaneous surface and in the extremities is weak and

---

*The article, "Diagnosis from the iris of the eye III", which Henry Lindlahr is referring to, appeared in the March issue, 1910 of *The Naturopath and Herald of Health* and was not included in this collection. —Ed.

sluggish and that as a consequence the inner blood pressure, especially in the brain, is abnormally high.

This means cold extremities, sluggish circulation in the portal system (stomachs, bowels, liver and spleen), swollen veins on the legs, hemorrhoids, neuralgias, toothaches, colds and catarrhs of throat, lungs and nose.

From this it is apparent that in order to cure these various ills it is necessary to re-establish the normal activity of the skin, and this is best accomplished by the nude air baths, cold water baths, light, porous or no underwear, massage, osteopathy, and by pure food free from all excess of uric acid poisons.

But I hear you say, "I cannot stand cold water, I might just as well die. So and so may stand it but it would certainly kill me. Unless I wear the warmest of clothing I freeze to death." Not so, Madam; keeping warm is not a matter of piling on clothes but of good skin action and reaction. We cannot make a weak enervated skin strong and active by coddling it and by burying it under piles of dense heavy underwear and clothes. People come to us in the middle of summer wearing one or more thick suits of underwear and then are shivering and catching cold in every passing breath of air.

A few weeks of cold water treatment, light, sun and air baths, massage and osteopathic treatment bring new life and blood into the surface and the skin takes on the pink and rosy hue of life. Snakelike they shed skin after skin of underwear, chest protectors, woolen stockings, gloves, overcoats and the dead surface cuticle of their bodies, and then begin to enjoy contact with the life giving elements. Like the Indian they can say, "My body all face". The cuticle of their bodies has become as active, alive and immune to heat and cold as that of their faces.

Many patients who came to us at first in such weakened sensitive condition are now taking regularly every day on the roof of our institution in the crisp January and February air, their nude air bath. They do this not because we advise them to do so, for we refrain from prescribing such heroic treatment, but because they enjoy the sport.

Regeneration of the third lung under a natural regimen is accompanied by a gradual decrease and often by a complete disappearance of the scurf rim. When the skin becomes active and alive find white lines become visible in the dark rim and these broaden out gradually into light patches.

*The name Scurf Rim was applied by German diagnosticians to the dark ring often visible in the outer iris of the eye, because it usually appears and is always intensified, after suppression of milk crust, scurf, sycotic and other eczematous eruptions on the head and bodies of infants and children.*

*Suppression of skin eruptions, mercurial inunctions, hot bathing, steam baths, heavy, dense clothing and anything else which weakens skin action tend to intensify the scurf rim.*

*The scurf rim is therefore a reliable indicator of the normal or abnormal condition of the skin. This becomes of eminent importance in diagnosis and prognosis when we consider that the skin is the largest and most effective organ of elimination.*

*If the action of the skin is inhibited by sudden chilling, uric acid precipitation, or by other paralyzing, enervating or occluding influences, the inner organs of elimination, in addition to their own, have to do the work of the skin, and become congested and overworked, and catarrhal conditions are the result.*

*For these reasons, we often say that we cure tuberculosis by the regeneration and cultivation of the "third lung", that is, the skin.*

*Not so, Madam; keeping warm is not a matter of piling on clothes but of good skin action and reaction.*

# DIAGNOSIS FROM THE IRIS OF THE EYE, ITCH OR PSORA SPOTS

## by Henry Lindlahr, M.D.

*The Naturopath and Herald of Health, XV (8), 449-454. (1910)*

In about 25 per cent of all human eyes can be readily discerned in various parts of the iris sharply defined dark brown spots ranging from the size of a pinhead to the size of a buckshot. These spots, the diagnosis from the eye calls itch or psora spots, because they appear after the suppression of itch eruptions and of psoric parasites (*pediculi capitis* and *pubis*).

The word psora was adapted by Hahnemann, the father of Homeopathy, from a Greek word signifying "itching", and he applied the name to certain skin diseases which are characterized by intolerable itching.

Probably no other problem in medical science has given rise to so much controversy as Hahnemann's much disputed theory of psora. It is therefore very interesting to observe in how far the eye confirms these theories and in how far it contradicts them.

### THE THEORY OF PSORA

For one hundred years *Similia similibus curantur*, the fundamental law of homeopathy, has been the only fixed point in the chaos of constantly changing medical theories and in a perverted form, under the guise of vaccination, antitoxin, serum and organ therapy, this great law of cure has been adopted even by the allopathic school of medicine.

Comparatively very few of his closest friends and followers accepted Hahnemann's theory of psora. This part of his teachings was unmercifully ridiculed by his opponents and silently ignored even by those who were believers in and exponents of the law of *Similia*.

Is it possible that the great genius of the art of healing, who in his chosen field stands unequalled for acuteness of observation and of reasoning, was right in one part of his teachings and entirely mistaken and imaginary in another?

After one hundred years of ridicule and controversy, the diagnosis from the eye confirms the essential parts of Hahnemann's theory of psora. For nothing in the entire language of the iris stands more plainly revealed than the signs of hereditary psora (scrofula) and of suppressed itch.

Briefly stated, the psoric theory claims that age-long persistent suppression of itchy, parasitic skin eruptions and of gonorrheal and syphilitic diseases has encumbered almost the entire human race with three well-defined hereditary taints or miasms. These were named by Hahnemann psora or itch, sycosis or gonorrhea, and syphilis. He further claimed that

Henry Lindlahr had published his own book on Iridology.

the greater part of chronic diseases had their origin in these hereditary miasms and that many acute diseases are merely external palliative manifestations of these internal latent, chronic taints.

## SCURF RIM AND HEREDITARY PSORA

Darkening of the iris color and the scurf rim stand for those conditions which Hahnemann called hereditary psora and which we have described as hereditary scrofula, and the name psora we have purposely reserved for those disease conditions which result later in the life of the individual from the suppression of scabies (itch) and of other psoric parasites. We have done this because the "itch or psora spots" are never seen in the eyes of the new born, but only later in life when psoric eruptions and parasites have been suppressed by means of sulphur, zinc or mercurial ointments, by hot water, steam or hot air bathing, or by any other method of suppression.

To recapitulate: darkening of the iris color and scurf rim stand for the long list of hereditary ailments which Hahnemann calls hereditary psora and which we call the "scrofulous diathesis". The dark brown itch or psora spots stand for the effects of suppressed itch and psoric parasites. We have stated in former articles of this series that blue-eyed parents suffering from suppressed itch, as shown by the itch spots in their eyes, usually have brown-eyed or "scurf rimmed" children, and these revelations of the iris confirm Hahnemann's statement that suppression of acute itch creates chronic constitutional psora and hereditary psora in the offspring.

Before we proceed in our study of the "itch spots" in the eye it will be very instructive and interesting to quote a few passages from Hahnemann's *Chronic Diseases* and to learn just what he means by psora and suppression of psora. This wonderful man will greatly rise in our estimation and admiration when we stop to think that he discovered by keenness of intuition and by marvelous powers of concentration and observation which we today see so easily and plainly revealed by the diagnosis from the eye.

When the microscope revealed a minute, ugly looking parasite as the apparent cause of the itch eruptions, Allopathy jubilantly declared that Hahnemann's theory of *Psora* was thereby finally disposed of. The little mite which is blamed for this disagreeable disease has been named by science, the *acarus scabies,* or *sarkoptes hominis.*

Under the microscope the parasite presents a ferocious appearance, having a body resembling somewhat that of a tortoise with the legs of a spider. His body is studded with strong bristles by means of which he braces and supports himself in the flesh of his victim when burrowing his tunnels into the lower layers of the skin. It is the prick of these bristles in the flesh and the work of his voracious maw which causes the intolerable irritation peculiar to the disease. The insect is devoid of eyes and of a nervous system; it is all mouth, teeth and stomach. The male is small and burrows in the surface layers of the skin, while the female is larger and digs its shafts deep down into the *cutis vera*, or true skin, where it taps and sucks the minute blood vessels.

Orthodox science says, "Itch is never found without the *acarus scabies*, therefore, the latter must be the cause of the disease." Since the discovery of germs and bacteria, Allopathy has extended this local and parasitic conception of disease so as to embrace almost every known pathological condition. As a natural corollary of this theory, germ killing has become the basis of modern medical science.

The diagnosis from the eye, however, conclusively proves that Hahnemann after all was right and that Allopathy is in error when it claims that the killing of the itch microbe and of the vermin which infests head and pubis effectually terminates these diseases.

For after killing of these parasites by means of sulphurous and mercurial ointments, sharply defined brown spots appear in certain parts of the iris and it has been conclusively proven that the areas in the iris displaying these psora spots correspond to the parts and organs of the body in which, after external suppressions, the psoric poisons have concentrated.

We are often asked, "How can you prove that the brown spots in the iris have any relationship to suppressions of itch parasites and vermin?" Our answer to this is, "The diagnosis from the eye and the development of chronic cases under natural methods of living and of cure conclusively of living and of cure under natural methods of living and of cure conclusively prove these facts." Instances like the following come under our observations almost daily.

## CLINICAL PROOFS

A case of itch has been promptly cured with sulphur ointment and within a year there appears in the iris of this person, close to the pupil (area of the stomach), a sharply defined dark brown spot, and from that time on, the person is greatly troubled with chronic gastritis and later on with ulcers of the stomach.

A mother is horrified to find on the head of her little girl some lice. Within a few days the hair is full of nits and the vermin have increased to an alarming extent. The mother applies coal oil, or mercurial ointments, and the "nasty things" disappear from the surface but not from the body. The psoric taints which Nature was trying to eliminate, now reinforced by drug poisons and by the deadly miasms contained in the bodies of the parasites themselves, recede into the interior and in place of being distributed throughout the entire body they now concentrate in some vital part or organ, and chronic headaches, epilepsy, chorea, asthma, nervousness, sexual perversity, etc., are often the result.

Several years ago a lady belonging to a wealthy and refined family came to us for a diagnosis of her case. The left iris displayed in the region of the cerebellum, a light brown spot, and I remarked, "You have suffered for many years with chronic headaches, nervousness, twitchings in the limbs and the muscles, and with dizziness." All of this she confirmed and wanted to know the cause of her lifelong suffering.

"As a school girl", I continued, "you were troubled with head vermin and your mother treated them in the usual way."

"Yes," she answered, "I remember distinctly, I was affected that way several times, but what has that to do with my ailments?"

I explained to her that not external filth alone but internal uncleanliness also favors the development of these parasites, that like all bacteria they subsist on constitutional poisons and act as Nature's scavengers which purify the system of scrofulous and psoric miasms. I also informed her that in many instances Nature Cure treatment had reproduced the old suppressions and warned her to avoid suppressive treatment, if such a healing crisis should develop in her case.

One day, after three months' of vegetarian regimen, Nature Cure and Homeopathic treatments, she complained about intolerable itching of the scalp.

A look in her eyes revealed that the brown psora spot was surrounded and interlaced by fine white lines, the signs of an approaching acute reaction. "You will have visitors very soon," I remarked.

"What visitors do you mean, doctor?"

"The same kind that your mother killed some 25 years ago."

Within a week after this conversation she entered my office laughingly and exclaimed, "Oh, Doctor, not one visitor, but a million; I am just alive with them." "All right," I answered. "Be thankful they have come. This means the cure of your chronic ailments. Do not use anything now but a comb and cold water."

"How lucky, Doctor, that you told me about this in advance. Without your warning I would surely have rushed to a drug store and have done the same thing over again."

Her old friends remained about two weeks and then disappeared as they had come. From that time on she was cured of the "terrible periodical headaches" and other nervous ailments which had troubled her since girlhood. Possibly this psoric crisis prevented the development of paresis in later years.

"Catching" in this case was absolutely out of the question, for she lived in the most refined surroundings and for three months cold water sprays and douches had been applied almost daily to head and body.

We are often asked the question, "Where do they come from—you do not believe that they come from the body itself?" We do not know, but we do know by frequent experiences that when the body begins to eliminate scrofulous poisons we need not worry where germs and microbes are to come from. As carrion attracts vultures, so the chronic miasms attract bacteria and parasites.

Occurrences like the one related answer the oft repeated question, "Why stir up these disease miasms—why not leave them where they are, if their elimination causes so much trouble?" If they are allowed to remain their presence mean much greater trouble in the future; like weeds in the field they grow and multiply unless pulled up by the roots.

## Cancer Grows In Psoric Soil

Furthermore, the psora spots in the eye solve to a large extent the mystery surrounding the nature and origin of malignant tumors, or chronic asthma and tuberculosis. If we find a vital part or organ affected by suppressed itch we know that such a person is in great danger of developing cancer, sarcoma or tuberculosis in the encumbered parts.

With two exceptions so far in our practice, every case of cancer which we have cured has developed itch eruptions as healing crisis. The two exceptions to the rule eliminated the psoric taints by means of furunculosis.

The almost uniform appearance of itch eruptions as healing crises, during the cure of cancer cases, is certainly of great significance. It throws new light upon the true causes of these dreaded diseases and wonderfully confirms Hahnemann's theory of psora. Knowing these facts, is it wise to avoid an insignificant healing crisis and to run chances of developing cancer in later life, or is it better to give the organism a thorough housecleaning in order to eliminate the morbid miasms and this to preclude the possibility of malignant tumors and of other chronic destructive diseases?

Medical statistics prove that during the last fifty years, among the common causes of death, cancer shows an increase of 400 per cent. This simply confirms our opinion that the more refined the old school of medicine becomes in the suppression of acute diseases and the more they contaminate the blood of our people with small pox, anti-toxin and other disease miasms the greater will be the increase in chronic destructive diseases.

In the following we give the history of another typical psora case and of its development under natural treatment. Mr. B. of Chicago (his name and address can be had on application) will be pleased to acknowledge the following statements: This man had been a chronic invalid ever since childhood, doctoring continually for all sorts of ailments, and growing worse instead of better. Four years ago he had become so weak that he was obliged to give up his profession and the doctors declared his to be a hopeless case.

Accidentally he met Doctor Lane, the author of the *Diagnosis from the Eye*. The doctor, after a superficial glance into his eyes, remarked, "Early in life you had the itch and it was suppressed. The poison then concentrated and located in small intestine, causing chronic intestinal indigestion, irritation and occasional diarrheas. You are now in great danger of developing cancer in the affected parts."

Mr. B. at once admitted the correctness of the diagnosis. He stated that while the doctors had treated him mostly for "stomach troubles", he had always felt and insisted that most of the difficulty was in the bowels. On closer inspection Dr. Lane made the statement that there were two distinct and separate itch spots, the one overlying the other, and that, therefore, the itch must have been suppressed twice. Mr. B. corroborated this also, saying he remembered distinctly that his mother had twice cured his itch eruptions with sulphur and mercurial ointment.

Dr. Lane then informed the patient that he could be cured easily and thoroughly by strict adherence to pure food diet and by systematic Nature Cure treatment, and he concluded by saying that, if his theory and diagnosis of the case were correct, itch eruptions would again manifest on the surface as healing crisis. This, however, would not occur until the organism had been sufficiently purified and strengthened by the natural regimen.

Mr. B., captivated by this remarkable diagnosis and prognosis of his case, entered with enthusiasm on the new plan of living and of cure. His improvement from the beginning was remarkable. After the lapse of two months, having passed through the first preliminary crisis, he returned to work and has not missed a day's labor for many years.

A year after he had entered upon the simple life I met him in Dr. Lane's office. The doctor gave me an introduction and demonstrated the case to me from the eyes and from the history of the patient.

Mr. B. reported remarkable improvement in every respect. Both patient and doctor, however, were somewhat puzzled because so far there had not been any manifestation of itch and because the spots in the iris had not changed nor diminished to any considerable extent.

## HOMEOPATHY, A BRANCH OF NATURE CURE

On inquiry I found that so far homeopathic remedies had not been administered and suggested that "psorinum", Hahnemann's great anti-psoric remedy, should be given a trial. The patient received one dose of psorinum C.M. Nine days after this he broke out on arms and body with the typical itch eruptions. At the same time he developed a violent intestinal crisis manifesting as severe colic and diarrhea. One day he reported in alarm that his bowels were passing away from him. On inspection it was found that these "bowels" were the decayed casings of his diseased intestines.

This simultaneous, external and internal crisis conclusively proved the relationship between suppressed itch, itch spot in the iris, chronic enteritis, itch eruption and internal crisis. The acute reactions lasted fourteen days. The scabies then disappeared and the bowels subsided into their natural condition and normal activity. The treatment during this crisis consisted of fasting and the usual cold water treatment, no medicines of any kind being given. After this thorough house cleaning, he felt greatly improved in body and mind and an examination of the iris revealed the fact that the uppermost layer of the itch spot had disappeared, but the lower and darker layer was still in evidence.

Six months afterward the patient, who had in the meantime continued in the right way of living and of treatment, received another dose of "psorinum", partly in order to stir up the remaining psora and partly to prove whether or not the first results had been merely accidental. Six days after he received the remedy, an acne form eruption appeared on his body. This lasted about three weeks and was accompanied by a severe catarrhal condition of the nasal and respiratory passages. This crisis also left him much improved in general health.

At the present date the remainder of the itch spot in the iris is very small and has paled into a yellowish color.

This remarkable case is instructive in many respects. It proves the correctness of the diagnosis from the eye; the efficiency of natural diet and Nature Cure treatment; the truths of Hahnemann's theory of psora, and of his law of *similia similibus curantor.* This is only one of many cases which can be cited as positive proof of the laws and principles laid down and demonstrated in these pages.

After reading this history of a psora case our friend Homeopath will be tempted to say, "Why bother with Nature Cure? After all, the Homeopathic remedy had to do the work."

No, brother Homeopath, "psorinum" alone did not do the work. It merely gave the final push and pull to the psora-encumbered cells which aroused them into acute activity. Nature Cure first had to purify and sensitize the organism before the Homeopathic potency could act. We always use the *similia* together with our other natural methods of cure, but we find that in many cases where the vitality is low and the organism heavily encumbered with disease and drug poisons, the indicated remedy alone is too weak to produce a reaction. When, however, the system has been sufficiently purified of its grosser encumbrances and when the entire body has been stimulated into vigorous activity, then a high potency of the similar remedy often does wonders.

True, Nature Cure means the harmonious combination of all natural healing factors in accordance with the fundamental laws of Cure and with the individual characteristics of the case. To treat serious chronic ailments with one 'pathy' or one method when many others are at our service is too much like pulling a heavy load with one horse when others are idle in the stable.

*The psoric theory claims that age-long persistent suppression of itchy, parasitic skin eruptions and of gonorrheal and syphilitic diseases has encumbered almost the entire human race with three well-defined hereditary taints or miasms.*

*Since the discovery of germs and bacteria, Allopathy has extended this local and parasitic conception of disease so as to embrace almost every known pathological condition. As a natural corollary of this theory, germ killing has become the basis of modern medical science.*

*The psoric taints which Nature was trying to eliminate, now reinforced by drug poisons and by the deadly miasms contained in the bodies of the parasites themselves, recede into the interior and in place of being distributed throughout the entire body they now concentrate in some vital part or organ, and chronic headaches, epilepsy, chorea, asthma, nervousness, sexual perversity, etc., are often the result.*

*With two exceptions so far in our practice, every case of cancer which we have cured has developed itch eruptions as healing crisis.*

*Medical statistics prove that during the last fifty years, among the common causes of death, cancer shows an increase of 400 per cent. This simply confirms our opinion that the more refined the old school of medicine becomes in the suppression of acute diseases and the more they contaminate the blood of our people with small pox, anti-toxin and other disease miasms the greater will be the increase in chronic destructive diseases.*

*Knowing these facts, is it wise to avoid an insignificant healing crisis and to run chances of developing cancer in later life, or is it better to give the organism a thorough house-cleaning in order to eliminate the morbid miasms and this to preclude the possibility of malignant tumors and of other chronic destructive diseases?*

# The New Psychology

## by Henry Lindlahr, M.D.

*The Naturopath and Herald of Health, XV (8), 458-461. (1910)*

In this great domain of medical science Nature Cure occupies a unique and isolated position, and the mere claim that it permanently cures at least 50 per cent of all so-called incurable nervous disorders, and of insanity, awakens incredulity where it does not draw down the wrath of our orthodox fellow physicians. Nevertheless, for years such cures have been made by physicians in excellent standing, and positive proof of the facts can be conclusively shown to anyone who cares to investigate.

## A New Classification

The diagnosis and classification of mental disorders given by the regular schools of medicine are not in exact conformity with actual conditions and are therefore very confusing and unsatisfactory. We shall give in a series of articles on the NEW PSYCHOLOGY our own classification of nervous and mental disorders and describe their causes, symptoms and cures from our own "Nature Cure" point of view.

To begin with, we divide all nervous and mental disorders into two great groups:

The Physiological Or Organic Group

The Psychological Group

Under the head of Physiological Insanity, we classify all those types of mental and nervous disorders due to abnormal organic changes in the physical brain and nerve matter; under Psychological, all those types which have been produced by mental and psychic causes.

Roughly speaking about one-half of all cases confined in our insane asylums belong to the Physiological group, that is to say, they are due to the presence of waste matter and poisons, or to abnormal changes in nerve and brain matter; and the other half, or Psychological group of disorders, are due to weakening and destructive psychological influences. Morbid encumbrances and decay of brain matter often open the way for disorders of the psychological type. The interblending of these two types produces many varieties.

We shall now give a brief description of each group and then proceed to analyze in detail various disorders belonging to these main types.

## Organic Insanity

A few cases of organic insanity are caused by injury to the brain, but the great majority are due to the action of morbid matter and of paralyzing or destructive poisons on the physical brain matter. These poisons in a few cases may have been generated in the body by unnatural methods of living, they may be alcohol, nicotine, caffeine or destructive acids, and paralyzing alkaloids which are the waste products of starchy and protein digestion. Morbid encumbrances and organic decay are frequently due to the suppression of scrofulous, psoric and syphilitic diseases. About 60 per cent of all organic cases, however, are due to the ever lengthening array of destructive drug poisons, such as mercury, iodine, quinine, arsenic, phenacetin, anti-kamnia, bromine, etc.

### ORGANIC DEFECTS

Organic defects are created in the following manner: Earthy waste matter often forms deposits in, and clogs and hardens the minute blood vessels of brain and nerve centers. Poisons and alkaloids of the uric acid type, or destructive drug poisons, cause obstructions, abnormal changes, decay and actual destruction of nerve and brain matter.

To this group of Organic or Physiological Insanity belong all nervous and mental disorders classed by the regular school of medicine as arteriosclerosis, paresis, *dementia paralytica,* senile dementia, *tabies,* paralysis agitans, locomotor ataxia, etc.

This entire range of diseases is looked upon by the orthodox medical profession as incurable. Nevertheless, we constantly prove in our practice that all of these cases can be alleviated and that one-half of them can be cured by natural methods of treatment, provided there is sufficient vitality left in the organism to respond to treatment, and provided that actual destruction or hardening of brain and nerve matter has not too far advanced.

The "regular" treatment of these disorders consists almost universally in the administration of the so-called "alteratives"; that is, of mercury, iodine, arsenic, strychnine and of the coal tar products as palliatives and sedatives. The diagnosis from the eye and the history of these types of cases, however, reveals the fact that almost without exception these diseases have been produced, in the first place, by the absorption of these same poisons earlier in life.

How then, can such cases be cured by the same poisons which produce them? Is it any wonder that "regular" science calls them "incurable" when "too much drugging" is all that ails them? Is it any wonder when they improve under Christian Science or any other negative treatment? Every case of locomotor ataxia, paralysis agitans and paresis which has come under our observation revealed the signs of "alteratives" in the eyes and a close inquiry into the history of these cases usually confirms the drug records in the eye.

It takes the mercury from 5 to 16 years to work its way through the bony structures into brain and spinal cord, and then its destructive symptoms begin to manifest. What is commonly called secondary and tertiary syphilis is nothing but mercurial and iodine poisoning. Syphilis and gonorrhea in themselves are easily curable by natural methods of treatment. If properly treated, without poisonous drugs, these taints can be completely eradicated from the system within four or five months' time. Not a single case treated by us from its incipiency—that is, before mercury was given—has ever developed any secondary or tertiary symptoms or hereditary diseases in the offspring. Many other types of organic insanity reveal the signs and histories of quinine, iodine or coal tar poisoning.

But we shall treat at greater length the subject of physiological or organic insanity in future articles. We shall now proceed to a consideration of psychological insanity.

### PSYCHOLOGICAL INSANITY

While the preceding statements pertaining to organic insanity may seem in many respects radical and revolutionary, our analysis of Psychological Insanity may be considered even more extravagant. I am very aware of the fact that anyone calling himself M.D. who dares to utter statements like the following is certain to fall not only under the ban of orthodoxy but also under the ban of the liberal but materialistic and agnostic elements in and out of the profession.

For instance, Brother Tilden, of the *Stuffed Club* will surely put us down among the same class of patients which we are now going to discuss. However, as a "Nature Cure Doctor" we are already so hopelessly "irregular and unscientific" that a few more sins added to our already long list of medical and scientific heresies matter but very little.

We have been strongly warned by good friends not to destroy the value of our "scientific" work by bringing in tabooed "spiritualistic" subjects.

To this we wish to say:

Firstly—While we recognize the verity of spiritualistic phenomena, no one can realize more fully than we the destructive nature of hypnotism and mediumship, the more so as a large part of our practice consists in overcoming the detrimental results of these practices.

Secondly—Knowing that the conditions and phenomena described in these articles are positive truth, verified by many years of practical experience and close observation, are we justified in withholding a knowledge which is of such vital importance to the public in general and to the victims of the hypnotists and of the séance room in particular?

Thirdly—Why not give ourselves wholly as we are? The phenomena of destructive psychism are so closely interwoven with all subjects pertaining to Life, Health, Disease, Death and Immortality that it would be very difficult to do justice to one phase of life's phenomena and at the same time hide and obscure other phases of equal or even greater importance.

Many good and wise men in the front ranks of the medical profession know the facts which I am going to disclose, but they refrain from discussing them publicly for fear of losing professional prestige and of being ostracized from medical societies. Before very long, however, whispered truths will become public property, and if the statements which we are about to make are really true, the sooner the public learns about them the better. Someone in the ranks of practicing physicians will have to open the subject for discussion.

All we have to say has been treated already in a masterly manner by the anonymous author of the *Great Psychological Crime*. Years of close observation and practical application of the principles disclosed in this remarkable volume have convinced us of the truths therein contained, and we would advise anyone interested in the subject of Psychology to carefully study this great work.

### THE CAUSES OF PSYCHIC DISEASES

The majority of psychological mental disorders are induced by negative, sensitive conditions on one or more planes of being. We mean by this that physical, mental and moral vigor and resistance have become weakened in some way or another and that as a result reason, will and self-control are benumbed and paralyzed to such an extent that the individual comes into abnormal contact with the lower spiritual planes of existence and lays himself open to hypnotic control by other intelligences in or out of the physical body.

The paranoiac, the delusional maniac, the true medium, etc., are frequently hypnotically controlled by other intelligences on the physical or spiritual planes of being.

The drunkard in delirium tremens actually seeing things. The snakes and other horrid creatures which terrify him are not altogether hallucinations of a distorted imagination. In his case the physical organism and its senses, under the deadening influence of alcohol have become so benumbed and paralyzed that the senses of the spiritual body are abnormally active. In other words, the victim of alcohol becomes clairvoyant on the lowest plane of spiritual life—the hell of the theologians.

Our physical material place of life corresponds, as far as location in space is concerned, to the lowest spiritual plane, and therein lies the awful danger of premature and abnormal psychic development through negative subjective processes. All such experiments are extremely dangerous so long as the individual is bound by his heavy physical body, and by heavy spiritual gravity, to the lowest place of spirit life.

The doctors who lately "weighed the soul" by observing and recording the loss of weight at the point of death were right in their conclusions. The spiritual body, mentioned by Paul and visible to the independent seer, is material just as well as the physical body, and, although this spiritual counterpart of the physical body consists of matter in a very rarefied form, it still occupies space and has some weight.

Those who, by a weakening of willpower and by subjective, negative processes of psychic development rashly expose themselves to psychic control and abnormal quickening of the spiritual organs of sense, come in contact with the slums and vicious inhabitants of the lowest planes of spiritual life.

To the religiously inclined who doubt these statements we would say that if these things are untrue, then the New Testament is false from beginning to end. If obsession was a fact in Nature 1,900 years ago, then it is fact today.

To the materialistic, skeptical scientist I should simply adapt the quotation and bid him remember, "There are really more things in heaven and earth, no medical Horatio, than have been dreamed of in thy philosophy."

Only he who has sincerely and earnestly investigated and tested these subjects has a right to speak and judge.

When I took incurable paranoiacs from a State Insane Asylum, the doctor in charge smiled at my presumption, and informed me that never in history of the institution had a case been cured. Yet we have permanently cured many such cases within from two to four months' time.

It is not to be wondered at, however, that these patients are incurable under the conventional treatment when we stop to consider that insane asylums are veritable "hells on earth", where ignorant and vicious spirits congregate to obsess and vampirize defenseless victims. The latter are usually rendered more negative and subjective by idleness, negative diet, solitude, confinement, constant intercourse with other insane, a vicious spiritual atmosphere, and by the paralyzing influence of sedative and hypnotic drugs which are negative in their effects on the human organism.

*The diagnosis and classification of mental disorders given by the regular schools of medicine are not in exact conformity with actual conditions and are therefore very confusing and unsatisfactory.*

*The "regular" treatment of these disorders consists almost universally in the administration of the so-called "alteratives"; that is, of mercury, iodine, arsenic, strychnine and of the coal tar products as palliatives and sedatives.*

*It takes the mercury from 5 to 16 years to work its way through the bony structures into brain and spinal cord, and then its destructive symptoms begin to manifest.*

*It is not to be wondered at, however, that these patients are incurable under the conventional treatment when we stop to consider that insane asylums are veritable "hells on earth", where ignorant and vicious spirits congregate to obsess and vampirize defenseless victims.*

# Is Medicine Behind Time?

## by Benedict Lust

*The Naturopath and Herald of Health, XV (12), 749-750. (1910)*

The *open-air treatment* which has been extensively practiced and advocated by the natural healing school for the last hundred years ever since that genius Priessnitz, first introduced it in his water cure treatments is of late being more favorably considered by some of the "advanced" medical practitioners who are daring enough to investigate the causes of the success of "irregular" practitioners all over the world.

So-called progressive medicine is as orthodox and narrow-minded to-day as it was hundred years ago, when Priessnitz dared to treat cases that were pronounced chronic and incurable, and by way of natural methods, such water-cure and open-air treatments they got well. Such success was preposterous then to the "regulars" who would only drug the poor patients, as it is ridiculous to them to-day, when a naturopath or an osteopath, or a chiropractor, or a neurologist succeeds with a confirmed chronic, after all medical school fool-doctors with their nasty drugs had failed. In spite of all the successful cures of the natural healing school, from Priessnitz and his followers down to Kneipp, and Still, and Palmer, and McCormick, in our days, medicine as a school and system, had only contempt and ridicule to offer the new school of healing. However, this bold and much-ridiculed imp, like young David of scriptural times, proved to be a veritable giant destined to slay the antiquated, arrogant, sluggish monster medicine. An ever increasing army of natural healers is diligently busy to spread the teachings and practices of the various systems of natural healing, and their followers are counted by the millions in all parts of the civilized world. In this very country of ours, there are about twenty million happy people who discarded drugs, and are following the various drugless, natural healing systems in vogue. While there may be some differences in minor ideas and methods, they all agree on the dangerousness and uselessness of drugs, vaccines, serums, anti-toxins, and mutilating operations of medicine. They are marching separately forward and onward, ever-ready to unite forces when called upon to fight the common old arch-enemy of natural healing and of personal liberty to choose our own physicians. The right spirit of solidarity fills them all, and thrills the hearts of those progressive millions of lovers of the natural way of living and curing.

True enough, ignorance, superstition, prejudice, and fallacies, upon which ancient medicine is founded, are hard to overcome and to root out. However, science, nature, and experience, the mighty fundament

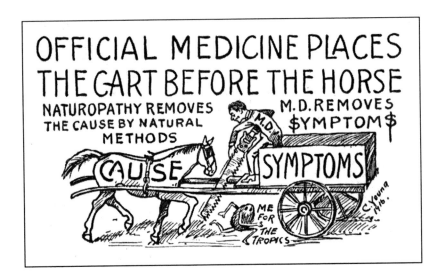

on which the School of Natural Healing stands, are the greatest powers known to us, and they are bound to win out in any struggle with the powers of darkness. Truth will win out, and it is ever victorious. And while it is true that one may fool some people sometimes, it is just as true that one cannot fool all the people all the time. And that is exactly what medicine found out. It realizes now that it had its days, and that its doom is set. People are observing the *results* of natural healing methods, and *results tell the story,* after all. Against *facts* all medical twaddle becomes ridiculous. To-day, millions of highly intelligent people have come to the conclusion that poor old medicine is a decided failure, and that to the School of Natural Healing belongs to the future.

Wide awake medical practitioners are realizing the true situation, and are quietly or openly adopting the natural methods of healing and treatment for which the people are clamoring. Unless they drop medicine altogether, and try to study the laws of nature, and free themselves from all medical notions and fallacies about the nature, cause and cure of disease, their reforming will not amount to much, and their efforts of mixing the natural with the unnatural methods of treatment will be more harmful than beneficial to themselves as well as to others.

In the children's department at the Philadelphia Hospital, they have been experimenting, for some time, with open-air treatment, and the results, although obtained under medical management, proved to be encouraging. Since the introduction of this method, even in spite of the fact that drugging and medical dieting still prevail, the mortality in certain diseases of children, was greatly reduced, so that this open-air-treatment is now permanently established at this department of the hospital.

But it took our medical friends at Philadelphia all these many years to find out the great value of the open-air treatment long since established by the School of Natural Healing. And it will cost many a thousand of lives more, before the drug-ridden medical schools will grasp the idea, and incorporate it into their course of study. Better late than never. Meanwhile poor suffering humanity depending on medicine dragging behind times will have to wait and foot the bill of medical prejudice, incompetency and backwardness.

While it is rather gratifying and deserving of encouragement whenever honest attempts at reform are made by members of the medical fraternity, one must rather be reserved in all such cases, since it is a matter of fact, that medical men in general are hard to unlearn so many useless and dangerous things before they can learn the most necessary essentials of the true science and art of healing and master the natural methods. Their previous medial education is usually a detriment and a drawback hard to overcome. Their mere shifting from one system of treatment to another does by no means give them the knowledge and efficiency so essential in their practice and success. It takes both time and efforts to unmake a medical and to make a true physician of the School of Natural Healing.

Of the truth of this fact, the Philadelphia incident is but another illustration. The medical superintendent of the children's department, who introduced the open-air treatment—and who, by the way, is professor of diseases in children in the Jefferson Medical College—in a report of his experiment, winds up with the following words: "Let us all join hands and preach fresh air; vote for open squares, endorse roof gardens, *have adenoids and tonsils removed.*" Here we have a good example of the true medical mixer of the natural and the unnatural. Think of it, this man after seeing the wonderful results of open-air-treatment, which reduce the mortality compared with that of the exclusive medical treatment; still recommends the useless and harmful mutilation of poor innocent children! That is the curse of half-truth! Formerly, these miserable medical butchers confined themselves more to the mutilating of the adults, by cutting out the "useless" thyroid gland, the "useless" appendix; and by unsexing the poor woman; but now, they commence already with the poor babies! Where will the cutting mania end? It is high time, that we put a stop to their entering our schools and ordering the adenoids and tonsils cut out of our children. There is no telling what we would have to suffer, if that famous Owen's Bill would become a law establishing a Public Health Departments under the management of these barbarous medical mutilators.* Let the past be our lesson, and prevent a perpetuation of

---

* The Owen Bill drafted by Senator Robert Owen of Oklahoma in 1910 had culminated in the establishment of the Federal Department of Public Health. —*Ed.*

vaccination, inoculation, and mutilation. Onward and forward the march of civilization goes, in harmony with nature, science and humanity; and not backward and downward into the barbarity of poisonous drugging, and the cruel tortures of operative mutilations of degenerated medicine. *Eternal vigilance is the price of liberty from all medical tyranny. Remember the Medical Trust!*

*So-called progressive medicine is as orthodox and narrow-minded to-day as it was hundred years ago, when Priessnitz dared to treat cases that were pronounced chronic and incurable, and by way of natural methods, such water-cure and open-air treatments they got well.*

*While there may be some differences in minor ideas and methods, they all agree on the dangerousness and uselessness of drugs, vaccines, serums, anti-toxins, and mutilating operations of medicine. They are marching separately forward and onward, ever-ready to unite forces when called upon to fight the common old archenemy of natural healing and of personal liberty to choose our own physicians.*

*To-day, millions of highly intelligent people have come to the conclusion that poor old medicine is a decided failure, and that to the School of Natural Healing belongs to the future.*

*And it will cost many a thousand of lives more, before the drug-ridden medical schools will grasp the idea, and incorporate it into their course of study.*

*While it is rather gratifying and deserving of encouragement whenever honest attempts at reform are made by members of the medical fraternity, one must rather be reserved in all such cases, since it is a matter of fact, that medical men in general are hard to unlearn so many useless and dangerous things before they can learn the most necessary essentials of the true science and art of healing and master the natural methods.*

# 1911

## THE "NATURE CURE"
### DR. MARGARET GOETTLER

---

## RULES OF BATHING IN THE AIR-LIGHT BATH
### BENEDICT LUST, N.D.

This ad appeared in 1911 in Benedict Lust's journal a year after the Flexner Report. Ironically, Andrew Carnegie, along with John D. Rockefeller, was a major sponsor of the Flexner Report published in 1910.

# THE "NATURE CURE"

## by Dr. Margaret Goettler

*The Naturopath and Herald of Health, XVI (4), 37-39. (1911)*

Following is a paper read by Dr. Margaret Goettler, of Pasadena at the first annual meeting of the Association of Naturopaths of California.

"'Not to know at large of things remote from us lies in daily life is the prime wisdom.' These words by John Milton suit me fully tonight, for I come so poorly prepared to speak that I will surely not go back for data any further than I can possibly help.

"Repeatedly we are asked, 'What is a Naturopath?' If you try to find the word in a dictionary, I fear you will have a difficult time. The expression is somewhat older than our association, and was conceived by Dr. Lust of New York and Dr. Schultz of Los Angeles.* These two are among the men who have brought ideas for which the word stands to this continent. The word is a translation of the German *Naturheil-methode*, which means 'the art of healing by and through nature', that is, air, light, water and earth; air, without which nothing can live; light, the greatest disinfectant there is; water, the nourishment of nature itself; and soil, imparting electricity.

"Some of the first and most prominent men in this movement have been: Kneipp (he of the barefoot walking fame), Rausse, Kuhne, Rikli—all these of Europe—and Trall and Rheinhold of New York, the last named in particular issuing excellent books. All have passed on for their reward, which they fully deserve, for these men have been true benefactors to mankind, true philanthropists, although none of them possessed, as my knowledge goes, much of any worldly means, but every fiber in them was yearning to do good to their neighbor. They were true Christians. They have also fully disproven the principle of 'stick to the point when it is narrowly taken'. One ought rather say 'hold fast to the line'. Most of these men were not college bred, with a number of years more or less wasted, but good, practical laymen, natural scholars and common-sense thinkers. For this reason some individuals try to belittle them, but they forget that the founder of manufacture of cotton was a barber, the screw propeller was invented by a farmer, the man to endow London with good water was a goldsmith, the inventor of the telegraph was a photographer, and John Hunter, the physiologist, was a day laborer.

"Neither is naturopathy something new, for the Greeks knew fully

---

*The author may have confused the person who coined the term "Naturopathy". John Scheel and his wife Sofia were the first to use the word, Naturopathy, in the promotion of their clinic. Please see the Scheel ad that appeared in *The Kneipp Water Cure Monthly* in 1901 on page 78.—*Ed.*

the value of air-baths. Arnold Rikli was the man to reinforce them in 1885. At present Dr. Winternitz is considered the greatest authority on hydropathy in Germany. He, although a medical doctor, became a scholar of Preissnitz. Preissnitz died in 1851.

"Kneipp took his ideas from Sigismund and Oscar Hahn, whose book was published as early as 1672. Kneipp added the use of non-poisonous herbs, as teas and baths. At the time of his death in 1897 he had 1,500 patients at his water-cure establishment at Wöerishofen, Bavaria.

"The most prominent men of recent date in the field are Lahmann, then Bilz, who has a magnificent sanatorium at Dresden, Kolb, Platen and some others. At all of these establishments the vegetarian diet and non-stimulating drinks are encouraged to bring about best results in addition to their mode of treatment, which consists of sun- and air-baths taken in parks especially provided for that purpose, or as a substitute for the sun-bath, the electric-light bath. Then vapor and herbal baths, hot and cold packs and gushes, massage, and electricity, light therapy, vibration, gymnastics etc. Dr. Medtzger, formerly of Amsterdam, now of Wiesbaden, is the best authority on massage. This mode also originated with the ancients, and is greatly used in Japan, where the blind are educated to manipulate the body. Reibmeyer is another authority on massage. Brandt, a major in the Swedish army, is another. Osteopathy and chiropractic are also branches of naturopathy.

"Someone has aptly said, 'How can we acquire patience if we never bore a burden? How can the individual acquire pity if he was never allowed to see suffering of others?' All of these men mentioned had their full share of persecution and prosecution. Kuhne, who taught the oneness of disease and made wonderful cures, died with a broken heart, and our men of the present time are not exempt. Dr. Lust of New York has to sacrifice much of his time and money in the courts of that city, and Dr. Carl Shultz, who brought Naturopathy to the western coast, has had an abundance of trials and tribulations. Had it not been for his determination and courage and his good wife's labor and devotion to the cause with the assistance of a capable third, George Dryden of San Francisco, who assisted in the political campaign, in addition to our friends who will speak later on, we would not be here to celebrate to-night. It was these people's freedom and conviction of thought that brought such success to the naturopaths of this state, the only state of the Union so far advanced.

"Naturopathy also encourages fasting, to clear stomach and mind; physical culture, to create deep breathing; and as to suggestion—every physician ought to be a suggestion to his patients for mind and body—an educator. This reminds me of what Father Vaughan says in his sermons from Shakespeare, "Shakespeare is a liberal education when we come to understand education properly. It means something more than the know-

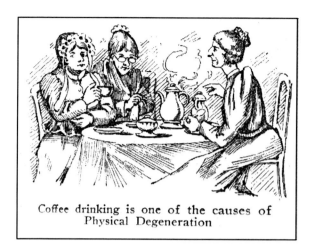

Coffee drinking is one of the causes of
Physical Degeneration

ing the dates and facts and figures, something more than a memorizing of rules and formulas. Education, when we come to understand, truly means, taking the first steps into God's great world. It is getting our bearings aright on the sea of life. To me, education is the lighting of a lamp by which we may read aright the enigmas of life, the unfolding of the human soul, whereby we may drink in the wonders and the mysteries and the laws and the beauties which the hand of God has painted all over the face of nature. True education is to know something of the heartaches, the death pangs, the anxious seeking, the bitter disappointments and the soul's yearnings of the human race, and so be able to attune our own hearts to be in harmony with God's great world around us."

"This is and should be the ambition of Naturopaths—to assist our patients mentally, as well as physically, to bring them closer to God or nature—call it which you like—to make plainer, nobler characters of them, to teach them that we are valuable as we make ourselves valuable to others, that there is no glory or true satisfaction in being a bull or bear of Wall Street, that true happiness comes only with a healthy mind and body, and such can be attained only by moderation in eating and drinking, abundance of sunshine, cleanliness in thought and body, and common-sense wearing apparel, such that will leave the body in proper poise where the Creator intended it to be.

"Personally, I am convinced that the vegetarian diet, if the combinations are made correctly, is the better one to develop the best mental and physical powers. Not that we have more strength, but most assuredly more reserve energy, never being overstimulated. I also endorse it from a humanitarian standpoint, and would plead with our women to give this matter more thought. To my mind it certainly takes the most proficient woman to conduct a home and kitchen intelligently and thereby influence and benefit not only her own family, but indirectly the different sections of the whole human family. Woman is and always has been the making or unmaking of man in general. If you get to be master of yourself and palate, hold your inner self in hand. After that, listen to nature. It is truly an easy matter to be well.

"Allow me to urge you to learn to know what naturopathy fully stands for; time not allowing me all that I would like to impress you with. Bear this is mind—Naturopathy does not treat symptoms, but goes to the root and tries to find the cause of mental and physical illness.

"Some will say, 'Oh, I would rather lead a short and merry life, eat and drink as I choose.' Without giving it a second thought, this may seem quite reasonable, but how can that individual tell us how long before he will have overfilled his system, becoming disabled, going about a burden to himself and others, wearing out two or three persons, before he is able to breathe the last?

"Naturopaths are no faddist, no extremists, or eccentrics. They simply refer you to natural law, and Nature will never be deceived."

---

*At present Dr. Winternitz is considered the greatest authority on hydropathy in Germany. He, although a medical doctor, became a scholar of Preissnitz. Preissnitz died in 1851.*

*Kuhne, who taught the oneness of disease and made wonderful cures, died with a broken heart, and our men of the present time are not exempt. Dr. Lust of New York has to sacrifice much of his time and money in the courts of that city, and Dr. Carl Shultz, who brought Naturopathy to the western coast, has had an abundance of trials and tribulations.*

*Bear this is mind—Naturopathy does not treat symptoms, but goes to the root and tries to find the cause of mental and physical illness.*

# Rules Of Bathing In The Air-Light Bath

## by Benedict Lust, N.D.

*The Naturopath and Herald of Health, XVI (5), 288. (1911)*

1.  Air-light baths should be taken not only on warm, sunny days, but also when the weather is cool and gloomy. In this case they have a very refreshing effect if combined with lively exercise. The air-baths should be begun in the warm season to become accustomed to them and must not be extended too long in the beginning.

2.  The air-light bath shall not be applied especially for the sake of causing perspiration, but to promote the influence of light and air upon the naked body. The whole body can hereby properly evaporate and draw in pure, healthy air by the pores of the skin.

3.  After undressing there must in cool weather strong exercise be taken. The cooler the temperature, the shorter must be the bath and the stronger the exercise.

4.  After having become accustomed to the air-bath, it can be extended as long and repeated as often in a day as one feels comfortable.

5.  Nobody must be chilled in an air-bath. If the motion of the body gives not warmth enough, the bath must be interrupted at once. One must dress again and try to regain the lost warmth by exercise, athletics, sanitary gymnastics, by running quickly, etc.

6.  His layer or position the bather must change in the sun about every ten minutes, as inflammation of the skin may easily be caused by sun-burning, which appears mostly in the heat of summer. If in spite of this protection the skin is being inflamed, the infected places must often be cooled by lukewarm, or cool water, the sunbeams be avoided and the air-bath taken covered with a shirt.

7.  Oversensitive persons can protect their head and neck by large straw hats, veils, etc., from the sunbeams.

8.  Nervous persons are much strengthened by short air-light baths, but they must expose themselves directly to the sunbeams on hot days moderately only, on account of their irritating effects.

9.  Sun-baths, i.e., the open lying in the sunshine effect greatly the change of substance matter and are therefore most useful in cases of gout, rheumatism, diabetes, obesity, etc. But they must not, on hot days especially, be taken for a longer time than one feels comfortable and must be often interrupted by bathing in the shade.

10. In sand-baths the warmth of the sunbeams and of the earth are

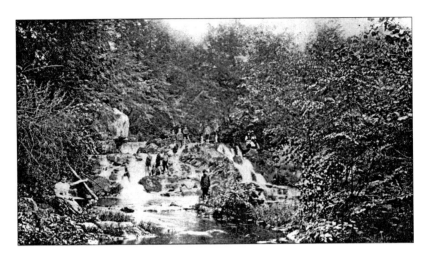

The air and light baths were central to the activities enjoyed at the Butler Yungborn.

stored up in common. They are very salubrious also by the magnetism of the earth, are greatly inciting, giving warmth and absorbing perspiration. But only the higher layers of the sand must be used which are thoroughly warmed by the sun. The sand-baths give also an opportunity for exercises with shovel and spade.

11. Rain-baths are extremely influential upon the nervous system and the brain. The head and neck must therefore be protected here also, and during the bath quick movements must be made, but it must not be extended too long. A fast walking and jumping can be here recommended. Nervous people may avoid them.

12. An application of water (a bath douche, a rain-bath, lavations, treading water, or running on a wet lawn) may be combined with the air-bath if a desire is felt for it; on cool days omit this. After the application one must not be standing about in a wet bathing-costume, but must change it and take exercise.

13. After every air-bath a perfect warming up must follow by a corresponding exercise.

14. The air-light bath brightens up the mind and acts exhilaratingly, especially when combined with gymnastics, athletics, sport and a humorous conversation. It creates a new enjoyment of life and work.

15. It is hardly necessary to mention that not only men, but also women and children, if possible, should daily take air-light baths. Even the very little ones should be accustomed to air-baths; they may on cool days bustle about in their shirts.

## Hints On How To Sleep Soundly
### Edward Earle Purinton

## Vibration And Health
### T. R. Gowenlock

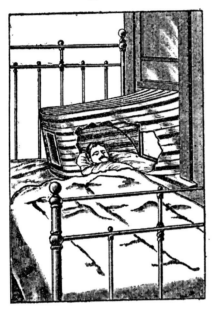
The window tent allowed it's users to breathe fresh air while they slept.

# Hints On How To Sleep Soundly

## by Edward Earle Purinton

*The Naturopath and Herald of Health, XVII (2), 75-81. (1912)*

### 1. Sleep Outdoors—Or As Near It As Possible

This suggestion is put first because it seems of first importance. Scientific articles pertaining thereto may be found in the *Cosmopolitan Magazine* of April, 1907, and in back files of *Health-Culture*. For the present let us quote verbatim a little essay by Julian Hawthorne in the *New York American*—Mr. Hawthorne being the one popular man writer, so far as I know, who can look squarely on two sides of a matter of health and see both without squinting. He writes thus,

"At the risk of being monotonous, I must once more call your attention to the importance of improving every opportunity to sleep in the open air. If you live in a tenement, you may perhaps contrive some sort of a shake-down on the roof—you will not be crowded there until hygiene comes to be more widely understood in this country. If you are in more sumptuous quarters in the city, you may rig up a bed-extension which goes through the lower part of your bedroom window, and allows you to sleep with your head actually out of doors. But well-to-do folks need not resort to such devices, for they are able to leave the city in the warm weather, and once there, there is no excuse for stifling yourself in a bedroom. There must be a balcony somewhere; or you may hang a hammock between two apple trees, or between the posts of the veranda. Sleeping in a hammock may not seem to come by nature, but a little practice will enable you to master the art. The open air itself is a medicine which puts one to sleep better than all the narcotics, and it makes your sleep so sound that you need less of it than indoors. Joaquin Miller, the Poet of the Sierras, has a fine verse about its effects on the plains, where, says he, you lie down and sleep for a few hours beneath the stars and wake at dawn with 'your fists full of strength'.

"I am talking for the benefit of those who have never tried outdoor sleeping. Those who have done so need no urging; they are only too anxious to get at it. The chief hardship has been returning to a bedroom in Winter after a Spring and Summer of luxury outside of it. For that matter, there is no real need of sleeping indoors even in Winter, though the arrangements of our modern civilization certainly do facilitate the practice. You will at any rate keep the windows wide open, and move the bed up so as to get the most of what air is going. I used to keep my head up to the open window when I lived down on Long Island, and I awoke one morning in a strange darkness, which turned out to be caused by a snowdrift which had formed over my face during the night; I had breathed two holes through it, and had never noticed the snowfall while it was going on. It is an excellent thing for the complexion, sleeping under snow; but I do not consider it desirable as a rule, because snow over your face impedes the access to your nostrils of the cold Winter air, which is better for the complexion as well as for everything else.

"If you have slept outdoors all Spring and Summer, you will have a better chance of getting through the Winter without sickness than you have ever had before. You will be astonished at the difference it will make in your robustness and animation. Nothing seems to hurt you, and you can live on mince pies and welsh rarebits and thrive. Now is the time to begin; and do not mind a little rain or wind; get under the lee of the house and sleep away, using a rubber blanket to keep your skin dry, and getting the blanket well up about your neck. The mother of Achilles made him invulnerable by dipping him in the enchanted river. Had she made him sleep every night in the great river of the open air, he would have been quite as immune. Begin to-night and keep it up and you will be an athlete and a picture of health before you know it."

As if in direct response to the foregoing advice, the following clipping from the *New York Globe* offers a bit of very human proof as to the wisdom of the course prescribed.

Insomnia? Do I know anything about insomnia? Is there anything about it that I do not know, I wonder?

I have walked miles and dieted until I was as thin as a rail and then I turned around and drank cream and olive oil until I had a figure like a sofa pillow.

I have gone resolutely to bed at 8 o'clock and got up at 5 regardless of whether I had slept or not. And I have stayed up until I actually dropped from fatigue and slept half the next day.

I have trained for an inebriate asylum by drinking stout and pale ale to make me drowsy, and I have drunk cold water until I deserved a gross of white ribbons from the W. C. T. U. *

I have ridden a wheel, toyed with dumbbells, and set up a punching bag which gave me a black eye upon our introduction.

And yet I slept not.

Then came a mild little friend whose advice I had never asked. She said, "Amaryllis, do you turn off heat and open your bedroom window before you go to bed?"

"Yes, it's open two or three inches from the bottom," said the insomniac. "And I always turn off the steam."

"If I were you I'd let it down from the top to within half an inch of

---

*WCTU refers to the National Woman's Christian Temperance Union (WCTU) which was founded in Cleveland, Ohio in November, 1874. ——*Ed.*

the sill and raise the lower part half an inch. Then draw the green shade if you like to keep out the light. Cover yourself well and go to sleep. If you are rheumatic or anaemic you'd better buy a flannel nightgown, and if you are subject to neuralgia make yourself a coquettish nightcap, but make your room as much like outdoors in temperature and atmosphere as possible. If you don't get rid of most of your nerves and all of your insomnia in a month, I'll buy you the finest brass bed and reading lamp on the market."

I smiled incredulously, and that night I followed directions as to the window; but didn't dress the part. Result: numbed feet, a cold in the head, and a stitch in the shoulder. The next day I bought a flannel gown and bed slippers.

I didn't get the brass bed or the reading lamp. In two weeks I had to admit I was cured. I bought my quiet friend a Humane Medal. It is of filigree and dangles from a bracelet, and is enameled with a poppy, the sleep flower.

All life is changed for me now. The days are joyous incidents in a fascinating play called "Life". I used to call it a dull round of care, and when it became dramatic I was apt to compare it to cheap melodrama. I suppose I had cob-webs in my head. Now, I'm filled to the brim with oxygen, and the world isn't either black or white or gray, as it used to be. It's a beautiful, serviceable, earthly, brown, shot through with the gold of the sun and the blue of the sky and the green of the woods a beautiful rainbow world, full of delights and surprises.

I used to lie awake and toss and have the blues; that is all passed. The years don't go marching wearily, monotonously past in a dull gray procession, bearing illness and poverty, loneliness and failure, before my burning eyes. I sleep. I don't think of all my dear dead friends and worry about the woman that ruined my new dress and the sneak thief that stole my pearl brooch. I sleep.

Dreams? Oh yes, I dream, but my dreams are more like visions than dreams. They are so restful. I see wet green hedges starred with wild roses, and the air is fragrant with honeysuckle and sweet with bird songs. I see sapphire seas at dawn with the sun coming up; rose and gold and a flight of swallows skimming back against an opal sky. I hear brooks singing in the dim green coolness of woodland glens.

They say dreams go by contrary you know, and I suppose that is true because when I wake up my room is like Greenland. The polar bears at the zoo would approve of my room for a den, and my family calls me the Eskimo. At first I used to dread to get out of bed. I wanted maids to come in and turn on the steam and close the windows and bring hot tea. But I got over all that. I wake now so full of exhilaration that I stand at the open window and take deep breathing exercises, and I really enjoy them.

I am ready to eat a big breakfast, a thing I never did in my life until lately, and I have my bath and am dressed and ready to tussle with the world in less time than it used to take to get into a bathrobe and moan for a cup of tea. Take my word for it, the greatest of all cures for every ill from pneumonia and tuberculosis to nerves and sleeplessness is sleeping outdoors if you can, or in an ice-cold and well-ventilated room if you can, if you haven't a roof or veranda that you can use as a bedroom.

### 2. SLEEP ALONE

By this I mean, have a room or tent or balcony all to yourself, with no other person near you enough for the breathing to be audible or the presence perceptible. The world of relationships is the waking world; when we sleep as when we die we enter the vale of solitude. As the soul grows it comes to place one's aura and atmosphere before the physical body or mental state and perfect sleep is impossible in the atmosphere of souls unattuned. Separate sleeping rooms are a *spiritual necessity* to unfolded individuals. No matter how congenial two friends may appear by day, when night comes and sleep descends there is always some disparity to the vision of the inner senses. So that presently one feels the suffocation of occupying not merely the same bed but the same room in common. This does not apply to the presence of a pet animal, such as a canary, a kitten, or a poodle. Rather a sad commentary on human nature that we cannot sleep in peace beside our best friend while the dumb brute we buy for a few pennies remains to us harmonious. Human beings are so variously and habitually unfaithful to self that the poorest animal is a truer companion than the most excellent man.

A mother may sleep with her babe, and both be the happier; but *only while her babe is helpless.* Super extended motherhood retards the soul in women more than any other one cause. And the feeling a mother indulges that she belongs to her children produces both weakness in her and selfishness in them. It is *not* natural to arise from one's couch at midnight for the purpose of rocking a baby to sleep. I say this with impunity, not having been a father. If you wise people who have children would only listen to us fools who haven't, what a model world this would be!

Physiologists claim that when two people occupy one bed the vitality of the stronger saps that of the weaker, and thus the arrangement is not hygienic. I think the fact differs somewhat; I think the soul of the weaker follows the soul of the stronger to a haven of refreshment appropriate to the stronger but not to the weaker, and thus the slumber of the latter is disturbed by a spiritual incoherence. This suggestion is only surmise but it helps clear the way for science. Every discovery had a dream as forerunner.

Certain it is that the fully-evolved soul shrinks from the touch of every human body save that belonging to the soul's affinity. The only natural slumber mates are ideal lovers, who can be both animals and gods together. And the lives of these are portrayed nowhere but in the sealed book of Perfected Humanity. The highest attainment possible to a man is to satisfy his sweetheart's ideal; the highest attainment possible to a woman is to attract a lover whose ideal she is! And the only slumber wholly guarded by the angels is the gift of oblivion Nature yields true lovers. Who but sweethearts understand how night holds the key to the portal of peace but Dawn is the usher through paths of power! In the heat and din and riot of noontime we may grit our teeth and mumble a stoic's vow; but when the shadows lengthen into twilight's soft caress, and when the sunrise challenges our motive for the day—ah, then we know we are lovers all in the deeps of the aching heart, and we look with eyes unseeing into the void of space, and we hark with ears benumbed for the lightest footfall, and we wonder if someone waits on the other side of chance with hope as weary as our own, a life as desolate. If only we knew that the way to draw oneself!

### 3. Consider The Character Of Your Bed

Nothing in common usage so needs reforming as the character of our beds, unless it be the character of our books. But as the only effective way to reform a book is to burn it, we shall confine our efforts to the scene of the bolster and counterpane. And here we have to thank modern science for much improvement in matters hygienic. I can easily remember when it wasn't considered good form among the elite of the neighborhood to leave a bed unmade longer than its occupant took to get half-dressed; they woke us up for the express purpose of arranging the coverlet in a geo-metrical fashion, and the housewife was forever disgraced if the pillows looked anyhow but glue to the headboard by a compass and hydraulic press. The power for the hydraulic press could have been generated from the tears of the martyr within. Now airing a bed does not mean letting an accidental breeze flirt a minute with a wrinkle in the top cover—it means stripping the whole business down to the springs and laying out each piece separately where the sun and wind can renovate it. This should be done every morning if time and place and strength should permit. Anyway from the habit of throwing back all the upper covers as far as they will go over the footboard and letting the air from the open window play freely between the sheets. You can almost tell how a man was brought up by watching how he leaves his bed in the morning.

Encourage the children to celebrate frequent pillow-fights. If they are the right kind of children, a very few sallies will suffice to rip the cases open and sift the feathers or whatever other sickly stuff is inside to the four corners of the room. Then will the pillow have achieved its highest destiny. If a little boy should ask me where "nightmares" are stabled, I would tell him in the bolster. Learn to sleep without a pillow; or at most let the anaemic thing be quite hard, and inconsiderable as to thickness. Feathers were for chickens to sleep in, nor for men. Before the age of feather beds women didn't cackle and men didn't crow; there may be some connection. We may note one exception in this matter of pillows—that made of pine is most beneficial either to rest the head upon, or to hang above the bed and breathe the aroma. The use of a pine pillow has been known to cure sleeplessness where all other means failed. To obtain one, address any souvenir store in Lake Placid, N. Y., or the Kalish Drug Store, New York City.

The spring of a bed should be thick, strong, and resilient; the mattress should be of felt, in one piece if available so as to offer an unbroken surface to the position of the body; the frame should be wide to permit of changed postures during the night; the sheets should be of fine linen and large enough to tuck in securely on all sides; the under covers should be thick and soft and plentiful, the upper covers thin but with a supply in reserve so that the grades of required warmth may be exact. The right amount of bedclothes is just enough to keep you warm with enough more at the foot to draw up in the night. Everybody who sleeps indoors is prone to bury himself in a seething mass of wool and cotton; in general the caution should be less and not more covering. I slept one whole winter before an open window in an unheated room with never more than one spread and a sheet over me. This was an extreme measure; it was better for the soul than for the body, but it cured me of a disposition to evade hardship and made me love the essential rigors of development.

The way a bed is made up has more to do with sound sleep than most people ever imagine. Get a hospital nurse to instruct your maid in the art and science thereof. I often wonder why men don't feign illness in order to be cured for properly; perhaps because their wives would attend to them and wives don't know how. How women can be so entirely hopeful yet so utterly helpless is enough to perpetuate a belief in miracles. You want to watch how good men get all of a sudden the day that women cease confusing their business of running a household with their profession of chasing a husband. The acme of human efficiency is to manage a sick man or a well woman.

### 4.  CHANGE YOUR MEAL HOURS

From some experience with the merits and demerits of human habitude I should judge that undigested or ill-digested food is responsible for about three-fourths of the sleeplessness that haunts civilized society. *There can be no insomnia without congestion*; the simple physiology of the matter resolving to excess of blood in brain or stomach. Food digests during the day but assimilates during the night, thus very thin people are martyrs equally and simultaneously to faulty assimilation and sleeplessness. Digestion is a vital process but assimilation a nervous, in this way one's temperament determines one's amount of flesh. Now sleeping soon after eating follows the blood from the brain but leaves the soul in the stomach, and this is not natural, for during slumber the soul instinctively moves toward the sky. A brief siesta after dinner may be salutary but only because we don't know enough to be quiet without it. Dinner should never come less than three hours before bed-time, a four hour interval is better still. If the heavy meal occurs at noon, then a frugal repast might well be served between seven and eight o'clock at night. Watch also the matter of digestion. At least six hours should elapse between the meal of midday and of evening; but if the noon luncheon was wrongly eaten, the stomach may be incapacitated for effective work at night. A bowl of glacial milk and a slap of discouraged pie swallowed as though the crack of doom were scheduled for three minutes hence may put the abused and benumbed stomach out of commission for the rest of the day. To be really hungry is to digest perfectly. Let us hope that someday the cheerful science of feeding ourselves may be as popular as the mournful art of symptomizing us is at this present absurd era of patent medicines and faith cure.

## 5. Study Foods, As To Choice, Preparation, Combination, Effect

I have to inject this advice in order to be conscientious, but in order to be merciful I anxiously entreat you not to pay the slightest attention to it. If you eat oranges, lemons, or other acid fruit in the evening—you won't sleep; if you put away meat, milk, nuts and cheese at the same seven o'clock dinner—you won't sleep; if you mix lobster, pickles and ice-cream in one frantic unmasticated riot; you won't sleep; if you warm your beverage with a boiling soup and cool your chowder with a freezing potation—you won't sleep; if you start to nibble candy before the pork and beans are served—you won't sleep; if you gulp soggy biscuits out of kindness to the cook or nip at this and that concoction to show you knew it was fit to eat—you won't sleep; if you do a hundred-and-one unnatural things at the table—you won't sleep. The science of dietetics is that system of counterfeit wisdom which teaches you to eat what you hate and should rather than what you love and shouldn't. When a melancholy brother announces himself a food-expert, I know either he needs the money or the looney-house is one man short. But if any rash reader, shouldering the entire responsibility, inclines to acquaint himself with these pepsin-pestleizers, the writer or the publisher of this magazine will point the way in fear and trembling and then vanish beyond recall.

A sample suggestion meanwhile. *Fresh salads* are the best soporific. Lettuce, watercress, nasturtium, endive, chicory, and the other bases for salad are distinctly sedative. Onions, asparagus, spinach, kohl-rabi, and allied vegetables also tend to induce sleep if eaten in the evening meal. Fresh apples and pears have the same effect. A little study along this line will amply repay the time and effort. I think that in this field, Eugene Christian of 38 W. 32d Street, New York City, is achieving the most for humanity. His book on Raw Foods I should judge more indispensable to marriage than the license.*

## 6. WATCH HOW YOU FACE

Many psychologists hold the theory that one should always sleep with the head to the north, inasmuch as the magnetic currents of the earth promote quietude when they flow parallel with the nervous system of the body. No harm trying. Of one thing be especially careful; see that the light does not strike your eyes as you wake in the morning. The best sleeping-light is none, or at most only what the stars offer. If we retired at dusk we should just naturally arise at dawn; but while the sun's good-night is habitually scorned, its good-morning looks like a frown. Another suggestion as to geography is to elevate the head of the bed slightly by supports placed beneath the frame; this facilitates retreat of blood from the brain.

## 7. GIVE YOUR PAJAMAS TO THE HEATHEN

If you can add a plug hat to the outfit, that will afford the lost dweller in outer darkness a complete idea of what civilization looks like. And you'll fare better without either absurdity-in-custom's-guise. A nightgown is quite as nonsensical as a night-cap, the only people who retain either are the ones that sin against Nature and would shun the sight of the penalty she marks with them. No great wonder, some people's untailored appearance is such that if they woke up in the middle of the night and happened to see themselves by the pale and languishing light of the moon, they would forthwith go into hysterics imagining they had witnessed a wraith, a gargoyle, or a sausage-factory. But if you can summon enough courage to look yourself in the face, I don't think you'll ever go back to the bondage of so unhygienic, uncomfortable, unartistic, and altogether indefensible swathing-device as a nightgown. Anybody who has to dress to go to bed is unhealthy, immoral, or a slave to tradition; in which case his conscience will keep him awake and no more said.

---

*Eugene Christian was an avid vegetarian and endorsed raw food which was quite controversial at the time. He published a book, *Uncooked foods and how to use them* in 1904. —Ed.

### 8. Lie Straight In Bed

I have known persons whose chief occupation by night consisted in a frantic endeavor to demonstrate beyond peradventure how near the human knees can embrace the human chin. This is no doubt an interesting experiment, but it might be prosecuted with equal benefit under somebody's tutelage other than Morpheus.  Somnolence is straight-backed. Particularly must the chest be held broad and free that the lungs and stomach may function to a vital depth and regularity.  The head should not be buried in a pillow that obstructs access to the air-passages; the nasal ducts should not be allowed to remain the least impeded by the presence of foreign matter, whether dust or mucous; the mouth should not be left open as if to keep talking still; but this is no doctor's compendium and sufficient has been said.  If you need some gentle invitation to assume a civilized posture in bed, during cold weather put a hot brick between the sheets where your feet are supposed to reside.  In case the wrapping comes on the brick so much the better—for the blood will have to leave your brain and cure the burn.  The natural position during sleep is to lie on the stomach, or half on the side.  Which side is immaterial if digestion had gotten well over.  And the principle thing is to stretch out so there can be no impaired circulation or active nerve-tension to disturb the equilibrium.

### 9. Employ Mechanical Means To Distribute The Blood

Among which may be mentioned, a crash towel for vigorous friction rub below waist; a massage roller or application of manual massage in like manner; hot foot-bath, hot sitz-bath, hot-compresses to spine, cold compresses to head, wet stockings under dry, worn in bed after the practice of Kneipp, woolen bed-socks and non-inflammable foot-warmers.  Cold baths of whatever kind should never be taken at night, as they induce wakefulness.  Indeed bed-time is the only time when hot bath should not be followed by the cold ablution.  Massage of the extremities is best performed by another person, since the effort of stooping send the blood back to the brain.

### 10. Take An Air-Bath

Even if your slumber be profoundly desired, you can still improve it by habitual exposure of the body to the air for a half-hour before retiring.  A gentle stream of cool, fresh air blowing directly over the body not only equalizes circulation and relaxes nervous tension but also quiets and renews the soul by the etheric influences of psychic and spiritual origin.  Never let yourself become physically chilled during this procedure; on the other hand you may so accustom yourself to the bracing effect of the atmosphere that the coldest night in winter is none too cold for comfort. For detailed explanation of air-baths, see [Adolph] Just's *Return to Nature*.

*I used to keep my head up to the open window when I lived down on Long Island, and I awoke one morning in a strange darkness, which turned out to be caused by a snowdrift which had formed over my face during the night; I had breathed two holes through it, and had never noticed the snowfall while it was going on.*

*Now airing a bed does not mean letting an accidental breeze flirt a minute with a wrinkle in the top cover—it means stripping the whole business down to the springs and laying out each piece separately where the sun and wind can renovate it. This should be done every morning if time and place and strength should permit.*

*At least six hours should elapse between the meal of midday and of evening; but if the noon luncheon was wrongly eaten, the stomach may be incapacitated for effective work at night.*

*The science of dietetics is that system of counterfeit wisdom which teaches you to eat what you hate and should rather than what you love and shouldn't.*

*Many psychologists hold the theory that one should always sleep with the head to the north, inasmuch as the magnetic currents of the earth promote quietude when they flow parallel with the nervous system of the body.*

# Vibration And Health

## by T. R. Gowenlock

*The Naturopath and Herald of Health, XVII (11), 713-715. (1912)*

If a tree should fall in the primeval forest and there should be no one around for a hundred miles, there would be no sound. But if you were to stand close by and see it as it plunged downward to the ground, you would be conscious of the sound.

A strange statement to make, you say? But it's the absolute truth. Sound is but a form of vibration and when we are not within the radius of the sound waves, we cannot be conscious of the sound. When the tree fell, it started sound waves which, radiating in all directions with the swiftness of forked lightening, struck upon the eardrum. That caused you to hear. But if you had not been within the radius of the sound waves, the vibrations would not have fallen upon the ear drum, and consequently there would have been no sound. The energy of the radiating sound waves would have been dissipated before they had a chance to affect your ear drum.

Do you think that this simple statement of fact is mysterious and weird? Before the many manifestations of the peculiar power and force of electric vibration, it pales into insignificance. For as vibration is the greatest force in the universe, so is electric vibration the greatest vibratory force—the great remedy for a thousand ills that afflict suffering humanity.

Vibration is life! Without it we would not be in existence! Life depends upon it! Your life and mine! And if vibration is life, then electric treatment properly administered, is its right hand man.

Would you know the secret of youth? It is vibration.

Why were the ancient Spartans such a strong and virile race? Why were they so hardy—able to stand all sorts of weather—endure so many hardships? Why, just because their life was one continuous round of exercise. And exercise is only another name for vibration or rather exercise is a form of vibration and electric vibration for that matter. You may cause electricity to be generated by friction. Ever scrape your feet [on] the carpet in the winter time and then go up to some friend and touch the tip of your finger to their cheek. What happened? You saw a tiny spark of fire shoot forth and a tingling sensation was felt by your friend. That spark was electricity. When you exercise you cause friction and the friction generates electricity. That's why exercise is so good for you—provided you do not over indulge in it.

What is electricity? Alas, we cannot say. Even the master minds of the century have failed to unfold and reveal its mysteries. The wizards of the realm of electricity are at a loss what to say. They are unable to fathom its weird mysteries. All that they know is that it is a form of vibration—that it is a tremendous power for good or evil just as we make use of it.

But even if we do not know just exactly what this tremendous force is, still we do know this much: electricity is able to cure many human ills. And electric vibration applied in the proper manner is one of the greatest boons to the human race that has been discovered since the curtain went up thousands of years ago on the greatest drama of the ages—the drama that is comedy, tragedy, melodrama and farce combined—the drama that we call life. Yes, electric vibration is the magic wand that is able to wave away our cares and pains and renew our youth again in a great degree. Men have searched for many years for the fabled fountain of life. They have found it! Their goal is reached! The electric vibrator has come into its own.

What is this electric vibrator? Men and women—it is the highest expression of human skill and ingenuity. A master mind has imprisoned that tremendous force, electricity—big with life and power, youth and beauty—in a little instrument the size of a man's hand—so imprisoned it that YOU can make it do your bidding.

There is no need for anyone to suffer from backache, headache, listlessness, or a hundred similar ills. You need not be affected with facial blemishes such as pimples, wrinkles, crowsfeet, blackheads and the like, or scalp diseases such as dandruff or falling hair. All skin affections, bruised, nervousness, etc., can be dispelled by the aid of this wonderful, miracle-working instrument, the electric vibrator.

Did you ever strike your shin? If you have, you will remember how you reached down and rubbed the sore spot. How that gradually as you rubbed, the soreness was rubbed away, in the same way you have hit your funny bone and rubbed it. If you think back you will recall a hundred times how when you bruised your skin or hurt yourself in one of a thousand different ways that you rubbed the injured spot.

Well, the electric vibrator goes about its work in much the same manner only with a far greater degree of helpfulness. It applies massage methods in a scientific manner without the possibility of harm to you, and massage incorrectly applied often works injury to you. No masseur, expert though he may be, can hope to attain the beneficial results that are attained by the use of the wonderful electric vibrator.

What then does this vibrator do to accomplish its end? It stimulates the circulation thus transmitting new life and energy into every vein, every little capillary. It starts the blood circulating by quickly alternating compression and relaxation of the nerve tissues. Thus fresh blood finds its way to every portion of the body. Perfect circulation means perfect health! Therefore, the electric vibrator—because it keeps the blood in

One of the many ads for vibrator devices.

perfect circulation—starts new life flowing through your body and gives you such perfect circulation that you fairly glow with energy. You go forth prepared to conquer worlds, feeling fit and fine for every problem that may confront you along life's journey.

No home should be without one of these marvelous instruments. The time is surely coming, and in the near future too, when no home will be considered complete without one. An electric vibrator will be as common as the powder puff on the dresser, or the nail file in the boudoir.

If you are troubled with poor complexion, if your natural beauty is marred by pimples or unsightly wrinkles, if you have that tired listless feeling that won't leave you, if your back aches or your spine seems weak; in fact, if you are troubled by any ill of a similar nature, take the advice of the author of this article and purchase an electric vibrator. They are inexpensive and cost less than [an] ordinary massage treatment. The electric vibrator can be used for anything where massage treatment is needed and what is more to the point, it is much more economical. Then you have the treatment at your own home. But buy the best machine. Some of the leading manufacturers are offering special inducements this month. The time is ripe for buying. Therefore purchase the electric vibrator at once. Strike while the iron is hot.

You cannot begin to imagine what the vibrator will do for you. The best of these wonderful instruments develop 2,000 vibrations a minute. Imagine such radiant energy at work. Every vibration that it sends forth is filled with life for you. And 2,000 every minute! Why, it will chase away those unsightly blemishes that spoil the beauty of your complexion in no time. And even if you not have a sickly complexion, you should be on the safe side and buy an electric vibrator just to prevent such blemishes. "A stitch in time saves nine," as the old saying has it. The electric vibrator will save you a lot of trouble and worry if you will only take the trouble to investigate it. It will keep you young and beautiful long after others, who are no older than you, but who have not learned the advantages of this wonder-working machine, are faded and worn out.

Oh, that I could impress upon you the true value and importance of the electric vibrator in preserving the general health. It is the greatest discovery that man has produced along such lines since the world was formed and the stars threw forth their light for the first time upon man's abode. It means life itself to you! A life that has a bigger and better outlook! It means health, a radiant health that knows no misgiving that helps you to go forth on life's journey with a calm and determined demeanor, knowing that you have at your elbow the great electric vibrator—the sovereign cure for your ills.

I have neither the time nor space to tell you all about this unequalled instrument. But any manufacturer will be glad to give you full details of their marvelous powers. And let me assure you that no one can over-estimate the important and good that this electric vibrator is capable of performing. Take the advice of one who knows from personal experience and get the electric vibrator without delay. It is a pleasure to use. Nothing can equal the tingling pleasure and that sensation that you derive from their use except it be the pleasant after effect. Don't put it off a minute! Every delay means the foregoing of relief from pain and care! Action now means added comfort to you! Action now means freedom from sleepless nights, constipation, backache, all facial blemishes, tired listless moods, and a host of kindred ills.

Do not imagine the electric vibrator is extremely expensive. Just now the prices are very reasonable indeed, and with a vibrator of reliable make comes a number of attachments which enable you to have many additional comforts such as electric baths, etc., right in your own home. For your health's sake, act now.

The electric vibrator does more than just affect the outer skin. It reaches forth to the vital internal organs, giving them new life and vigor. The fresh blood floods away all waste tissue and builds new clean fibre in its stead, stimulating the entire body.

---

*If a tree should fall in the primeval forest and there should be no one around for a hundred miles, there would be no sound.*

*There is no need for anyone to suffer from backache, headache, listlessness, or a hundred similar ills.*

*Perfect circulation means perfect health! Therefore, the electric vibrator—because it keeps the blood in perfect circulation—starts new life flowing through your body and gives you such perfect circulation that you fairly glow with energy.*

*You cannot begin to imagine what the vibrator will do for you. The best of these wonderful instruments develop 2,000 vibrations a minute. Imagine such radiant energy at work.*

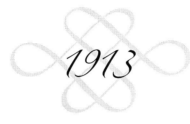

*1913*

## The Use Of Phrenology In Medicine
Eleanor Van Buskirk, M.D.

Jessie Allen Fowler (1856 -1932) followed her father and mother's medical footsteps and also became a phrenologist, succeeding her father as the editor of the American Phrenological Journal. In 1911, she sat as the editor of the "Phrenological Section" in *The Naturopath and Herald of Health* for 3 years (1911-1913).

# THE USE OF PHRENOLOGY IN MEDICINE

## by Elinor Van Burskirk, M.D.

*The Naturopath and Herald of Health, XVIII (6), 412-414. (1913)*

On speaking of the use of phrenology in medicine, the doctor said in part:

"The physician begins his preparation by studying organic structure. He spends long days and much midnight oil over his anatomy, his physiology, and his organic chemistry, for the whole process of metabolism is simply a question of chemical reactions carried on within the human body. Then he studies physical disease and its many methods of alleviation, including mental and nervous diseases. I am now speaking strictly along physical lines. His college gives him his diploma, and after hospital service he puts up his sign, and probably the very first case he has will probably be one of the most unusual ones in the whole gamut of human ills; or, worse still, one he never even heard of at all!

"But a very short time goes by when he discovers the biggest problem he has to meet has been very inadequately handled in his curriculum, and unless endowed by nature with great intuition he feels his equipment unsatisfactory. What is the trouble? Not the ability to cope with disease itself so much, for he has been well prepared, as the ability to meet the ever-varying personalities accompanying those diseases. He has studied the four great types of disposition—the choleric, the melancholic, the sanguine, and the phlegmatic—as taught him by the latest psychologies, and he is perfectly willing to grant many things inscrutable and past finding out, or known only to God, as the schoolboy says—for as yet he is familiar with only one part of man—the animal man.

"In his dilemma, if he is a truth-seeker, he makes further studies in psychology and philosophy to help him—perhaps even the study of mentation, which opens up such a vast field for the student. Here he finds variable chaos, for all labyrinths with ways that are dark and confusing and with vast aptitude for losing the way, his field is the most intricate, for there are mental charlatans as well as in other walks of life, and those who understands pre-eminently for mental science are usually coldly critical and unfeeling. What do they lack? They forget the Life itself, which is the spiritual and essential part of us. When I say Spirit, I mean the life, the part that always was and always will be—what we consider the real I. There are those who divide the individuality into seven divisions, but three is much more practical and leaves us happier.

"Until the physician realizes that human nature has three aspects instead of one he will not be of the highest efficiency, for it is the deviation from harmony in the chord of life that brings to him his life's duties.

"What has all this to do with the use of phrenology in medicine?

"Phrenology is a system which teaches the faculties of the mind are manifested in separate portions of the brain, modified by temperament, the doctrine that the mental powers are indicated by developments of the brain upward, forward and backward from the medulla, which are measured by cranial diameters and distances from the opening of the ear, and not from 'bumps'.

"How, then, can this be of service to us as physicians?

"I think no one present at a meeting of this kind will deny the first duty of a physician to his patient is to make a diagnosis of his case. The true physician is one who desires to heal his patient. Recalling our constitution as being a triple one, he must discern which part is the one whose functions are abnormal, then the cause or causes for the same. This is not always easy—in many cases very difficult—some even past finding out. How do we do this?

"One of the primal postulates of biographical evolution is that 'Form is a tract left by Life'. We first observe the physical structure or **Form**, knowing the builder was **Life** or **Spirit**, and after many experiences we can tell from form the proportion between the mental and spiritual and the physical in the individual before us, and hence can determine which is apt to suffer with its consequences upon the whole, destroying its harmony—for health is harmony, while disease is lack of harmony.

"The idea of the trinity of life is a very fascinating one to me. The number 3 stands for '**Expression**'. The physical gives form, or instrument of expression, without which life is not manifested. In phrenology we have the three temperaments—the motive, vital and mental. Every human accomplishment is dependent on a harmonious action of our three natures. Every deed is first an **idea**, then a **will** to perform, then the physical **act**. Ideation, willing, doing may be termed the great trinity of human endeavor that will bring us our desires if manifested intelligently. This is why I cannot agree with my mental friends who say 'All is mind.' Mind is a very essential part, but not the whole. Mind must be expressed through the physical instrument to make a poised, balanced life—strong, ready and efficient. Is it reasonable to suppose that a crippled or deformed or diseased body can allow expression in full measure? The bodily states react on the mind and spirit, as well as vice versa. I never knew mentation alone, **without some expression,** to have practical results. It doesn't buy food or clothing or shelter—which are necessary things while in the body—without touching the material plane at some point.

"But I have seen many victims of subjective thinking, uncontrolled, lose their reason, when, if they had expressed their thoughts through the hand, both mental and physical would be improved and the balance kept. It is the one-sided lives where the crises come. The phrenologist sees this, and if he has influence he can stimulate the latent parts to activity, saving the whole.

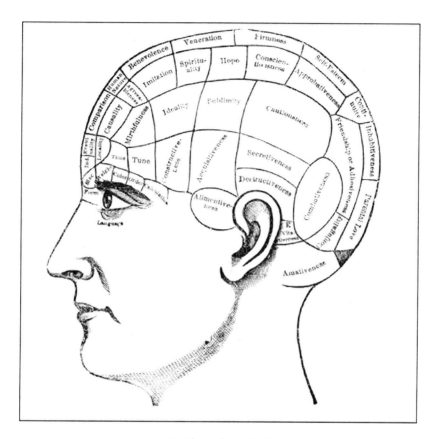

The Phrenology Skull.

"Recently a 20-year old girl came into my office with such a case of pseudo-laryngitis that she could not speak. I found the cause to be a negative suggestion, whereupon I made a stronger positive one to her, and she left me using her voice. Cause not physical, cure also not physical.

Case of emotional breakdown: Cure stimulated courage and the ability to obtain perspective to look beyond the present and to replace old emotion. In last analysis, a spiritual case.

"Case of broken femur: Cure, mechanical.

"Besides enabling us to classify life, phrenology also teaches, through physiognomy, the strength or weakness of the internal organs from their corresponding poles in the face. Thus we can read the weak heart or lungs before we use the stethoscope.

"The use of phrenology is as multiform as there are people, for Nature never repeats herself, and there are no two just alike. Hence the unending fascination of its study and use. We see the great contrasting types—the vital, with the desire to please, beautiful in form and feature; and the fierce, impulsive, vindictive nature, equally a part of human nature and bound to express itself in its own way. The eagle cannot help being an eagle any more than the dove can help being gentle, each fulfilling its primal urge and each good when understood, each with its purpose, all parts of one great whole, entitled to consideration. When we take this view we understand more, and come more quickly to the point of helpful service.

"Phrenology is the one science along mind culture lines that gives the true place to the physical part of the trinity. It denies nothing, but recognizes all, pointing out lines of least resistance, leading to fulfilment and peace.

"In conclusion, let me quote the following lines:

Let there be many windows in your soul, that all the glory of the universe may beautify it. Not the narrow pane of one poor creed can catch the radiant rays that shine from countless sources. Tear away the blinds of superstition; let the light pour through fair windows, broad as Truth itself and high as Heaven. Tune your ear to all the worldless music of the spheres and to the voice of Nature, and your heart shall turn to truth and gladness as the plant turns to the sun. A thousand unseen hands reach down to help you to their peace-crowned heights; and all the forces of the firmament shall fortify your strength. Be not afraid to thrust aside half-truths and grasp the whole."

*When I say spirit, I mean the life, the part that always was and always will be—what we consider the real I.*

*Until the physician realizes that human nature has three aspects instead of one he will not be of the highest efficiency, for it is the deviation from harmony in the chord of life that brings to him his life's duties.*

*Phrenology is a system which teaches the faculties of the mind are manifested in separate portions of the brain, modified by temperament, the doctrine that the mental powers are indicated by developments of the brain upward, forward and backward from the medulla, which are measured by cranial diameters and distances from the opening of the ear, and not from 'bumps.'*

*Ideation, willing, doing may be termed the great trinity of human endeavor that will bring us our desires if manifested intelligently.*

# 1914

## THE SCIENCE OF KINESIOLOGY

### DR. FREDERICK W. COLLINS

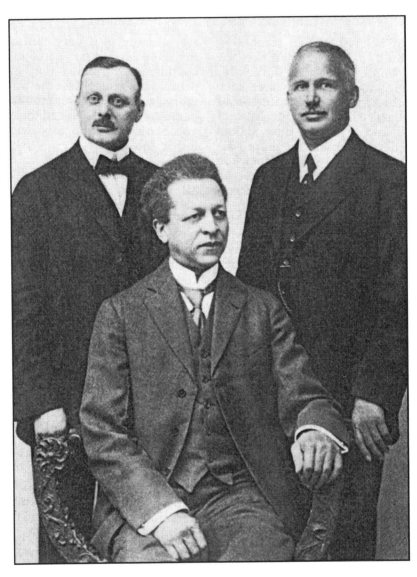

In 1920, Dr. Frederick W. Collins [left] was a Candidate for Presidency of the United States and Drs. Amzazon Ira Lucas [seated] and Benedict Lust supported his nomination.

# THE SCIENCE OF KINESIOLOGY

## by Dr. Frederick W. Collins, Hoboken, N. J.
### President of the Hudson Osteopathic Association

*The Naturopath and Herald of Health, XIX (1), 14-16. (1914)*

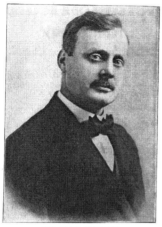

DR. F. W. COLLINS
Candidate for the Presidency of the United States
on the Platform of the Constitutional Health
Medical Liberty Issue

Kinesiology is the science of move-ments.

Kinematics is the science of motion.

Kinesitherapy [sic] is the movement cure; the treatment of disease by gymnastic movements and similar means.

We will start with Kinesiology, the science of movement.

The first thing we are inclined to say when we are told the earth moves is that we do not feel the earth moving, but the answer to that is easy. When you are in a train in a station, you sometimes cannot tell whether the train is moving or not, except, perhaps, by looking at another train standing at the other platform, and sometimes you think your train is moving, until you see that the platform is quite still. It was the moving of the other train that made you think your train was moving. So is proves nothing to say that we do not feel the earth moving with us. If you are traveling in a train, or on a boat, or in a balloon, or on the great earth of ours, you have only two ways of judging whether you are moving or not. One is by feeling the movement under you, and the other by noticing that things outside seem to be moving past you. Now, certainly we cannot feel the earth move under us, but this is simply because the movement is so smooth. When you are inside a very big boat, you cannot tell whether the boat is moving if the sea is smooth. If you shut your eyes in a balloon on a calm day you cannot tell that it is moving—often you cannot tell even if your eyes are open. When we feel that a car is moving under us, that is only because its movement is jerky. Every time a car moves a little more slowly, our bodies go on moving forward at the old rate, and then are slowed up with a jerk; then, when the car goes on a little faster, our bodies are left behind a little, and then are jerked forward. So we know that the car is taking us where we want to go. The more smoothly the car travels, the less we can feel it traveling. What would happen if the earth suddenly stopped moving?

If suddenly the earth did stop moving, as a car pulls up sharp, or as you pull your arm up sharp when you throw a ball, what would happen to us? When a car stops suddenly, all the passengers are jerked forward. When you pull up your arm sharply to throw a ball, it is thrown forward ever so far. Why can we not the feel the earth going round?

The answer to this is that we are going round with the earth, and, as we are moving round with it exactly the same rate and exactly the same direction, we notice nothing. If you were in a train and did not look out and the train moved at a constant speed in a straight line, and gave no jolts at all, you would not know it was moving; but, if it suddenly went more quickly or slowly, you would feel its motion. So, if the earth were suddenly to go round very quickly—say, so as to make a day of six hours instead of twenty-four—we might feel that it was going round because our bodies might be affected, as they are when a train suddenly give a jolt as you get in, and find yourself in someone's lap.

The real lesson that we can learn from this question is that the only kind of movement which we can feel is relative movement—that is to say, movement of one thing as compared to another.

Motion cannot be weighed; it cannot be handled or tasted, but it is very real as we know. We know, too, that there are many kinds of motion, and, of course, it does not do to say that heat is motion unless we add that it is a very special and particular kind of motion, quite distinct from any other. We believe heat is a special to-and-fro motion, which we have learnt to call it with other relative motion.

What is inertia?

We probably know what we mean when we say that anyone is inert. It means that he does nothing "of himself" but has to be made to do anything he does, and that he is even then only passively acted upon, not active. Inertia is thus the name given to the property of matter by which, in the question of motion, it is inert. If at rest, it remains at rest until something acts upon it. If moving, it goes on moving, changing neither its speed, until something acts upon it. In other words, the first law of motion, which explains why a bicycle keeps upright, is the law of inertia. It says that, so far as motion is concerned, matter is passive, resting unless something moves it, and moving unless something brings it to rest. This inertia, or passiveness, or tendency to go on doing what is being done, is also, a vibration, of the atoms or molecules of which matter is made. We cannot say in what direction, or at what speed anything is moving, or even that it is moving at all, except as compared with something else. If, however, we admit this, still it is possible that we may measure relative motion, and compare I think, the first law of mental motion. Our minds do not move unless and until something moves them; and when we have got "into a groove," as we say, we are apt to stay there until something

Dr. F. W. Collins founded a College of Naturopathy, Chiropractic and Osteopathy in Newark, New Jersey.

jogs you out of it. We have specially to remember what people usually forget—that inertia, of matter or of mind, is shown in the going on until something interferes, as much as in resting until something interferes.

In Kinesitherapy [sic], the movement cure, "The system (though practiced under various and different names) is the oldest in the healing art, and scarcely any has become so popular and won such general recognition. It was practiced by the priests, or in healing institutes, which served for this scientific purpose. The ancient Greeks and Romans, too, had a great regard for it as a valuable method of healing and combined it carefully with hot-air and other baths. Herodicus and Democritus, two of the most famous ancient Greek physicians, recommended this form of treatment. Hippocrates, the ancient father of medicine, advocated it and made especial mention of the fact in one of his writings. Though a French physician named Pare endeavored rehabilitating Osteopathy in the Sixteenth Century, it was Dr. Mezger of Amsterdam, who received the chief credit of placing it on a sound physiological foundation in Europe."

Osteopathy found its way to the United States in the Nineteenth Century, when in 1874 Dr. Still announced himself as the discoverer and he established the first school of Osteopathy in America.

Dr. Davis gives 71 moves; Dr. Murry 96. Prof. Jones 34 moves. Dr. Barber 46 moves. Dr. Kellogg 78 moves. Dr. Cohen over 40 moves. Bernarr McFadden over 300 moves. Dr. Schultz 60 moves. Dain L. Taskes in his New Book just out, third edition, revised 1913 has 90 moves.

On page 519 in Taske's new book, in speaking of *Glucokinesis and Mobilisation*; many efforts have been made to develop a method of treating fractures, that will not only insure a reasonably perfect union but will avoid the serious sequela incident to the use of casts, splints and extension apparatus. No single method of treatment is applicable to all forms of fractures, but there are certain principles, underlying the art of manipulation, which are applicable in the treatment of certain forms of fractures. The use of a form of massage, by Dr. Just Lucas Championniere, in the treatment of fractures is a new development in the art of manipulation. He calls his method "glucokinesis", painless massage. It is so different from massage. As generally understood by masseurs, that none but physicians, who understand the phenomena in tissues involved in fractures can use it intelligently. It consists in stroking the injured part very gently, in the direction of the venous circulation and the muscle fibers. This stroking is rhythmical and continuous for about fifteen minutes. The stroking is so gentle as to seem quite ineffective. The first principle is, "Never be afraid of rubbing too gently, or of giving too small a dose of mobilisation; always fear that the massage is too heavy and the movement too great." The result of this stroking is the relief of pain in the injured part and a coincident relaxation of the muscles involved in the fracture. This relaxation of muscles allows replacement of the fragments. Mobilisation consists of minute "doses" of passive movement in all of the joints above and below the fracture. The "dose" should cause no pain to the limb. The application of Prof. Lucas-Championniere's methods has been excellently described by Dr. James B. Mennell in his work on the *Treatment of Fractures by Mobilisation and Massage*, Publisher, MacMillan and Co.

Dr. Burgess says if you don't get results you are not doing it right.

What have we learned from this lecture on kinesiology, that we should avoid all jerky movements, all motion that tends to roughness, to retain poise and power and give kinesitherapy [sic] for results.

I have tabulated about 200 moves and from these have arranged ten general treatments, so that a patient taking a course of treatment will receive specific treatment for the complaint and the general treatment to follow will receive different moves at each treatment.

> *Motion cannot be weighed; it cannot be handled or tasted, but it is very real as we know.*
>
> *In Kinesitherapy [sic], the movement cure, "The system (though practiced under various and different names) is the oldest in the healing art, and scarcely any has become so popular and won such general recognition.*
>
> *It consists in stroking the injured part very gently, in the direction of the venous circulation and the muscle fibers. This stroking is rhythmical and continuous for about fifteen minutes.*

## THE SCIENCE OF CURE
### WILLIAM FREEMAN HAVARD

Complex homeopathic remedies were first created and used by Emanuel Felke, who was famous for his clay and nature treatments. Naturopaths were quick to recognize the importance of these complex homeopathic remedies in their own practice.

# THE SCIENCE OF CURE: A POSITIVE METHOD FOR THE RADICAL CURE OF DISEASE

## by William Freeman Havard

*The Naturopath and Herald of Health*, XX (10), 600-604. (1915)

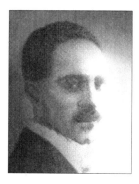

William Freeman Havard.

Every homeopathic physician is constantly receiving requests for information as to the differences between homeopathy and all other forms of medical treatment. The impossibility of giving satisfactory and comprehensive reply to everyone so inquiring must be apparent.

This article is designed to meet and answer the most frequent and important questions that naturally occurs to the layman. It is with the hope that the information herein contained may prove valuable and enlightening to many seekers for improved health that these pages have been prepared by the writer.

Homeopathy is a system of treatment based on the law of nature, that "Like cures like", as expressed by the homeopathic motto, *Similia similibus curantur*.

Careful and extensive experiments have proved that this is the quickest, surest, safest, and only scientific method for the use of drugs in the treatment of disease.

By this method each patient receives his individual, specific, curative medicine, selected upon the basis of an exact similarity between the symptoms of the patient and the symptoms which the medicine will cause when given to a healthy person in large doses.

The reason for this, contrary to what is generally believed, is that drugs are curative only for symptoms and diseased conditions like those which they can cause. Medicines used in this way not only give quick relief, but the relief is curative and lasting; and, owing to the special way in which such medicines are prepared, poisonous drug action never occurs.

## SPECIAL ADVANTAGES

Among the principal advantages of homeopathic treatment are:

1. Better control of disease and consequently less pain and discomfort.
2. Greater freedom from complications and bad after-effects.

3.  Large saving in doctor's, nurse's and druggist's bills, as well as great saving of time lost from work.

4.  Impossibility of the formation of drug habits.

5.  Comparatively certain in nearly all forms of disease and improbability of the development of cancer, tuberculosis, Bright's disease, diabetes or other serious forms of disease later in life.

6.  Better subsequent health of patients who are treated homeopathically and enjoyment of a longer life than would otherwise be possible.

To unfold these advantages more in detail:

In acute illness correct homeopathic treatment either stops the course of disease within a few hours, or causes it to run a much milder and shorter course than is ever possible when not treated at all, or when treated by other methods.

In the more severe forms of disease, pain and discomfort are markedly less; recovery is quicker; convalescence is more thorough; and the chances of escaping an untimely death are, at least, three times better with homeopathy than with other methods.

As a result of the quicker control of sickness, the earlier recovery, and freedom from complications, the expenses due to sickness are always markedly less with homeopathy than with other forms of treatment.

Cancer, tuberculosis, insanity, chronic kidney trouble, and other fatal forms of chronic disease, seldom or never develop in persons who have previously had the benefit of homeopathic treatment. The reason is that the tendencies toward such diseases are previously driven out of the body by correct treatment applied to the lesser ailments.

On the contrary, by the customary forms of medical treatment, the various illnesses of childhood and adult life are seldom, if ever, really cured; and, nearly always, the seeds of chronic disease are driven back into the body, where they germinate and finally develop into some one of the serious ailments under discussion.

The foregoing applies especially to the local suppressive treatment of diseases of the skin and mucous membranes, by which eruptions and discharges are dried up or suppressed with strong ointments, injections, douches, etc. Such conditions are nature's attempt to get rid of internal disease by forcing it out of the body to the surface, where it will be least harmful.

Naturally, patients dislike such symptoms, and usually prefer local treatment, which will dry up the eruption or discharge and drive it back into the body again. Getting rid of an eruption or discharge in this way, however, is in its ultimate results, analogous to closing a city's sewer outlets.

Everyone knows the serious results which follow the suppression or driving inward of the eruption of scarlet fever or measles; and yet seemingly but a few have the foresight to perceive that the penalty exacted by nature is just as certain in all other forms of disease. The only difference in results is in the time of their appearance, which is governed by the rhythm of the disease, like scarlet fever, the bad results of suppression appear quickly. In a chronic, slowly progressing disease, like eczema, the bad results may not be noticeable for weeks or months. Otherwise there is no difference; the results are just as bad as certain in one instance as the other.

The forcible lowering of high fever with ice baths or strong drugs, and the breaking up of colds with large doses of quinine, are also suppressive in character and always harmful. Recovery following such measures is only an evidence of the strong recuperative powers of the patient, and health is often seriously and permanently damaged by such treatment. The "scattering" of inflammations and swellings with local applications of iodine, camphorated oil, and other strong drugs is also harmful and just as foolish as would be the scattering over an entire farm of weeds in one corner of a field.

With correct homeopathic treatment, such eruptions and localized ailments are not suppressed or driven inward by local measures; but disappear as a result of internal medication, and because the internal disease which caused them has been cured.

When comparing the quickness of action of methods, if a fair comparison is to be made, the character of the various diseases, the time of their existence, and the precious health of the patients should be taken into account. It is also essential to consider whether it is the true curative action of remedies, or only the temporary stoppage of certain symptoms which should be compared. In a chronic ailment of several years' duration it would be foolish to expect a cure within a few hours, such as we might expect, for instance, in an acute condition like a cold in the head. If only temporary relief of pain in chronic neuralgia is wished for, a strong dose of morphine or acetanilid will stupefy the nerves, so that no pain will be felt for the time. It would be futile, however, to compare the temporary, poisonous, non-curative action of such drugs with the actions of homeopathic remedies which induce a lasting cure, without either poisoning the patient or risking the formation of a drug habit.

## HOMEOPATHY IN SPECIAL DISEASES

### FOR WEAKNESS AND LOSS OF APPETITE

The homeopathic physician obtains, by careful questioning, all the other symptoms, including those of an individualizing nature and prescribes a medicine which would cause similar symptoms. A medicine selected in this way, when properly administered in small doses, will overcome the weakness and loss of appetite and cure the other symptoms as well. A medicine so selected also removes constitutional tendencies to disease; and for this reason patients so treated are always much healthier afterward than before.

For conditions involving weakness and loss of appetite, most physicians prescribe tonics containing strong doses of such poisonous drugs as nux vomica, strychnine, arsenic, quinine or iron, and apparent benefit from which is purely temporary, artificial and harmful in the long run. Patients so treated are never in as good health afterward.

### FOR CONSTIPATION OR DIARRHOEA

The homeopath gives small doses of medicine, which are capable of causing, when given in strong doses, constipation or diarrhoea of exactly similar nature. When accurately selected, such drugs, in small doses, are positively curative.

For constipation, most physicians give cathartics or laxatives which relieve only temporarily, and always make the patients more constipated and more in need of laxatives than ever before. For diarrhoea, the average physician usually gives a prescription containing opium; which, while it is constipating for the time, is never really curative for diarrhoea and is always more or less harmful.

### HOMEOPATHY IN CHILDREN'S DISEASES

Not only is there little trouble in getting children to take homeopathic medicines; but, when these are used, recovery from dangerous illness is almost certain, remarkably quick and free of complications.*

One of the most principal advantages, also, is that children who are brought up under the supervision of homeopathic physicians enjoy much better health later in life; tendencies to disease, which exist in every child, being eradicated by homeopathic remedies given during and following the various ailments of childhood.

### HOMEOPATHY IN WOMEN'S DISEASES

In no other way is homeopathy more brilliantly successful than in the treatment of diseases peculiar to women; most of the expense, discomfort and embarrassment connected with the usual forms of treatment, as well as most of the surgical operations, being rendered unnecessary.

---

*The Homeopathic Journals of the 19th and early 20th century provide ample evidence of the efficacy of Homeopathy during the fatal epidemics that ravaged North America. —Ed.

Neither surgery nor local treatment ever removes constitutional disease which usually precedes and makes possible the various troubles in the organs of women. On the other hand Homeopathy will nearly always cure both the constitutional disease and the local trouble without an operation. Even when an operation is imperative, such an operation does not remove the original cause of disease. In this instance, Homeopathy will generally bring about a cure of the original cause of the trouble and the patient is thereby enabled to enjoy good health afterwards, which is usually impossible with surgery alone.

## HOMEOPATHY IN OBSTETRICAL WORK

The expectant mother, when treated by a competent Homeopath before and during pregnancy, can always be sure of a more comfortable period; and easier confinement; a quicker and more perfect recovery, with less danger of complications; and a stronger and healthier baby. Vomiting, indigestion, miscarriage, dropsy, kidney disease, convulsions and other trouble of pregnancy can always be controlled and usually prevented by homeopathic treatment.

There are certain tendencies to various forms of constitutional disease in every one; but, to a large extent, these can be removed from the mother and from the unborn child by homeopathic treatment of the mother before and during pregnancy.

## HOMEOPATHY IN SURGICAL CONDITIONS

Patients who are fortunate enough to have homeopathic treatment seldom need operations. At least, ninety per cent, of present day operations could be rendered unnecessary by the intelligent choice of the physician.

In conditions which have progressed so far as to render an operation imperative, not only is complete recovery almost certain, but the after effects are, at least, twice as good when a homeopathic physician and surgeon are working in harmony. The very best surgeon obtainable is seldom competent to treat a case medicinally; because his interest, his education, and his training have been almost exclusively surgical rather than medical.

It may be that a person is certain to die unless operated upon; and also, that he is very liable to die in spite of an operation, owing to the shock following all operation, especially in those who are severely weakened by disease. Under such circumstances, homeopathic remedies overcome weakness; control shock; and relieve all forms of dangerous and disagreeable symptoms, without, in any way, interfering with the work of the surgeon. It is, therefore, important that a homeopathic physician should be consulted in all surgical cases before an operation is decided upon.

## Homeopathy In Chronic Diseases

It is possible for nearly all chronic sufferers to be cured by a systematic course of homeopathic treatment by physicians who have specialized in this kind of healing.

Even in the last stage of organic disease, when the vitality is exhausted and death is unavoidable, homeopathic treatment prolongs life, prevents suffering, and renders death painless without stupifying the patient with morphine. It is most important for those who are nearing the end to continue in full possession of their faculties, for the settlement of estates, the drawing of wills and for religious reasons.

## Homeopathy In The Diseases Of Men

The working of nature's laws makes no distinction for age, sex or the mortality of individuals. Ailments which result from the sowing of wild oats can be radically cured by a course of individual specifics. The usual methods of treating such diseases with strong doses of poisonous drugs continued over long periods are seldom curative. This is proved by the poor health of such men subsequently, as well as the ill health of the wives and children who come later.

## Homeopathy In Diseases Of The Mind

The following quotations are taken from the book, *Mental diseases*, by Dr. W. M. Butler, Professor of Psychiatry, New York Homeopathic Medical College:

> The brilliant results achieved demonstrates that Homeopathy is as successful in mental disease as in the other ills of humanity. The homeopath needs no assistance from opiates, hypnotics, and anodynes (habit forming drugs). Desperate and apparently hopeless cases are often restored to perfect health of body and mind. When the cure is fully accomplished, it remains permanent.

Every homeopathic physician is able to verify these statements from personal experience. The superiority of homeopathic treatment has been publicly demonstrated in those State hospitals for the insane now under the control of homeopathic physicians.

## Scientific Correctness Of Homeopathic Treatment

Even the thoughtless boy knows better than to thaw his frostbitten fingers before a fire. He knows that a gradual thawing in ice water or melting snow is preferable; and he also knows that something of the baneful result of heat at such a time, either from hearsay or from never-to-be-forgotten experience.

Also, those people whose work causes them to be frequently subject to burns knows that the pain and inflammation following such accidents are markedly relieved by holding the burnt part close to the fire; and while the pain may be temporarily relieved by cold water, that it becomes much worse afterwards.

Now, why is ice-water best for frostbite, and why is heat best for recent burns? Is it possible for such to be anything else than examples of the "Law of Similars" by which physicians should be governed in the treatment of all forms of disease? The recently advocated treatment of bacterial diseases, such as blood-poisoning, rheumatism, tuberculosis, etc., with vaccines (which are solutions of dead bacteria or their toxins) is nothing more than a modified form of Homeopathy, which originated with, and has been in use among Homeopaths for the last fifty years, although no credit is given to the originators by the recent discoverers. Homeopaths have the advantage over other physicians in knowing how, when and where to use these agents, as a result of many years of experience since vaccines are useless in the majority of ailments, and are frequently harmful in the strong dose usually advocated.

Since all physicians acknowledge the harmfulness of contrary methods in frost-bite and burns, as well as the value of similarly acting vaccines in bacterial diseases, why do so many of them still continue to use drugs and other remedial measures according to contrary methods which are just as harmful, unscientific and useless as would be the application of heat for frost-bite or cold for burns? Is it because of prejudice, ignorance, indifference, or laziness that they refuse to study and apply the logical extension of the "Law of cure" in the general treatment of disease?

*Homeopathy is a system of treatment based on the law of nature, that "Like cures like," as expressed by the homeopathic motto,* Similia similibus curantur.

*By this method each patient receives his individual, specific, curative medicine, selected upon the basis of an exact similarity between the symptoms of the patient and the symptoms which the medicine will cause when given to a healthy person in large doses.*

*On the contrary, by the customary forms of medical treatment, the various illnesses of childhood and adult life are seldom, if ever, really cured; and, nearly always, the seeds of chronic disease are driven back into the body, where they germinate and finally develop into some one of the serious ailments under discussion.*

*Homeopaths have the advantage over other physicians in knowing how, when and where to use these agents, as a result of many years of experience since vaccines are useless in the majority of ailments, and are frequently harmful in the strong dose usually advocated.*

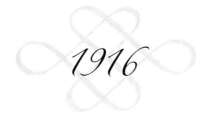

# 1916

### GYNECOLOGY MINUS THE KNIFE
DR. E. K. STRETCH

---

### NAUHEIM TREATMENT, CARBONIC ACID BATHS
JOSEPH HOEGEN, N.D.

---

### THE IMPORTANCE OF NUTRITIVE SALTS
DR. RICHARD PETERS

---

### NARCOTICS AND THE OSTEOPATH
DR. LAWRENCE E. KAIM, PH.D., D.O., D.C.

---

### A COMPARATIVE ANALYSIS
WILLIAM FREEMAN HAVARD

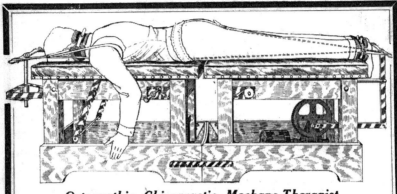

Osteopathic, Chiropractic, Mechano-Therapist, Naturopathic, and Medical Practitioners

# TAKE NOTICE

The most useful and practical scientific device ever offered to the medical profession

# Dr. Broberg's "Chiro-Traction" Massage
(TRADE MARK)
# Adjustment Table and Stretcher

A machine most vital to the success of the progressive up-to-date practitioner for the specific treatment of disease and the removal of its cause; for the correction of spinal curvature; the correction of deformities; for the correction of posture; for dislocations; for the permanent lengthening of the body and the administering of exercise for the symetrical development of the physique and the creation of physical energy.

*Some of its exclusive and important features*

Substantly made of solid oak; or birch-mahogany finish.

Upholstered in finest quality "muleskin leather." Colors: brown or red.

All mechanical parts are made of iron and steel, oxydized finish.

The table is made in two equal sections, with connecting rods to make it any length desired.

Upper part of table is provided with springs to protect the ribs or chest of the patient.

Lower part of table constructed so as to prevent the least friction against the body of patient while under traction.

Upper and lower part of table are both adjustable, on either side, to any position

desired, while patient is being treated.

The table may be used either with or without the motor for stretching purposes; for ordinary plain adjustments, or for massage and general treatment.

Size of table (when not extended or elevated for any special purpose): 65 inches long, 16 inches wide and 22 inches high.

*PRICES: By Freight or Express, F. O. B., New York*

| Table Complete, with Stretching Attachments | $100.00 |
| With Direct-Current Motor | 140.00 |
| With Alternating-Current Motor | $150.00 |
| Without Stretching Attachments or Motor | 60.00 |

*5% off for cash with order. Sold on periodical payment plan, if desired.*

WRITE FOR FULL PARTICULARS, and Dr. Riley's article on "Therapeutic Value of Stretching the Spine", and practical plan how to build up your practice and make Dr. Broberg Table and Stretcher quickly pay for itself in increased business. No obligation, WRITE TO-DAY.

## CHIRO-TRACTION COMPANY
Suite 828, Marbridge Bldg., 1328 Broadway, New York

Traction and chiropractic tables were popular amongst the early Naturopaths.

# Gynecology Minus The Knife

## by Dr. E. K. Stretch

*Herald of Health and Naturopath, XXI (1), 40-42. (1916)*

### Dysmenorrhea, Painful Menstruation

Under this heading we classify difficult and painful menstruation from a great variety of causes, all of which are due to lesions affecting the flow of vital fluids to the female genitalia, and modified by the temperament, environment, diet and general conditions of health. From a medical point of view the mechanical causes are lost in a maze of secondary effects, i. e., a case of painful menstruation applies for treatment, due to misplacement of the uterus, the obstruction and clots of blood causing pain, would be diagnosed from a medical standard as dysmenorrheal from prolapsus, anteversion, retroflexion, etc., of uterus. While Osteopaths admit the local disorder, they go a step further and locate the **cause** of this condition in the spinal area governing these parts.

The pain may be of any intensity from a slight feeling of discomfiture to intense pain which in some cases will lead to fits of mental aberration, and may occur before, during or after the flow.

### Home Remedies

In recommending the following treatment it is with the idea of encouraging the individual to self-help and the general improvement of health, but advise that physician, who will assist nature in her work and not one who will treat in the way that leads to operation, be consulted when in doubt. The first three methods are to alleviate the pain.

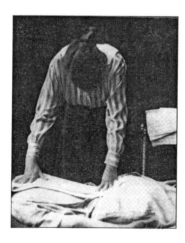

Fig. 1.

### Hot Packs (Fig. 1.)

Have patient to lie face down on bed or couch with the spine bare, and apply towels that have been wrung out of hot water, to which may be added one ounce of Epsom salts to the quart of water. See that the water is boiling hot and the towels are wrung out carefully so as not to burn the patient. Leave the towel on for from three to five minutes and then apply another in a like manner the same length of time. This should be repeated three, or four times, followed by a towel wrung out in cold water, for one half minute. After the hot packs use lumbar traction.

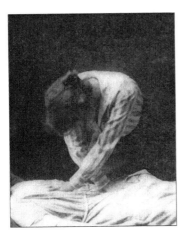

Fig. 2.

### Traction (Fig. 2.)

With the patient in the same position as for the hot packs, let the operator, any member of the family can serve in this capacity, as there is no need for the patient to expose any other part of the body than the spine. Mothers, daughters, sisters can do this as well if not better than a male member of the family. Stand close to the patient feet well together with hands crossed, the right hand resting on the sacrum, or base of the spinal column, and the left hand on the spine, a hands breath below a line drawn between the lower border of the scapula or shoulder blades. Press firmly downward with both hands and at the same time force the left hand towards the head and the right to the feet. Relax both hands and repeat this operation six times. Do not use any more force than the patient can bear with comfort.

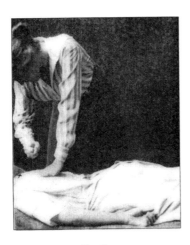

Fig. 3.

### Concussion (Fig. 3.)*

Locate the seventh cervical, called Vertebrae Prominens, so named because it is the most prominent of the first group, that is, it sticks out more than the rest, by finding the most prominent vertebrae on or near a line drawn across the tops of the shoulders. Count downward three bumps or spinous processes and place the fingers on the sides of these processes as shown in figure 3. With the other closed hand strike the fingers a series of short snappy blows for about one-half minute, follow by one half minute and repeat for five or ten minutes.

---

*Caution: Where there is any suspicion of functional heart trouble, use this method only on the advice of an Osteopath.

## Diet

Food is the matter taken into the body to supply nourishment and replace the worn out tissue. This subject had received the earnest thought of many students and scientific investigations show the importance of diet in health and exercise.

Unfortunately the practitioner meets with a deep rooted objection on the part of the patient to any change in the amount or character of his or her diet, due to, vicious habits, false ideas, lack of will power, poisoned systems demanding more poison, criticism of friends and relations, fear of losing weight, etc. All of which can largely be blamed upon the attitude of the Medical Profession on this question. So you will see that the individual needs must be considered in each case but to those willing to work along these lines I ask that they start with a breakfast of fruit only and with meals and which meat is served to eat a combination salad or raw vegetables instead of potatoes and bread. Many diet experts will condemn this as a small beginning. All I ask is for the trial of this simple rule and watch the good results, then seek to advise suitable to your case, as every case is individual.

To the skeptical, start three days before the expected time of next period and eat raw fruits three times a day, drinking plenty of water, nothing else, observe the effect.

Leaving aside the question as to what class men belong to, namely; omnivorous, vegetarian, carnivorous, fruitarian etc., chemically, we know that the raw fruits and vegetables are rich in minerals that are so necessary for the building up of the body cells and increasing the natural ability of these cells to function or work in their particular capacity, i.e., promote osmosis, which is the passage of fluids through a membrane—cells receive nourishment and throw off waste matter through the cell walls or membrane. Thus by supplying the fluids of the body with minerals in the form they obtain the fruit and vegetable life, we find that the activity, resistance, health, yes, the very life of the cells improve. Clinically, it is found that this fruit and vegetable diet supplies the solvents which dissolve and help to throw off the waste matters that have accumulated in the body.

*Have patient to lie face down on bed or couch with the spine bare, and apply towels that have been wrung out of hot water, to which may be added one ounce of Epsom salts to the quart of water.*

*Do not use any more force than the patient can bear with comfort.*

## NAUHEIM TREATMENT, CARBONIC ACID BATHS

by Joseph A. Hoegen, N.D.

*Herald of Health and Naturopath, XXI (1), 61-62. (1916)*

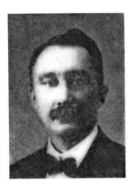

Joseph A. Hoegen, N.D.

Careless and intemperate partaking of food, lack of proper exercise in the open air, result in circulatory obstipation or stagnation, imposing a serious and unnecessary burden upon the sanctuary of vitality—the heart. It seems almost unbelievable, when we listen to the menus of our patients; many starting in with a heavy breakfast, which in many cases would be too much for a regular dinner meal. "Well, doctor, I am hungry in the morning, and my stomach needs this to satisfy its cravings." Nonsense and habit. Generally those who have passed the middle age of life are usually the first to fall to these temptations, thereby becoming victims to arterial degeneration and heart failure.

The saying, "a man is as old as his arteries" implies that most of the morbid or unhealthy processes known as degenerations are connected with diseases of these vessels, distinguished by the deposition of waste, which coat the arteries, thereby hindering their elasticity and contractile power. Many arteries of the body are more inclined to morbid processes than others. Gout and Bright's disease are associated with changes in the walls of the small arteries, and since these changes are due to defective elimination on the part of the kidneys, these organs also suffer in consequence.

We may have general arterial degeneration as well as local, affecting the large or small arteries, all the coats, or only one of them. The entire cardiovascular arterial system is greatly affected through the failure on the part of the emunctories to rid the body of its waste. They arise from defective metabolism, due to irregular modes of habit, sedentary occupations, dietetic errors, and other mental agitations of health, to which middle aged persons are subject.

Much can be done in the beginning of high arterial pressure with a course of Nauheim Baths of a moderate temperature, combined with strengthening exercises as devised by Dr. Theodor Schott. These effervescent carbonic acid baths have shown a remarkably gratifying beneficial effect. By their use, incipient decompensation, insomnia, and all neurasthenic conditions are greatly improved. The baths are not indicated, where patients suffer from a loss of compensation.

The effervescing carbonated bath produces a sensation of warmth to the skin, caused by the prickling of the gas bubbles, and the body of the patient assumes a healthy red color, due to the distention of the cutaneous capillaries. The pulse becomes full and strong, the heart beat is regular and the breathing easier and more composed.

Metabolism is increased by the improved circulation, which means improved cell nutrition, greater cell activity, which in turn accelerates glandular activity throughout the body, and thus the toxic products of circulatory stagnation are quickly eliminated.

The Nauheim Bath consists of a salt water bath properly carbonated. The body of the patient is covered with minute bubbles of carbonic acid gas that form rapidly on the immersed surface and when disturbed, are quickly replaced by new ones. I generally begin the baths with a temperature of 95° F. [35° C.], keeping the patient in the bath from eight to ten minutes, believing, that a short immersion stimulates and a long one depresses. The next day, the bath is reduced one degree and then for two or three days the bath is omitted. The temperature is gradually reduced to about 78° F. [26° C.], but not over a degree at a time, and the duration of the bath is so gradually prolonged. Care should be taken, that the patient is immersed up to the neck in the bath.

A series of baths consists of about 21. No exertion should be made by the patient in preparing for the bath or in leaving it. A rest for half an hour is essential after the bath, and no massage or exercise is advisable immediately after the bath, but may precede it.

*Much can be done in the beginning of high arterial pressure with a course of Nauheim Baths of a moderate temperature, combined with strengthening exercises as devised by Dr. Theodor Schott.*

*The effervescing carbonated bath produces a sensation of warmth to the skin, caused by the prickling of the gas bubbles, and the body of the patient assumes a healthy red color, due to the distention of the cutaneous capillaries. The pulse becomes full and strong, the heart beat is regular and the breathing easier and more composed.*

*The Nauheim Bath consists of a salt water bath properly carbonated. The body of the patient is covered with minute bubbles of carbonic acid gas that form rapidly on the immersed surface and when disturbed, are quickly replaced by new ones.*

## THE IMPORTANCE OF NUTRITIVE SALTS

**by Dr. Richard Peters**

*Herald of Health and Naturopath, XXI (5), 304-308. (1916)*

The importance of minerals and their salts in nutrition has been investigated and properly placed by modern biological researches. However, it would be unjust in considering these facts, not to mention the pioneer work of Liebig and his immediate followers. It cannot be denied that J. V. Liebig, in his discourses about food stuffs, always pointed out the importance of salts in foods. Also Carl Voit recognized their importance. That is proven by the *Reports of the Bavarian Academy of the Sciences*, in which Voit in December, 1869, reported the investigations of his pupil, J. Forster. To him belongs also the honor of having used the name Nutritive Salts for the first time in his scientific works, which he published in 1875. (*Zeitschrift für Biologie*, Bd. 9. 1875.)

Strange to say that then, the conception of nutritive salts for decades disappeared from scientific literature and the salts were often looked upon as a more or less unimportant part of food stuffs. Later, when their importance for the building up of organs and tissues was recognized, there was no clear idea concerning certain salts.

Meanwhile the scientific works of a man became known; a man who could not get the recognition of his confreres which was due him, on account of his peculiar position toward scientific medicine. This is the Psychological Chemist, Julius Hensel, who, in his *Makrobiotic*, (Hensel, Julius, *Makrobiotik*. 3rd Edition, Leipzig, 1904) described in minutest detail the importance of the mineral salts for the proper functioning of the organisms, in which work he also laid the foundation for a "Mineral Salt Therapy", which has found full recognition by modern authorities.

It was also Hensel who first called attention to the fact that our field and garden fruits are lacking in mineral salts, and from this he concluded the necessity of augmenting this lack, especially in vegetable foods, by adding corresponding salt mixtures. In any event, Hensel's Works, even if they contain some now obsolete views and errors, gave the impetus to further scientific investigations along the lines laid down by him. The physicians Schuessler and Lahmann have unmistakably founded their theory and practice on Hensel's theories and profited by his experience.

In his capacity as chemist, Hensel observed the differences, in residual ashes of the secretions and excretions of the organism, as to their composition, a matter about which then the knowledge was very defective. Today we all know the mineral percentage of human excretions. The great differences between the ash percentage of pathological excrements and that of healthy beings is also well known.

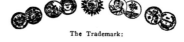
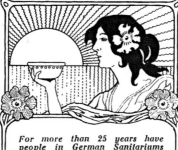
Julius Hensel produced a line of products containing Nutritive Salts such as cocoa and oat flour, coffee substitutes and others. Hensel Nutritive Salts were promoted and sold by the homeopathic company, Boericke & Tafel.

Ury and Alexander have investigated these results scientifically and published their conclusions. (*Deutsche Mediz. Wochenschrift,* 1904. Nos. 36, 37.) But also in the healthy, important differences are found, which must be laid solely to differences in nutrition. We will only mention the researches of Blauberg, (M. Blauberg, *Experimentelle und kritische Studienüber Säuglingsfäces,* Berlin, 1897) and Grundzach, who came to the same conclusions, even though their methods were apparently different and not absolutely free from objections.

Our organs and tissues, even the different cells, are dependent upon inorganic materials if they shall do their work effectively. We know that the preservation of certain parts demands also certain modifications of the minerals. Regarding the heart, L. Herman, (L. Herman: *Lehrbuchder Physiologie,* 14. Auflage 1910) has proven this conclusively. Especially Potassium and Calcium play an important role besides Sodium in connection with Chloride.

The presence of mineral salts in the organism is subject to such a strict law, that Hirth speaks of it as an absolute regulation of first order, because no compensation can be found for it in the sense of Rosenbach. As there is no substitute for oxygen, so there is none for salts among the foods and energetics. Animals, as well as plants, die when salt is absolutely withheld from them. Forster has delivered the proof for this statement, and his animals died in a short time when they were kept on salt-free foods. Even Bunge could not disprove Forster's claims by Lunin's experiments which he caused to be made. He, as well as all other physiologists, recognizes the necessity of the child organism, to have salts constantly with the food. Yes, he even believes that the young organism gets too little of it. Only for the adult body this ingenious scientist and some other physiologists consider the necessity of salt taking as not proven in the same measure. However, he contradicts himself by admitting that the adult organism demands salt influx at certain times, especially to reproduce semen, and in women during the time of menstruation, pregnancy and lactation.

That also the adult organism suffers during salt depletion, has been proven by many experiments on animals, and especially by the well-known experiments of the so-called hunger artists Cetti, Succi and Breithaupt (Senator, Zuntz, J. Munk; *Bericht über die Ergebnisse des an Cetti ausgeführten Hungerversuches,* Berl. Kl. Wochenschrift, 1887, S. 428. Also L. Luciani; *Das Hungern,* Leipzip, 1890) in which were found considerable changes in the mineral metabolism.

To be sure, the salts in the food stuffs are not the same quantitatively, and perhaps neither qualitatively, for the growing body as for the fully developed one. Forster pointed out that one part of the salts is found in close combination with the body substances in the organs and as necessary parts of the body juices and blood. Another part is found dissolved in the juices according to Forster. The first mentioned he considers the real body salts, the latter the surplus salts, which are liberated by katabolism [catabolism] and oxidation of combustible matters, or they have combined with the products of decomposition. Probably the salts taken by the adult become such of the second type, while in the child body the reverse is correct.

However, that a regular supply of salts is necessary in the adult organism is not only proven by their presence in the secretions and excretions, but much more by the fact that it was possible to turn away death from salt hunger in animal experiments, or in correct diseased conditions due to lack of salt. Also, the indisputable results obtained by the relatively young mineral therapy are proofs of the necessity of the mineral salts for the economy and proper functioning of the organisms on the one hand, and of the fallacy on the other hand, that the relatively small amount of minerals necessary is more than adequately supplied by the food we take. This latter mistake has been widely spread and is also found in some text books. The remarks of Albu and Neuberg (Albu und Neuberg, *Physiologie and Pathologie des Mineralstoffwechsels*, Berlin, 1906. S. 29) are very much to the point in this connection. For the healthy individual this is true; that is why he remains well. But on the other hand, there are just as often disturbances in the body causing a negative balance in albumen, and fat and carbohydrate metabolism. If the supply of minerals were always sufficient, then no anomaly in the mineral metabolism would take place, of which there are so many different kinds and also some grave ones.

This view has been proven beyond a question by experimental critical researches. As some cases of pathologic metabolism must be laid to disturbances in quantitative inorganic supply, so also other cases must be recognized as the result of disturbed resorption and assimilation.

Lime [calcium] is one of the most important mineral food stuffs. Combined with phosphates and carbonates and fluorine, it represents one of the essential constituents of the bones of the skeleton, the solidification of which it produces. It is met in all other organs and tissues, even if only in small percentage. The action of lime, taken with food, upon the bones is never direct, but it is a nutrition and irritant for the periosteum which, under normal functioning, makes bone development possible. Also, in the making of blood and in the coagulation of blood and plasma, the lime salts play an important part. Lime is also found as a preventative against tissue irritation: as lime excretion, e. g., calcareous tubercles, excretion in inflamed lymph glands; in the walls of old abscesses and in the lime capsule of intra muscular trichinae.

According to Bunge, next to iron, lime is the mineral which has been oftenest proven to be lacking in our food; for, aside from cow's milk, most foods are poor in lime. In pregnant women and nursing mothers, the want of lime is especially great, the fetus or suckling demands more than the mother can usually give. The skeletal tissue is largely cartilaginous and is, consequently, almost devoid of lime salts. That which forms during the nursing period is bone tissue, which is necessary not only for the additional growth of the skeleton, but also as substitute for the cartilage of the fetal period.

In pathological conditions, especially in chronic malnutrition, an increased lime excretion is found in the urine. On the other hand, an increased lime retention is found in arteriosclerosis. The supposition that all pathogenetic causes are based upon lack of minerals necessary to combine with or dissolve lime seems to be well founded.

In the much disputed rhachitis [rickets] question, this result has been reached: the cause is to be found in a disturbed lime metabolism which causes an increased excretion of lime salts into the intestines. The rhachitic skeletal changes are consequences of this generally disturbed metabolism, caused by a qualitative, often also quantitative, insufficient opposition, when increased resorption, especially of the mineral parts of the bone tissue, is present. That the skeleton of rhachitic children contains less lime salts than that of the healthy child is notorious.

Similar conditions are found in osteomalacia, which, by most authorities, is considered a disease of metabolism which may be induced by lime insufficiency in the food on account of lacking absorption of food lime, through diminished alkalescence of the blood due to lactic acid, etc., in the blood (which was found in the urine or blood of patients suffering from osteomalacia), or lastly, from phosphoric acid anomalies. This lime is also of essential importance to the nervous system, is clear when we consider the proportion of ca. [calcium] in the cortex ceribri, the irritability of which is increased when the quantity of lime is decreased.

In close connection with lime, we find in the organism magnesium; in no animal or human organ is it entirely absent, yet its presence is only slight (e.g. compared with lime only as 1:9), but hardly less important as a chemical agglutinant. Magnesium is found plentifully in the striated muscle tissue and especially in the gray substance of the cerebro-spinal tissues. It seems to have an especial affinity for the nucleins [nucleoproteins], for it is found abundantly in the sperm and, as an integrate ingredient, it is also found in blood and lymph.

The absorption of magnesium takes place in the small intestine, its excretion mainly through the urine, though partially by the intermediary route of the colon. Considering the important influence that magnesium has upon cell life, it must be recognized as an absolutely necessary mineral for the organism which must not be absent.

That sulphur must be an essential ingredient to our food, is known especially to the veterinary surgeons. Animals which do not get sufficient sulphur in the food lose their hair. The sulphur consumption of the body is no small one, per diem about 2.5 grams of sulphuric acid. We meet sulphur in especial close combination with the albumin molecule. No albumin without sulphur, therefore, neither a cell, tissue nor organ without sulphur. It is found in greatest abundance in epithelial tissue, for which it is as typical as lime for bone. The eminent importance of sulphur is seen from its constant presence in protoplasm. It is eminently important, even in minute quantities, for the vital functions in protoplasmic albumin and therefore minute disturbances of the sulphur balance in the albumen molecule must of necessity be followed by pronounced consequences. The importance of sulphur salts in the blood for normal digestion and for liver function is well known (sodium taurocholate). The excretion of sulphur as sulphuric acid through urine and feces, as well as by growth of nails and hair, demands restitution, which means a quantity equal to 3.5 grams of sulphuric acid, according to Hammarsten. Especially in young individuals, the sulphur consumption is relatively greater, and therefore, the necessity of more food containing sulphur.

Iron, present in the system to the amount of about four grams, plays a most important role as oxygen carrier in the composition of the blood. It is very important in a physiological sense, not only because of its function in the making of hemoglobin, but also on account of its general effect on tissue metabolism of all organs. It is even found in the bloodless cornea. Rightfully, it must be considered a nutrient.

In its capacity as an oxygen carrier, develops oxidizing powers, i.e. it acts as a katalysator, oxidizing without being oxidized itself.

While the action of iron as to its hemoglobin building property is beyond a doubt, nevertheless, its mode of absorption has not yet been clearly proven. Abderhalden proved the presence of iron, which had been fed in small quantities, in the intestine walls and in the lymph channels. According to present views regarding intermediary metabolism of iron, it enters the viscera by the way of the portal circulation (liver and bile).

Of the greatest importance as well for the growing as for the mature organism is phosphorus. Combined with alkaline earths it takes an important part in the growing of the skeleton and is in this form found in almost all tissues. Without phosphorus, nerve tissue of any kind is impossible, in which it is present in the form of glycerophosphoric acid, while in bone tissue it is found as calcium phosphate. In both instances, it plays the role of a building material. That it takes part in tissue building, is evidenced by the fact that a suckling in the first year accumulates about 50-60 grams of phosphorus. In organic combination it is found in the proteins, in nuclein and lecithin and in the phosphatins, and in the glandular organs: liver, spleen, and thymus. Through the investigations regarding phosphorus metabolism, we know that the body retains phosphorus with the greatest energy. Every disturbance in the quantitative proportion of phosphorus considering its importance for cell life must be of vital significance for the existence of the cell.

Natrium, especially as Sodium Chloride, forms about half of the salts dissolved in the blood serum. Therefore, it is clear that the loss of these salts in the organism must cause disturbances of health. An important function of natrium in our body is to be found in the fact that it chemically binds the surplus acids. It is a regulator of our life functions. The glandular organs need for normal functioning also a certain percentage of natrium to influence their secretory action. Natrium chloride stimulates the secretion of gastric juice, hydrochloric acid. The natrium proportion of the blood is usually constant, for by temporary retention of sodium chloride the system maintains its blood isotonia.

Kalium is found especially in the form elements of all kinds, the cells; as kali phosphate it represents the main part of the minerals of the red blood corpuscles, the muscles and the organ albumen. Like sodium, kali acts as an acid regulator in blood and body juices. Furthermore, alkalies are media for transporting the carbonic acid in the blood and act as solvents of many albumen in the juices of the body. The antiseptic and conserving power of kali is due to its dehydrating property.

Silicic Acid, so long under-estimated in its importance for tissue building, is found especially in the connective tissue, according to some authorities, like H. Schulz, in a great measure, in the embryonal connective tissue of the umbilical cord, in the epithelial tissue and in the lens. According to Runkel, it is always present in the pancreas. The proportion of silica is especially great in the hair, constituting here about 40 percent.

Fluorine participates in the formation of bones and teeth as calcium fluorine; it is also present in the blood and in the milk. The proportion of fluorine in the organs named, is minimal, to be sure (for bone and teeth about 0.05 to 0.1 percent), but in its sphere of action it has a very pronounced physiological importance.

Manganum [manganese] is intimately related, chemically speaking, with iron, but so far it has been found only in small quantities in the human system, but it undoubtedly plays an important role in the blood making of the organism.

The physiologist finds it impossible to think of red corpuscles without iron, the skeleton without lime, the nervous tissue without phosphorus. And so he knows, also, that quantitative changes in the mineral supply and mineral combinations are bound to cause disturbances in the vital functions of the cells and cell groups. Our organs receive all quantitative changes in their constituents as irritations, and they respond to such changes by changes of their function according to the intensity of the irritation. These reactions, in their manifold character, are so well known and recognized from our practice, that it seems hardly necessary to call special attention to their manifestations. The point to be made is solely this, that a lack in mineral combinations is bound to be followed by disturbed vital functions of more or less importance.

We are therefore forced to recognize the minerals as foods and we cannot consider them as food additions, as is held by Voit and Bunge, which might be valuable to life, without adding to the organism strength. With Hensel and Forster we must accept them as real Nutritive Salts, for they are absolutely necessary food elements, as builders of cells and tissues, and the small quantity necessary cannot be taken as a measure for their importance. But they are much more, they are powerful carriers of energy, and due to van t'Hoff's *Theory of Solutions* can be measured as such.

While the energy of albumen, fats and carbohydrates, measured in calories, is converted into heat, the energy of salt solutions manifests itself in pressure and motion, and can be measured in atmospheric pressure. The possibility of determining according to well-known laws, the motion difference in the organism due to osmotic pressure of salt solutions, may serve as an indicator of the importance of the salts.

If we pour carefully a stratum of water on a salt solution, we will soon find the entire salt solution of equal concentration. The salt particles have wandered from the solution upwards into the clear water. This motion phenomenon—called diffusion—appears in a different form, if we part salt solution and water by a semi-impervious wall. Since this wall is not keeping back the water, but certainly the salts, the salt molecules, striving to get from the solution into the water, cause pressure against this wall, called the osmotic pressure of the solution.

According to the laws relating to gases, which van t'Hoff proves to be applicable to the osmotic pressure, the latter can be measured, and we know that a 0.1 per cent sodium chloride solution exerts a pressure a hundred times greater than albumen solution. It therefore follows, that almost the entire osmotic pressure of a certain food is due to the salts contained in it.

The literature on the subject proves further, that equal masses of energy of different salt solutions act in various ways. As mentioned before, the inherent energy of salt solutions may manifest itself in motion or pressure. This is determined by the degree of permeability of the dividing wall, which is quite different in the different organs of the human system.

If this solution contains various salts, then the osmotic pressure will be different in the different places, according to the unequal permeability of the tissue walls; different in the stomach and also different in the particular sections of the intestinal canal. But we have not only to reckon with the pressure of the different salts, but also with the pressure of the products of dissociation of the salts, the free ions.

These phenomena give a solution of the action of the salt combinations, and at the same time they prove the importance of these combinations for the act of digestion. It is easily understood that death from salt starvation, in the case of Forster's animal experiments, as well as in his later experiment objects, was not only due to absence of anabolism, but also due to lack of the necessary pressure and motion manifestations.

But this does not yet exhaust the description of the action of salts. According to modern biology, salts in solution act also as electrolytes.

It is well recognized that electro-chemical transactions play an important role in modern biology. The scientific investigation of Loeb, Hamburger, Koranyi, Koppe, Pauli and others have made many things clear. It would lead too far, should I only mention the very extensive literature on this subject. Professor Ostwald has done this in a very instructive and clearly arranged way in his *Grundriss der Allgemeinen Chemie*, (4, Auflage, 1909). Recently the teaching of the electro-chemical workings of the organism and the principles of the electrolytic circulation have found a staunch advocate in George Hirth, and he has found a great many followers among scientists who accept his view. His views (*Der Electrochemische Betrieb der Organismen*, IV, Aufl., Muenchen, 1911) are expressed in this one sentence: The dynamics of organic action is not only brought about by the combination of chemical and physical powers, but that the latter are essentially electrolytic. With the convincing keenness he proves his views, according to which the solutions of salts in the blood are not the ultimate aim, but only preparation to reach the main object: to enter the nerve cells and connecting media as true electrolytes. The proof for this is not new. As previously stated, Rosenbach pointed this out earlier, but Hirth also established the necessity of an optimal electrolytic circulation for all organs in order to prevent disturbances of their function. Under these views the salts gain a sovereign importance for the prophylactic hygiene as well as for therapy. It is interesting to know that lately ministers of war of different States have considered the supplying of the soldiers in manoeuvers and on long marches with Sodium solution (with small additions of calcium and kali), in order to prevent heat stroke and dysentery. Also the eminent pharmacologist, Prof. Hugo Schulz, of Greifswak, Germany, (*Vorlesungen über Wirkung und Anwendung der anorganischen Arzneistoffe*, Leipzig 1907), has for years called attention to the manifold therapeutic action of inorganic combinations.

After these deductions, we will understand Albu and Neuberg, (*Physiologie und Pathologie des Mineralstoffwechsels*, Berlin, 1906) when they sum up the total knowledge of the present time concerning the physiological importance of the salts in the organism in these theses:

1. They are cell and tissue builders and play an important role in the anabolism of the organism.

2. They act as intermediaries of the osmotic tension in the cells and tissues, in blood and body fluids and are carriers of energy.

3. They regulate the reaction of the blood and the tissue fluids, as well as many actions of fermentation, especially in the intestinal canal.

4. They act as "katalysators" for a number of chemical processes.

5. They are intermediaries of the continual processes of autochthonic [indigenous] in and of toxification of the living protoplasm.

6. They direct, to a certain extent, detones [sic] position and assimilation of organic substances.

This proves what Hensel taught decades ago, that the salts are of vital importance. The supply of the same must therefore be constant in all phases of development. Aside from light and air they are the most important preservers of human life, and none would dare to dispute the hygiene and therapeutic priority of the trinity "Sud-Oxygen-Salts." [sic]

Experience disproves the claim that the ordinary food supply contains enough salt in every case. With predominanting vegetable diet, the want of salt is especially strong, as seen in the salt hunger of herbivorous animals. We will only mention the desire of horses and cattle to lick salt, and the wandering of roaming animals to salt springs in water and rocks.

Add to this the conclusive evidence that our field and garden fruits are poorer in nutritive salts (due to the fact that the soil is overworked and usually not properly resupplied, as many authorities along these lines teach) than such which come from virgin soil. This explains the lack of tissue resistance and low vitality (low opsonic index*) of the people in general, in spite of their sufficient, ever abundant, consumption of albuminous, fat and carbohydrate foods. They suffer from subnutrition. The logical consequence of this observation is the systematic supply of the lacking salt combinations. Table salt alone cannot be sufficient for any length of time, even if we have to give to sodium chloride the place of first importance among the salts.

Scientific investigations will have to establish the proportion of the other salt combinations for the rational nutrition at the different ages, taking into consideration the various conditions of the people, as Hensel has done with signal success. At any rate, here a great field is offered to exact scientific research.

In hygiene we will not be able to do without additions to foods which are lacking in salts. This will naturally lead to an extension of the dietetic therapy along the lines of nutritive salt additions in proper doses, in different pathological conditions, which so far have not been very amenable to ordinary therapeutic measures.

---

*Opsonic Index is the ratio of the phagocytic index or opsonin of a tested serum of a person with an infectious disease to that of opsonin in the blood sample of a healthy person. —Ed.

For further information send for free literature to the *Hensel Chemical Works*, Sioux City, Iowa, and see their ad in this issue.

---

*To be sure, the salts in the food stuffs are not the same quantitatively, and perhaps neither qualitatively, for the growing body as for the fully developed one.*

*Lime [calcium] is one of the most important mineral food stuffs. Combined with phosphates and carbonates and fluorine, it represents one of the essential constituents of the bones of the skeleton, the solidification of which it produces.*

*Furthermore, alkalies are media for transporting the carbonic acid in the blood and act as solvents of many albumen in the juices of the body. The antiseptic and conserving power of kali is due to its dehydrating property.*

*The physiologist finds it impossible to think of red corpuscles without iron, the skeleton without lime, the nervous tissue without phosphorus. And so he knows, also, that quantitative changes in the mineral supply and mineral combinations are bound to cause disturbances in the vital functions of the cells and cell groups.*

*The point to be made is solely this, that a lack in mineral combinations is bound to be followed by disturbed vital functions of more or less importance.*

# Narcotics And The Osteopath

## by Dr. Lawrence E. Kaim, Ph.G., D.O., D.C.

*Herald of Health and Naturopath, XXI (7), 390-391. (1916)*

In calculating the effect or desired result of certain Narcotics or other poisonous drugs, these important conditions must be taken into serious consideration i.e.—*local* and *remote*.

The *local* effect may be due to *ordinary* chemical action or to *specific* action of the substance employed, which are unfortunately various. For example—the *local specific* effect produced in the sentient extremities of the nerves, as is felt on the local application of Prussia Acid, Aconite, etc.

The *remote effects* are those **influencing organs at some distance from the part,** to which the substance has been applied.

These may be *common* or *specific*. *Common,* such as the constitutional indication of fever, however produced.

*Specific,* like the effects of **Opium contracting the pupils, producing constipation, over and above its** *local* **influence in relieving pain.**

Various narcotics and poisonous drugs produce but little local change, although their *remote effects* are very remarkable. For example—Belladonna and its active principle Atropine in whatever form they may be introduced into the system, by swallowing, hypodermic injections or direct application to the eyeballs—paralyze the ciliary nerves and so cause dilatation of the pupil and accommodation of distant vision. Many have **both** *local* **and** *remote* **action,** as is but illustrated by the influence of Cantharides (Spanish Fly) upon the part to which they are applied, in producing blisters *locally* and their *remote effect* on the urinary organs, there producing strangury and sometimes bloody urine.

The *remote* action of the poison may be **due in almost every case to absorption,** either in the veins or lymphatics.

The part played by the nerves in producing the *remote* effect is not clear, but undoubtedly many of the symptoms recorded in anomalous cases have been due to other influences. An illustration is the great tendency to convulsions of various kinds in many instances. This is just what is seen in ordinary practice, where **local irritation may give rise to various reflex phenomena—but if very intense or occurring in a remote subject, may induce convulsions.**

I will not dwell upon the different experiments, by which the absorption of poisons into the circulation have been proved, as it is rather a complex study and of no material value, as far as our part is concerned.

It must, however, be borne in mind, that **certain substances, effect** certain organs in particular, even when they attack more than one. For examples:

- Opium, Morphine, Alcohol—especially effect the brain
- Nux Vomica, Strichnia [strychnine]—the spinal cord
- Curare, injected—the motor system of the nerves
- Digitalis—the heart and kidneys
- Stramonium—the lungs
- Arsenic, Antimony—the stomach
- Mercury—the liver
- Cantharides—the urinary organs
- Belladonna, Atropine—the eyes
- Ergot—the uterus, etc.

In all these, the **action is complex,** yet the organs named, seem to be specially selected for the production of their respective effects. Also it must not be overlooked that a patient may die from shock of a powerful poisonous drug, just as he would from a mechanical injury.

## MODIFICATION OF ACTION OF POISON

The same poison does not invariably act in the same way, even when a number of people are attacked at the same time. **The most important modifying agency is the quantity or dose.**

Many substances which are deadly in large doses are exceedingly useful in small quantities. The mechanical stage of aggregation is of consequence; *solid* being usually much less active than *liquid* or a *gas* and a *pure soluble* substance much more than active than one, *mixed with foreign insoluble substances.* Still more important is the chemical constitution of the poisonous agent.

I spoke of the poisonous effects of absorption of the poison and **absorption implies solution, therefore, the more soluble the compound, the more speedy the effect.**

Again, while compounds, insoluble in water or some of the juices of the body, are inert, **if they are soluble in the gastric juice, they give rise to characteristic symptoms.** For instance—Calomel* is absolutely insoluble in water, yet, note what a powerful action it has, after it comes in contact with the fluids of the stomach.

The mental and bodily condition of the patient plays a very important part and must be carefully considered, when Narcotics are concerned. Thus in excited maniacs and in certain convulsive disorders, doses of

---

*Calomel, mercury chloride was the standard of care since the 19th century until 1960s. —Ed.

*Sedatives*, **which ordinary individuals may result seriously, may be given without producing any visible effect** and some act contrary and aggravate the condition, as the writer had occasion to observe many times, while connected for a number of years with institutions and hospitals, where such cases where treated.

Again the action or effects of Narcotics are governed by certain existing conditions—Habits, age, sex, temperament, idiosyncrasies, (individual peculiarities) mental and physical state of patient, condition of stomach and contents, (whether full or empty) the quantity of blood in the vessels, etc.

Children bear opiates badly, while they can stand comparatively large doses of Arsenic, Belladonna, Ipecac, Mercurials, Squills and purgatives.

The dose for children under 12 years must be **diminished in proportion** and the ***Rule of Young***, is almost universally adopted. This rule is— **the proportion of the age, to the age,** increased by 12; thus at 2 years, it would be $1/_7^{th}$.

Example: Divide the age by the age:

$$\frac{2}{2 + 12} = \frac{2}{14} = \frac{1}{7}$$

at 21, full doses may be given.

Thus purgatives, diaphoretics and diuretics must usually be given to children in larger doses and **Narcotics in smaller doses** than called for by the *Rule of Young.* For instance, a baby 6 months old will often **not be affected by 1/4 the adult dose** of Castor Oil or **1/6 the dose** of Calomel, but **will not bear well more than 1/25 the dose of Opium.**

Ad for the Chicago College of Naprapathy.

# A Comparative Analysis*

## by William Freeman Havard, N.D.

*Herald of Health and Naturopath, XXI (7), 479-482. (1916)*

### Analysis Of Manual And Mechanical Methods

Numerous requests have come to us for an article dealing with the comparative merits of the different manual and mechanical systems of treatment. This is an extremely difficult task because each and every system has its own conception of the cause of disease and as a consequence has devised a different method of treatment for the specific correction of this *cause*. It is the variance of ideas on the part of the exponents of Neuropathy, Osteopathy, Chiropractic and Naprapathy** which today is rocking our drugless boat.

This is a subject which the student must approach with a broad and open mind remembering that complete understanding comes to him only who is without prejudice.

Years of experience with the use of the various systems of Manual and Mechanical Therapeutics has led us to the conclusion that they are all of the utmost value to the drugless physician if properly employed but the effect of such treatment must be thoroughly understood before any attempt should be made to use them. Much harm can be done to a patient by the misapplication of mechanical therapeutics.

Before employing any form of adjustment or correction to the human body the physician should submit the patient to a thorough analysis. A spinal examination for the location of a *lesion* is not sufficient to enable the physician to establish a cure. Some readers who have had considerable experience in this line of treatment may say that this is an unnecessary statement but times without number we have seen Osteopaths and Chiropractors proceed with their treatment with no other information of the patient's condition than his symptoms and the location of the lesion. They never stop to reason whether the symptoms and the lesion are indications of a compensation for a disease cause farther removed or whether they are the result of primary conditions.

We would not attempt comparative analysis of these symptoms without first laying a foundation on which to base our appreciation of them. A simple outline of pathological processes and disease causes may be sufficient for this purpose.

---

*This article was a part of a series written by William F. Havard entitled, *The Therapeutic Melting-Pot.* —Ed.

** Naprapathy is a specialized hands-on manual therapy that was founded by Oakley Smith, DC, DN in 1907. —Ed.

However if we do not thoroughly understand the action and reaction of the body we are likely to mistake signs and symptoms of disease for the disease itself.

Let us ask the question, "When is a diseased body cured? Is it with the disappearance of the distressing symptoms?" It is a recognized fact that symptoms and signs are the result of the reaction of the body to some form of irritation and are brought about by circulatory changes. These irritants or causes may operate from without or from within the body and in by far the higher percentage of cases the disease promoting elements operate from within.

Disease causes may be enumerated as hereditary, the accumulation of morbid waste matter in the system, drugs and poisons, trauma and the lowered resistance of the body due to sexual abuse and faulty oxygenation of the blood through breathing impure air. Laying aside for the moment such causes as trauma, drugs, poisons and sexual abuse we find that the other causes all operate from within and their action produces circulatory changes with a train of symptoms that leads us to the classification of diseases.

We may safely say that disease processes are caused by the accumulation and retention of foreign matter and morbid waste products in the body. In hereditary conditions the system may develop sufficient resistance to overcome and eliminate the taint. In cases of gradual accumulation of irritants through dietetic abuse, faulty oxygenation, etc., the body develops a tolerance for such and does not react to the irritation until the lymphoid structures fail in their neutralizing action and the liver can no longer oxidize them.

Germs and disease virus introduced into the body would bring about no more than a mild, temporary reaction in a body that was free from morbid waste products.

We may say that an individual is cured of disease when the causes of disease processes have been thoroughly eliminated from the body and not with the subsidence of symptoms. Most any therapeutic methods applied for the purpose may be used to check symptoms, allowing the disease to continue to smolder in the system.

If we have the proper conception and understanding of disease causes it will not be difficult to find the proper uses for our mechanical systems of treatment. Here is where some of us will disagree but anyone may gain understanding who will work with an open mind.

We are now going to make a statement which will cause the prejudiced individual some annoyance. Systems of manual and mechanical treatment correct only secondary or contributory causes of disease and symptomatic conditions, with the exception of traumatic cases. Even in the latter cases many of the serious results are due to the presence of irritants within the body. There is no doubt, however, but that this correction will be permanent and assist in the process of cure if the proper methods are employed to bring about increased elimination of morbid waste products and to raise the patient's power of resistance to the point of reaction.

We cannot be reminded too often that disease is a process, not a thing and as a consequence cure must be a process and cannot happen instantaneously. A headache may disappear with the adjustment of a cervical vertebrae or through the mechanical inhibition of the occipital nerves but the cause which produced both the headache and the *subluxation* remains.

In whatever part of the body a disturbance occurs there is an attempted compensation in some other part. Whenever we have inflammation or increased activity in one part we must have a compensatory constriction and a lowered activity in some other part. Likewise, wherever we have decreased function of an organ we have a compensatory hyperactivity in some other organ. Many symptoms or even those conditions which are listed as diseases are not such at all, but are the result of attempted compensation on the part of the body. For example let us take thyroid hypertrophy. Many treatises have been written on this abnormality but few investigators have found the true cause for it.

The thyroid belongs to a system of glands which function for the purpose of supplying special substances to nourish and tone the nervous system. The substances are called the internal secretions. To this system of glands belong the ovaries, the testes, the suprarenals [adrenals], the thyroid, the pineal and some physiologists claim that the pancreas and spleen produce internal secretions. Alteration in the function of any of these glands may cause considerable disturbance in the nervous system. To a measure they compensate for one another. In action on the part of any one of them may produce increased action on the part of one or more of the others. Their activities seem to be regulated by the quantity of their secretions in the circulation.

Observations and experiments bear us out in the assumption that the generative glands are the basic organs of this system and most disorders resulting from faulty internal secretion can be traced to a disturbance of function in the generative glands. To give the data and reasoning on this subject would require more space than the purpose of this article would permit.

In most disease processes the seat and cause of the trouble is obscure and the symptoms present themselves in the area of compensation rather than in the original part affected. A differentiation between acute and chronic disease processes will help us toward better understanding. An acute reaction is an effort on the part of the body toward greater elimination and indicates increased activity. Chronic disorders are the result of failure of the body to successfully overcome irritation and indicate lowered resistance and decreased activity.

Hyperthyroidism is increased functional activity of the thyroid gland and leads to a hypertrophy of the gland. In reality this condition is not a disease except in cases where it is produced by the introduction of abnormal substances into the body. It is an attempted compensation on the part of the thyroid for a lack of the proper substances in the blood to nourish and tone the nervous system. The most successful treatment we have ever administered for this condition was not directed to the thyroid gland directly but to the basic organs of the ductless system, the generative organs. However where the gland has passed from the functional stage to that wherein there is a proliferation of connective tissue treatment must also be directed to the thyroid.

Local treatment directed to the gland or its nerve mechanisms during its state of hyperactivity or hypertrophy is likely to result in the suppression of function and lay the foundation for serious nervous disorders later in life.

A case which came to our attention will serve to illustrate this point. A single woman, twenty-five years of age, suffering from exhaustion, fainting spells, extreme nervousness. Examination showed digestive disorders and exaggerated heart and stomach reflexes. The entire length of the spine showed marked hyperesthesia and the lightest palpitation produced tonic contractions of the muscles of the back. Heart irritable and irregular.

During the examination we noticed a tendency toward exopthalmia and the diagnosis from the eye showed a lesion of the thyroid. On being questioned the young lady said that up to the age of 14 she had a swelling at the base of the neck and that she had painted it with iodine every night for a month or more at the end of which time the swelling disappeared. Examination of the thyroid showed it to be atrophic. Nervous symptoms began to manifest themselves at the age of 16 and continued to the present. She had been under osteopathic treatment and the symptoms had been relieved but returned after a few months. Medical treatment—tonics and stimulants, quinine, strychnine, arsenic. The urine showed a high percentage of triple and amorphous phosphates. Our chain of circumstances was then complete and the young woman's present condition could be clearly traced to an abnormality of internal secretions which became exaggerated at the age of puberty. The hypertrophy of the thyroid was a compensatory condition and its suppression with iodine without the correction of the cause brought on the disorder of the nervous system. Local, specific adjustment and concussion has the same effect—suppression.

During all these years the young woman's nervous system had been deprived of its normal nourishment which should have been supplied by the ductless glands, and the tonics administered (quinine, strychnine, arsenic) were a further aggravation of the condition.

The great fault with symptomatic treatments is that in about 99 percent of cases it proves to be suppressive. The symptoms which are the result of compensation are suppressed and the real disease process continues in the system until it completely undermines the health of the individual, whereas if the correction had been applied to the cause of the trouble at the beginning a real cure could have been obtained.

To explain this subject in detail would require the writing of a large volume and such would be necessary in order to establish a standard from which to judge the merits of our system of manual and mechanical therapeutics. The cause of disease must be clearly determined as well as value and relation of symptoms, before the application of any form of treatment can be appreciated.

*Systems of manual and mechanical treatment correct only secondary or contributory causes of disease and symptomatic conditions, with the exception of traumatic cases.*

*We cannot be reminded too often that disease is a process, not a thing and as a consequence cure must be a process and cannot happen instantaneously.*

*In whatever part of the body a disturbance occurs there is an attempted compensation in some other part. Whenever we have inflammation or increased activity in one part we must have a compensatory constriction and a lowered activity in some other part.*

*Many symptoms or even those conditions which are listed as diseases are not such at all, but are the result of attempted compensation on the part of the body.*

*An acute reaction is an effort on the part of the body toward greater elimination and indicates increased activity. Chronic disorders are the result of failure of the body to successfully overcome irritation and indicate lowered resistance and decreased activity.*

*The great fault with symptomatic treatments is that in about 99 percent of cases it proves to be suppressive.*

*Systems of manual and mechanical treatment correct only secondary or contributory causes of disease and symptomatic conditions, with the exception of traumatic cases.*

## NATUROPATHIC DIAGNOSIS
### WILLIAM FREEMAN HAVARD

---

## SLEEP AND EFFICIENCY
### OSCAR EVERTZ

JULY 1918—PAGE 683

# WE WANT YOU

To Enroll for a

*POST GRADUATE COURSE*

in the

## Lindlahr College of Natural Therapeutics

We offer

**Three Summer Courses**

beginning

**JULY EIGHTH**

First TWO WEEKS' Course, July 8 to 20, on Advanced Methods of

## DIAGNOSIS

Iridiagnosis, Basic, Spinal, Laboratory and Biodynamo - Chromatic Diagnosis, Practical and Clinical Work.

Second TWO WEEKS' Course, July 22 to August 3, on

## NATURE CURE

Philosophy and Practice,

Nature Cure Philosophy, Massage, Movement Cures, Curative and Corrective Gymnastics, Dietetics, Practical Work.

Third TWO WEEKS' Course, August 5 to 17, on

## NEUROTHERAPY

Principals, Structural Analysis, General Movements and Treatments, Specific Treatments and Adjustments, Reflexology—vaso and viscero motor reflexes. Practical Work.

**These three courses comprise the complete Science and Art of Natural Therapeutics. Write for detailed information and Enroll Now.**

**LINDLAHR COLLEGE OF NATURAL THERAPEUTICS**

**525 So. Ashland Blvd., Chicago, Ill.**

Ad for the Lindlahr College Of Natural Therapeutics.

# Neuropathic Diagnosis

## by William Freeman Havard

*Herald of Health and Naturopath, XXII (3), 151-153. (1917)*

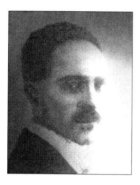

William Freeman Havard.

The V.M.R. (Vaso-Motor Reflex) taken on both sides of the spinal column shows the relative degrees of activity in the various regions of the spinal cord. From a chart of the nervous system showing the location of the vaso-motor and viscera-motor centers in the spinal cord, one can determine what mechanisms are involved in the disorder. For example, if your reflex shows hyperactivity of the dilators, the region controlling the activity of the stomach is in a state of inflammation. The V.M.R. shows the areas of disease and the areas of compensation, but will not always show the exact organ or part diseased. The reading of the reflex must be followed by a digital examination.

### Palpation Technique

Have the patient lie on his side on a treatment table or couch with a pillow supporting his head. Take your position facing the patient and proceed to palpate the side of the spine which is uppermost as this side is free from strain and more relaxed. Allow the finger tips to slide off the spinous groove to come in contact with those muscles which overlie the lamina of the vertebrae. This group of small muscles is known as the erector spinae and they receive their nerve supple from the segments of the cord opposite which they lie; consequently, from the law of reflexes, they become good indicators of the condition of the segments of the cord in which their centers are located, (the vaso-motor centers controlling the caliber of their blood vessels).

The conditions which can be determined by palpation are:

- Heat
- Hyperesthesia
- Hypertonicity
- Hypotonicity
- Passive Congestion or Infiltration
- Atonicity
- Atrophy

Excessive heat in a region or segment of the spine indicates inflammation or excessive dilation of the arterioles of that area, which means increased activity of the parts receiving nerve supply from that segment. Hyperesthesia indicates active congestion, and usually accompanies heat. Hypertonicity of the erector spinae muscles without heat or tenderness indicates hyperconstriction of blood vessels in the area of the body controlled from the segments of the spine opposite which the hypertonic muscles lie. Hypotonicity of these muscles indicates a lowered activity of the constrictor mechanism to the blood vessels of the corresponding part of the body.

Passive Congestion or Infiltration in these structures indicates constrictor fatigue in the corresponding organs or parts.

Atonicity indicates both constrictor and dilator fatigue.

Atrophy indicates dilator fatigue or paralysis, but may follow prolonged hyperconstriction.

To be able to accurately determine the exact degree of tone, etc., residing in these structures and to differentiate the various conditions enumerated above requires constant practise. The practitioner should keep accurate charts of his findings and compare them from time to time to note the changes which are taking place in his patient's condition. After examining both sides of the spine, the patient should be given a general physical examination in order to corroborate the evidence shown by the spinal analysis.

The presence of heat and hyperesthesia in any segments of the spine indicates an inflammation or hyperactivity of the organs or parts supplied with nerve fibers (V.M.) from these segments, and if very pronounced, indicates an acute disease process.

Hypertonicity existing in any region is for the purpose of maintaining the blood pressure where there is excessive dilatation of blood vessels in some other part of the body. In other words, a hyperactivity of constrictors to the blood vessels of some region of the body is a compensatory condition. A local or a general hyperconstriction may, however, take place, due to the action of some specific irritation at the constrictor centers, such for instance, as would be brought about by the action of strychnine. The other conditions found along the spine, such as hypotonicity, passive congestion or infiltration (without heat or soreness), atonicity and atrophy are all chronic in character.

TREATMENT

In a general way we may say that the treatment required for most passive or chronic conditions would be a stimulation of the segments so involved in order to increase the reflexes and likewise to increase the circulation to these sections of the cord, while the treatment of active conditions or acutely involved areas would be inhibition. It would, however, require an understanding of the philosophy of Neuropathy in order to apply these measures correctly.

### PHILOSOPHY

Realizing that all disease manifestations are brought about through changes in the circulation and alterations of nerve activity, neuropathy takes for its basis the laws governing circulation and nerve activity. It does not deny the "pressure theory" of disorders, but sees in these conditions the results of prolonged irritation preceding the subluxation, "lesion" or ligatite,* except, of course, in disorders of traumatic origin.

### LAWS OF CIRCULATION AND BLOOD SUPPLY

1. Every cell in the body will maintain a state of health, provided it receives the proper quantity and quality of food material—oxygen— and has its waste products promptly removed. (It must be understood that this law leaves out of consideration the effects from trauma and extremes of temperature.)

2. Every cell demands and receives blood in proportion to the degree of its activity.

3. The activity of cells is increased or decreased in proportion as their blood supply is either increased or decreased. This third law applies to conditions under which the circulation has already become altered as a result of irritation.

### LAWS OF ACTION AND REACTION

The cause of all disease is abnormal irritation, and there are definite laws governing the manner in which the body acts under irritation. The first response to an irritant is manifested by brief constriction of the arteries of the part affected, and the reaction from this constriction is a dilation of the same vessels, the degree of which is determined by the strength of the irritant and the degree of responsiveness in nerve mechanisms. In other words, we might say that inflammation is the natural reactive process which the body induces in order to procure the elimination of abnormal substances from the body. While such a process is in progress, it involves a deal of compensatory action in order to maintain the body constants, (temperature, pressure, density). The first and most necessary compensation is the one which occurs in the endeavor to maintain the circulation through the affected part by keeping up the force or pressure behind

---

*Ligatite is a term from Naprapathy that referred to ligaments that became constricted or tighten. —Ed.

the circulation. For this reason, a group of arteries equal in number to those of the area undergoing dilation are required to constrict, and this is exactly what happens under such conditions. Consequently, where one part of the body is inflamed, the blood vessels of some other part must be constricted. Where such compensation fails, the heart is called upon to maintain the blood pressure circulation by increasing the rate of its beat. The failure of this compensation results in a chronic disease condition of the part originally affected, for where the circulation cannot be sufficiently maintained to uphold the inflammatory process and bring it to a successful conclusion, and where the circulation to the part becomes obstructed, the cells are compelled to live surrounded by their own waste products, and consequently their activity becomes reduced, the nerve mechanisms become fatigued, and a degenerative process sets in.

### PRINCIPLES OF NEUROPATHY

The principles of neuropathic treatment may be cited as follows:

1.  To maintain compensation in body;
2.  To maintain the circulation, and restore a balance wherever it has begun to fail;
3.  To remove obstructions of whatever character that are interfering with the circulation or nerve action;
4.  To increase the patient's general vitality and raise his power of resistance.

Where such a procedure is followed, the natural forces of the body are given the fullest and freest scope to bring about an elimination of disease products and disease tendencies and to institute a process of reconstruction or regeneration.

---

*In other words, we might say that inflammation is the natural reactive process which the body induces in order to procure the elimination of abnormal substances from the body.*

*Consequently, where one part of the body is inflamed, the blood vessels of some other part must be constricted. Where such compensation fails, the heart is called upon to maintain the blood pressure circulation by increasing the rate of its beat.*

# SLEEP AND EFFICIENCY

## by Dr. Oscar Evertz

*Herald of Health and Naturopath, XXII (7), 250-252. (1917)*

Many people do not know how to sleep. The way in which you sleep plays an important part in your mental and physical efficiency. You cannot be at your best when you arise in the morning, if you have not had a night of good sound sleep.

Your mental attitude and your thoughts at the time you retire have much to do with the restfulness and benefits of your sleep. Let your last thoughts at night be not on how tired you are and how troublesome your day's work has been, but on how well you will sleep and how fresh and fine you will feel in the morning.

The thoughts which you carry over from waking to sleeping will greatly assist or interfere with Nature's work of restoring and rebuilding your worn out body and brain. This is because the Conscious Mind has a positive influence over the Subconscious. Every thought which we think has some power over the cell-processes of the body, and this is especially true of our thoughts just before we fall asleep.

Cheerfulness acts like a tonic while we sleep, whereas worry or despair acts like poison. No matter what happens, "Keep an even mind". The mother who sings her child to sleep does just that—harmonizes and soothes the mind of both herself and her little one. The man who sings at his work does the same thing—keeps himself even-minded. He is sure to do more and better work because of it. Evenness of mind spells *efficiency* because he who is unruffled is able to produce a maximum in results with a minimum of effort and energy. Therefore *efficient sleep* means that we make it as easy as possible for Nature to do her best for us during "the still watches of the night".

During "a good night's sleep" we renew our lease on life. Literally, we are reborn and new, fresh breath breathed into us for the next day's work.

In order to go to sleep we "let go" of the physical part of ourselves, and give free play to the physical or involuntary part. This is what happens when we "drop off to sleep". So, long as the body is active, the nerves tensed, the mind alert—you cannot begin your trip to Slumberland. While your senses are at work, you will be conscious all over, and then sleep is out of the question. When you are conscious you cannot at the same time be unconscious, and to be asleep means that you must for the time being, be profoundly unconscious.

It is a mistake to TRY to go to sleep. To try to do a certain thing means to make a conscious effort and that is just what you must avoid doing in order to fall asleep. Sleep involves complete loss of consciousness. Any sleep-formula which requires mental activity is a delusion and a snare. To count one hundred sheep jumping over a fence, one at a time, and other similar methods of inducing sleep, are effective only insofar as they produce monotony of thought and disinterestedness, or indifference of mind. Some people may have fair results with such a formula, while others will be driven further from sleep, the more they try to induce it.

During the waking hours, there is proportionately more blood in the brain than in the rest of the body. So long as you use your brain, the heart will pump the needed supply of blood to the head. Naturally, this makes the brain active and alert. The farthest thing from an active brain is sleep.

Before sleep will come to you, the surplus blood must be withdrawn from the brain. This you can accomplish in various ways. Try eating a light lunch (no pies, pastries, etc.) a little while before retiring. An apple or some raw fruit, which you know will agree with you; a glass of warm milk or any food which will tend to stimulate digestive activity and thus bring an added blood-supply to the stomach and away from the brain. Ten to fifteen minutes of mild physical culture exercises or a warm bath also will be found helpful. The idea is to distribute the blood over the entire body and by that means relieve the brain so the sleep can come spontaneously.

## How To Relax The Mind

It is not difficult to relax the mind although here is where most sufferers from insomnia have their main trouble. They cannot "quit thinking". The simplest and by far the most reliable method of relieving mental tension is by an attitude of indifference. To overcome insomnia, just say to yourself, "I don't care whether I sleep or not". At first you may find it hard to believe that this can be done, but a few trials will soon convince you.

Be at peace with yourself and all the world. Leave all of your troubles and problems outside your bed. Do all of your thinking before you get under the covers. Sleep is too precious to sacrifice for a tangled skein of worry-thoughts. Nature demands that you relax your mind as well as your body during sleep. This is overlooked by many people and for this reason alone they are troubled with sleeplessness.

A very effective way of relaxing both body and mind at the same time is to employ Deep Breathing. Lie flat on your back and unlimber your entire body. Make everything limp and heavy from the head down to the feet. Then fill the lungs "from the bottom up". Take good full breaths but do not stain or "pack" the breath. Be sure and exhale slowly and evenly. Have the lungs completely empty before each inhalation. Mental indiffer-

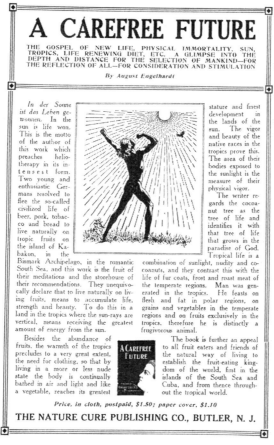
Ad for *A Careful Future* by August Engelhardt.

ence and deep breathing combined will enable you to fall asleep quickly and sleep soundly and restfully through the entire night.*

## How Much Sleep Do You Need?

What is the proper amount of sleep for me? This, like most matters of diet and hygiene, each one can best determine for himself. Ordinarily, it is no doubt true that manual workers need more sleep than mental workers. Where bone and muscle are used up during the day, it is obvious that it would require Nature longer to restore the wasted parts than when only

---

*Deep breathing has always been assumed the correct way to relax the body. However, the work of Konstantin Buteyko, Claude Lum and others have established a clear link to deep breathing and hypocapnia causing sudden vasoconstriction and other health problems. —Ed.

brain and nerve tissue is consumed. It is for this reason that sufferers from insomnia are seldom found among those who do heavy physical labor.

No doubt there are many who sleep too much, just as there are a great many who eat too much. The proverbial eight hours may or may not be your exact allotment. Weather conditions, climate and other factors also are to be considered. Yet, to believe very firmly that a certain exact number of hours are required, will tend to set up a sleep-habit, and then you will be thereafter ruled by this habit rather than by what your nature really needs.

When you lie down, let your thoughts be that you will have a good night's sleep, and will awaken as soon as you are thoroughly rested and restored. By educating your inner nature in this way, you will not hinder efficient sleep. Soon you will find that you will unconsciously have adjusted your sleep habits to a normal standard, one which is best for you, regardless of whether it be eight hours, more or less. Then you will be master of your sleeping hours as well as of your waking hours, insomnia will have left you for good, and you will measure up to efficiency standards in both mind and body.

---

*Let your last thoughts at night be not on how tired you are and how troublesome your day's work has been, but on how well you will sleep and how fresh and fine you will feel in the morning.*

*Cheerfulness acts like a tonic while we sleep, whereas worry or despair acts like poison.*

*Be at peace with yourself and all the world. Leave all of your troubles and problems outside your bed. Do all of your thinking before you get under the covers. Sleep is too precious to sacrifice for a tangled skein of worry-thoughts.*

*No doubt there are many who sleep too much, just as there are a great many who eat too much. The proverbial eight hours may or may not be your exact allotment.*

*1918*

## Zone Therapy
J. S. Riley

## Radiant Light In Naturopathic Practice
Per Nelson

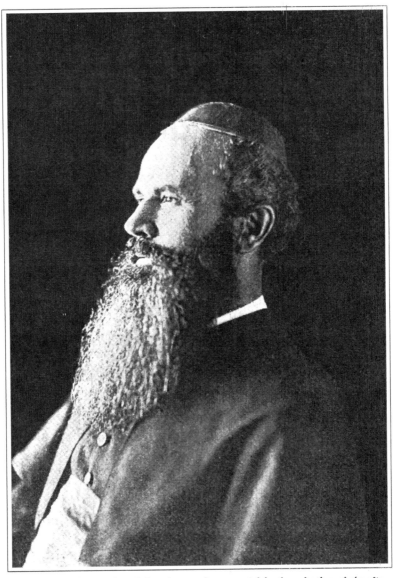

The late Rev. Albert Stroebele, who was instrumental in the selection of the site for the "Yungborn" at Butler, N. J. He was a regular contributor to the pages of the "Herald of Health and Naturopath," and revised the manuscript for the translation of "Return to Nature," promoted the Naturopathic Ideal by making new friends for the cause wherever he went. A Monument to his memory and honor was erected on the grounds of the Yungborn in Butler, N. J., and unveiled in the presence of a large gathering of his old friends on Sept. 15th, 1916.

# Zone Therapy

## by J. S. Riley, Ph.C.,

*Herald of Health and Naturopath, XXIII (5), 265-267. (1918)*

In the first part of this lecture, we invite the reader's attention to a brief study of the zones of the body. This being Zone Therapy, we must have as clear an understanding of the term Zone as can be given.

To this end, observe figure 1 from the left and figure 2 from the right. In these figures, you will see the markings for the ten zones of the body. Now put your thought, if not your imagination, to work a little more, in order to see that some organs of the body lie partly or wholly in certain zones as marked off or included by these lines.

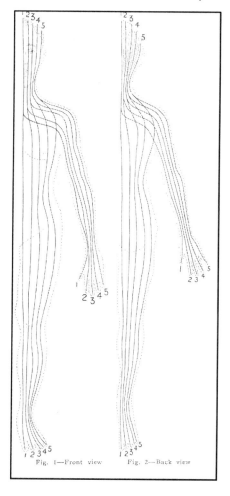

Fig. 1—Front view    Fig. 2—Back view

Now, another step, and believe that proper manipulations on the outer joints of the fingers and toes will produce an effect on the organs or parts included in the body zones into which the finger lines lead, or the toe lines.

Certain other appendages and prominences will affect the zones also. For instance, the tongue is in all zones, and proper manipulation of the tongue will affect any and all organs of the body. It is simply marvelous what may be done to the voice by treatment of the tongue. We will show how this may be done later on in this series of papers.

Take also the seventh cervical vertebra, and see what zones of the body and head may be reached through judicious zone treatment of this region. Someone may say this is only an application here of Abrams' method of Spondylotherapy, to which we reply that this principle of Zone Therapy to this region of the spine was well known ages before this distinguished Doctor and Spondylotherapist had an existence on this planet.

Observe that this seventh or prominent cervical vertebra lies in the same zone with the nasal passage, bronchial tubes, heart. What of it, you may say. Just this, that it will surprise you how readily you may cure colds, whooping cough, asthma, heart disease, with the simple treatment we are here going to illustrate to you.

The writer has cured so many cases of heart disease of the most serious character, apparently hopeless cases of asthma, and the worst cases of colds, whooping cough, etc., that he speaks dogmatically on the subject. With great certainty do we speak, and from wide experience. We know it can be done.

Take a case of heart disease, incurable under medical treatment, and just place your hand over the vertebra prominens; and give moderate concussion strokes with other hand for thirty seconds, and then rest for thirty seconds. Then repeat the strokes for thirty seconds, and again rest the same length of time. Keep this up for six or seven or eight minutes daily, or twice a day at first, if convenient, and all heart trouble will disappear in a few weeks, at most.

Take a child suffering with a whooping cough, and let the nurse or mother give this simple treatment three or four times a day with babe lying face down on her lap, and there will hardly be a paroxysm after the treatment is begun. You may make it a little better with some spinal adjustment in connection, but this alone is sufficient. If preferred, a hammer of wood of small size may be used, but the hand for small child is our preference in whooping cough. Any other cough may be broken in the same way, using heavier instrument for older people, if preferred. Asthma may be treated the same way.

We will next notice a cure of colds, la grippe, etc., from manipulations of the finger tips. This will, indeed, be a typical illustration of Zone Therapy, and is really more than marvelous. The writer has lost a number of patients by telling them this simple method. Formerly, when they were suffering with colds of any kind, they would come in for regular treatment as we usually give it with the heavy concussion and spinal adjusting, but now they only need to make this simple manipulation over the thumb and finger next to it, and soon cure the cold.

Note figure 3 for position to squeeze or manipulate the joints in making this treatment. Just clasp the finger and thumb at the outer joints with the thumb and fingers of the other hand. You may include the middle finger also, if you wish. Manipulate and squeeze thus for about a minute, and then perform the same manipulations on the joints of thumb, first and second fingers of the other hand, going from hand to hand for seven or eight minutes, and repeat a few times during the day. Often one day

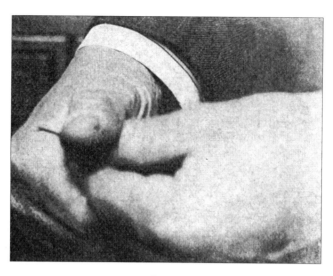

Fig. 3.

is sufficient, and sometimes one treatment only, if taken in the beginning. You may sit in church or at the moving pictures and cure a cold.

Pressure on the tongue also has a powerful effect on a cold. To treat from the tongue, protrude the tongue through or between the teeth, and bring the teeth together gently on it for a few minutes. Or tongue may be placed as far as possible under the upper or lower lip, and gentle pressure made with the teeth for a few minutes. This may be done while the finger manipulation is going on, and the one will aid the other.

For a long time we have used this method of curing colds and we do not remember of ever seeing it fail. A trial is sure to convince the most skeptical. Put it to the test under the most adverse conditions and see if you are not more than pleased with the results. It is very simple, indeed, but experience has led us to believe that nothing is surer than this simple zone therapy method of treating colds of every kind.

Catarrh of the head will disappear along with treatment also and eye troubles of many kinds will be helped. There are other manipulations that are very effective for colds, but we like the above the best, and will not illustrate any other at this time. If anyone should try this method and fail, we would be glad to hear from such a one, as our own practice has led us to believe the method to be infallible.

The same cure for the heart may also be made for goitre, with but little variation, but this subject, being of such extraordinary importance, will receive special attention in the next paper, together with some Zone Therapy work equally as startling.

We invite criticism from our readers.

## Radiant Light In Naturopathic Practice

**by Per Nelson**

*Herald of Health and Naturopath, XXIII (5), 469-473. (1918)*

Light is by no means a "cure all" or a panacea for all human ills as claimed by some profit-getting light cabinet manufacturers and certain "one-sided" enthusiastic practitioners of this branch of the healing art, but when properly applied in conditions where this form of therapeutics is indicated, it is indeed one of the most powerful means in bringing about a cure.

A knowledge of light therapeutics is therefore indispensable to every up-to-date, progressive, drugless therapist.

### The Phenomena Of Light

Many theories regarding the phenomena of light have been advanced by scientists from different parts of the world. The theory that is most supported by scientific men today is the so-called undulatory theory, which assumes that light, the same as heat, is caused by vibrations of molecules of bodies and that these vibrations are transmitted by the medium known as luminiferous ether. This medium, which extends through space, is capable of penetrating bodies, and that it exists in the intervals between the molecules of bodies.

It is further believed that the molecular vibrations of luminous bodies are imported to the neighboring ether and propagated through it by a succession of spherical waves.

The correctness of this theory seems to be substantiated by the fact that latter-day scientists have even been able to measure the frequency and wave lengths of the different rays emanating from the spectrum. Thus the frequency of the red rays has been estimated to be about 450,000,000,000 a second and their wave lengths about 700/1,000,000. The frequency of the violet rays has been estimated to be about 850,000,000,000 a second and their wave length about 400/1,000,000. Thus is will be seen that the wave length shortens relatively as the frequency increases. The wave lengths of the middle spectrum (green and yellow) are said to be about 500/1,000,000, and their frequency has been estimated to be about 600,000,000,000.

Sunlight contains, as far as we know today, at least nine different rays: the ultra-violet, violet, indigo, blue, green, yellow, orange, red and infra-red, of different frequency and wave lengths, of which the seven, the violet, indigo, blue, green, yellow, orange and red are capable of affecting the retina of the human eye. The ultra-violet and the infra-red rays can only be manifested by their effects on living tissue and by their effect upon sensitized plates. The ultra-violet, violet, indigo and blue rays are usually referred to as **actinic** or chemical rays, as they are the only rays that have any pronounced chemical effect on the tissues. The green and yellow rays produce intense light and are therefore called the **luminous** or light rays. The rays from the lower spectrum, the orange, red and infra-red, are called the **thermal** or heat rays. These rays have greater penetrating power and are therefore more capable of producing more heat than any of the other rays of the solar spectrum.

The reader should bear in mind that the light rays do **not** possess any heat until transformed into such by overcoming resistance in penetrating opaque bodies, such as the tissue structures of the human body. This explains why the red and infra-red rays, which have a low frequency and a great wave length, and therefore penetrate deeper into the tissues are capable of producing more heat than the actinic and luminous rays.

Quicke, a careful observer and well known writer on medical subjects, has noticed that haemoglobin gives off its oxygen more readily under the influence of light, especially the sunlight, or any light resembling the sun, such as the light produced by the electric arc.

Light treatments are therefore of value in all diseases where increased oxidation is desirable.

## THERAPEUTIC LAMPS

Several therapeutic lamps are on the market. These may be classified in **three groups:**

> **1st:** The Arc lamp, which has the same spectral composition as the sun.
>
> **2nd:** The Finsen lamp, which produces almost pure ultra-violet rays.
>
> **3rd:** The Incandescent, or Leucodescent lamp, which produces mostly thermal and luminous rays.

## THE ARC LAMP

Sunlight is not only the best sterilizing, disinfecting and hygienic agent we have, but also one of the best means of restoring functional activity.

It is, indeed, a true "elixir of life". To understand the great action of solar light on human well-being, one has just to compare the robust farmer or outside worker with the pale and bloodless factory worker, deprived of the life-giving, health-preserving, vibratory energies radiating from the solar spectrum, or to look into some of the cures brought about by this simple God-given remedy in some of our naturopathic sanitaria and health resorts.

The arc light is not only a "substitute" for natural sunshine, having the same spectral composition and the same effect on the human organism, but is **fully equal or better than sunlight** in that it can be used any time at any place and under any atmospheric conditions. The chemical rays produced by the arc light have a great affinity for oxygen and carry this into the tissues. It has been observed that these rays, which otherwise have very little power of penetration, when combined with the heat and light rays from the electric arc, seem to be carried deeper into the tissues than if they are given separately from the heat and light rays as is the case when the Finsen light is used.

The arc light should therefore be preferred in all diseases where increased oxidation is desired and of course, in conditions where the bactericidal effect is sought.

It should also be remembered that the ultra-violet rays given off from the arc light produce nerve reflexes through their slight irritation of the peripheral nerve endings in the skin and is therefore a powerful stimulant to cellular activity and a great factor in eliminating disease toxins from the body. In diseases such as tuberculosis of the lungs, bronchitis, anemia, nephritis, neuralgia, or in a general run-down condition, the arc light is very much to be preferred.

### THE FINSEN LIGHT

We have in the preceding paragraphs mentioned the great bactericidal effect of the ultra-violet rays. We will now describe them more fully. The therapeutic effect of the ultra-violet rays was first observed by a Danish physician, Dr. Niels Finsen of Copenhagen, who invented a therapeutic lamp which eliminated the luminous and thermal rays and gave out almost pure ultraviolet rays. Dr. Finsen employed these rays in the treatment of various skin affections in his institution in Copenhagen and brought about many a cure with this simple remedy. His light treatment of lupus [Tuberculosis of the skin] is regarded in advanced medical circles as the most astonishing discovery in the field of therapeutics.

Not only has this grave and obstinate affection been conquered but a large number of other skin diseases yield readily to this treatment. After visiting Denmark, Alexandra, then Queen of England, introduced one of these lamps into the London Hospital, where it has been used with invariable success. (The Finsen light is therefore known in England as the London Hospital lamp.) Several of these lamps have since then been installed in different hospitals in England as well as in other countries, producing wonderful results in nearly all skin diseases.

Several improvements have been made on this lamp in this country and we have today two modifications of this lamp on the market, one where the ultra-violet rays are produced by an iron arc and another where the rays are produced by passing an electric current through a mercury vapor contained in a rock crystal tube or burner.

According to statistics made by the Danish investigating committee who investigated 800 cases of lupus treated at the Finsen Institute in Copenhagen, the following figures were given:

- Cured, 407 cases (51%)
- Nearly cured, 193 cases (24%)
- Much improved, 89 cases (11%)
- Slightly improved, 40 cases (5%)
- 71 cases (9%) lost for statistics, as either treatment was discontinued or results could not be considered for lack of accurate information in regard to their condition when the above summary was prepared.

Similar results were recorded in the St. Göran's Hospital in Stockholm, Sweden. In their report, which is reproduced on page 68 in Dr. William Bernham Snow's book, *The Therapeutics of Radiant Light and Heat and Convective Heat*, (New York 1909, Scientific Authors' Publishing Co.), the following figures are given: Of 32 completed cases of lupus, 17 were cured, 10 almost cured, 4 improved and 1 hardly influenced.

These are certainly gratifying results, when we consider that lupus is the most dreaded and disfiguring of all skin diseases.

Other skin diseases, such as tinea, eczema, psoriasis, furuncles, carbuncles, alopecia, epithelioma, acne, impetigo, ringworm and many other yield readily to this form of treatment.

### THE INCANDESCENT LIGHT

The light cabinet fitted with a number of incandescent light bulbs is perhaps the most common form of light-therapeutic appliance used in this country. The first light cabinet was designed by Dr. Julius Mehls of Oranienburg, near Berlin, Germany, in 1892 and is widely used in his country, as well as here. As a pure perspiratory stimulant, the light cabinet has no equal. The therapeutic indications of vigorous sweating, however is limited to a small number of diseases. The writer has seen great harm done by the vigorous overstimulation of the sweat glands, and it has often happened that patients, after having taken this form of treatment for any length of time, could not perspire in a natural way without some "external" or "internal" stimulation by light or medicine. Practitioners of this branch of the healing art should always remember that prolonged and frequently repeated treatments by light or any other powerful stimulant may tend to overwork and thus weaken or destroy the delicate sweat-glands. Sweating and elimination of disease matter are two different things and

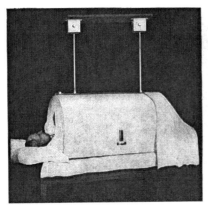

Cabinet "G" Attached to Ceiling.

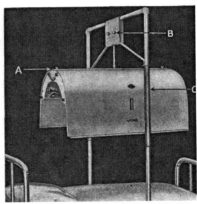

Cabinet "G" Easily Movable.

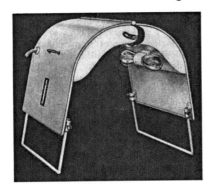

Cabinet "I" Open Position.

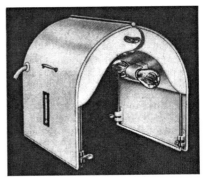

Cabinet "I" Collapsed.

that toxins cannot be "forced" out of the body by any artificial stimulation of the sweat-glands.

Dr. Lindlahr, the famous Nature Cure practitioner in Chicago, has made similar observations. The following is taken from his book, *Nature Cure, Philosophy and Practice*:

> We can now understand why the flushing of the colon with water, laxation by non-poisonous herb remedies **and forced sweating**, cannot be called natural means of cure. These agents irritate the organs of elimination into forced activity, without, at the same time, arousing the cells in the interior of the body to natural elimination.

> Dr. Lahmann made a series of experiments which prove these principles in regard to sweating. His chemists gathered the natural perspiration of certain patients produced by ordinary exercise in the sunshine. These secretions, evaporated and analyzed,

contained poisons powerful enough to kill rabbits. Produced in sweat-boxes, the profuse perspiration of the same patients, when evaporated and analyzed, contained only a very small amount of toxins, showing that artificial sweating does **not** eliminate disease matter; that sweating and elimination of disease are two different processes; that we cannot force the organism to elimination by irritants and stimulants; that the system eliminates morbid matter only in its own natural manner and when it is in proper condition to do so.

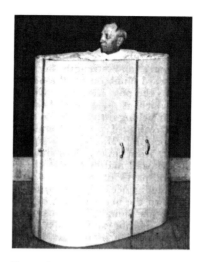

Two cabinet sections combined for Sitting Cabinet.

The above expresses the writer's views on this matter and he sincerely hopes that the reckless use of the light cabinets in many institutions will soon be discarded and that the arc light, which is the only substitute for natural sunshine and the best stimulant to **cellular elimination**, gets the advanced place it deserves.

The **local** application of incandescent light, however, is very beneficial and if the general light cabinet has been misused and its therapeutic effect overestimated, it can truly be said on the other hand that the **local** light cabinet, the 50 candle-power incandescent or leucodescent lamps have not been used as much as they deserve. The local application of light in congestion is very beneficial. When we apply light to a small part of the body, the blood will rush to this part in order to carry away the excessive heat, thereby preventing injury to the tissues. Hyperemia will thus be induced with all its beneficial results. The local application is therefore to be recommended and should be used in all cases of local congestion and capillary stagnation. The incandescent light does not produce any ultra-violet and very few other chemical rays and has therefore no direct bactericidal effect. Its effect is chiefly thermal and no solar erythema or sunburn is produced by this light.

If colored screens are used, the local incandescent light may serve a double purpose, in that it can be employed for both, sedative and stimulating treatments. By passing the light through a red glass screen, for instance, only red light is allowed to pass through, the other rays being absorbed by the red glass. The same is true of all other colors; if blue glass

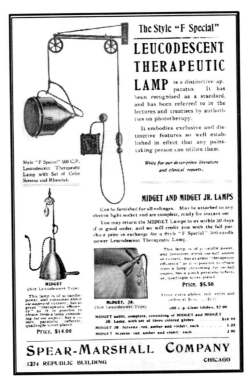

Ad for the Leucodescent Therapeutic Lamp.

screens are used, only the blue rays are permitted to penetrate. Thus, light passing through a blue glass screen is white light **minus** ultraviolet, violet, indigo, green, yellow, orange, red and infra-red, and **not** white light plus blue.

The red rays, on account of their low frequency and great wave length, penetrate deeply before they are all transformed into heat by absorption. The red light is therefore a very good stimulant and should be used where a stimulating treatment is indicated.

Dr. Finsen has proved that smallpox can successfully be treated by red light. Smallpox patients were placed in rooms with red windows and red wall paper. Light treatments by means of a small candle-power, red incandescent light, were given three times a day. The result of this simple measure was wonderful, pus formation being prevented and no scars formed. Similar observations have been made by Professor Schlanger of Germany and others.

The blue and violet rays are sedative and should be used where sedative treatments are indicated. In the London Hospital, the blue light has been used as an anesthetic with varying results.

The incandescent light is useful in all circulatory disturbances and in the following diseases: lumbago, neuritis, neuralgia, neurasthenia, arteriosclerosis, chronic dyspepsia, indigestion, obesity, diabetes, nephritis, lithemia [excess uric acid in the blood], local congestions and inactivity of the skin.

In diseases such as acute and chronic articular rheumatism, acute and chronic muscular rheumatism, gonorrheal rheumatism, acute and chronic gout, arthritis deformans, sciatica, traumatic and tubercular synovitis, muscular atrophy, sprains and strains, pleuritic, muscular adhesions, ankylosis, etc., light treatments will prove to be of value, but better results may be obtained in these conditions if superheated, dry air of a temperature of 400° to 450° F. [204° to 218° C.] is applied by means of the dry-hot-air apparatus.*

All light treatments should be followed by a cold spray or if local, by application of a 40% alcohol solution.

---

*Sunlight is not only the best sterilizing, disinfecting and hygienic agent we have, but also one of the best means of restoring functional activity.*

*The therapeutic effect of the ultra-violet rays was first observed by a Danish physician, Dr. Niels Finsen of Copenhagen, who invented a therapeutic lamp which eliminated the luminous and thermal rays and gave out almost pure ultraviolet rays.*

*The local application of light in congestion is very beneficial. When we apply light to a small part of the body, the blood will rush to this part in order to carry away the excessive heat, thereby preventing injury to the tissues.*

*The red rays, on account of their low frequency and great wave length, penetrate deeply before they are all transformed into heat by absorption.*

---

*The temperatures of 400° - 450° F seem humanly impossible. —Ed.

# 1919

## WHAT MORE?
### BENEDICT LUST

---

## WHY THE ALLOPATH IS UNPOPULAR
### GILBERT PATTEN BROWN, PH.D., D.P., D.C., N.D.

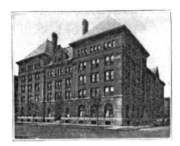
Ad for the National College of Chiropractic, Chicago, Illinois.

# WHAT MORE?

**by Benedict Lust**

*Herald of Health and Naturopath, XXIV (4), 166. (1919)*

There was a time when the average person would not entrust an acute case to a drugless healer. The remark was frequently made by such persons, "Your methods are all right for rheumatism and other chronic conditions but what could you do for a case of diphtheria or small-pox or in fact any acute disease?" Then when we at last won the confidence of our patients and they allowed us to demonstrate on acute cases, the M.D., who had previously ignored us, spoke his little piece and incidentally let the pet cat out of the bag. He offered the information that acute diseases are self-limiting and with good nursing a patient would get well anyway, even without our treatment. We are willing to corroborate that testimony but the dear people have not yet gotten past the stage where the M.D. can scare them half to death. They still cling to the old superstition that an acute disease is a calamity, filled with menace and lurking death—such is the power of suggestion. In witness, whereof, we ask you to look back over the newspapers and periodicals for November and December, 1918. Yes, acute diseases are self-limiting. They run a definite course and terminate in recovery where conditions are made suitable. Medicine, serums or other unnatural measures have nothing to do with the recovery but very often are responsible for the failure of patients to recover. The natural thing for an acutely sick person to do is to recover—it is decidedly unnatural for him to die from an acute disease. Treatment can either assist or hinder the recovery, depending on whether it conserves or lowers the patient's vitality. Those who recover from an acute disease under allopathic treatment do so in spite of the treatment. Drugless treatment for acute disorders is just good nursing and we are not ashamed to say so, but mind you I said good nursing. The history of the "flu" epidemic bears out our contention that allopathic treatment is gross interference with nature's methods of cure, for almost without exception: cases recovered without any particular treatment, cases recovered under natural treatment, but a large proportion of cases died under allopathic treatment.

What does the Old School have to say about it? Not a word. It keeps very mum—possibly thinking up some new scheme to distract public attention from its failures. Be on the lookout for a new scare.

Natural Healing has proved itself worthy under the most trying and adverse conditions—compelled as it was on the one hand to beseech the public to give it a trial and on the other hand engaged in constant warfare with organized medicine backed by government. First, it got only those cases which had turned aside from medicine in desperation; cases termed hopeless—incurable chronics—and it demonstrated cures. Then it was entrusted with the severest of acute disorders—and it demonstrated the highest percentage of cures.

What else can we do to prove that our principles are true and our practice a godsend to a poisoned race? Must we work miracles before we can hope to be accepted as a necessary factor in society and are freed from ridicule? Must we raise the dead before the poor befogged public will recognize who is who in the healing art? It is a sure thing that the public will raise hell when it at last learns the truth and finds out who has been fooling it and preying on its ignorance for so long a time.

*We are willing to corroborate that testimony but the dear people have not yet gotten past the stage where the M.D. can scare them half to death.*

*Yes, acute diseases are self-limiting. They run a definite course and terminate in recovery where conditions are made suitable. Medicine, serums or other unnatural measures have nothing to do with the recovery but very often are responsible for the failure of patients to recover.*

# Why The Allopath Is Unpopular

**by Gilbert Patten Brown, Ph.D., D.P., D.C., N.D.**

Life Member of International Medical Freedom Association

*Herald of Health and Naturopath, XXIV (9), 441-442. (1919)*

Not long since a bright young schoolteacher in the Athens of America said to one of the professors of Harvard University, "Will you please tell me, professor, why the allopathic physician is becoming so unpopular among the masses of our American people of late years?" His reply was, "We are living in an age when people think for themselves." This question is almost as ridiculous as the one asked by another educator, "Who was Stephen Decatur?" To be exact one need not ask questions these times, but listen and read, and reason will do the rest.

There is no other one society so dangerous to the welfare of the general public as the American Medical Association. This organization is composed of allopathic physicians whose duty it is in the name of their association to prey on public sentiments and play politics to promote the business relations of its members in the places of their respective abodes. Materia Medica is a blind science. It is therefore not an exact one, nor ever was it such. Its forte is to deal chiefly with drugs. It is a dying institution. It sees the "handwriting on the wall". It is a deplorable fact that drugs killed more people than bullets ever did. The Allopaths are *registered* in their respective States to *practise medicine*. Many of them are honest men as far they know the real meaning of the word. They can kill you with *medicine* and the law protects them, and then after you are dead, they can sign your *death certificate*, and you nor any of your kith or kin have any redress, and still they want further protection by the passing of more *medical laws*. These scientific and political experts work while the rest of us sleep. This is the case pure and simple of the more law there is the less liberty the masses have. The more ignorance there is in society the greater call there is for the medical physician. Let us therefore make our education brave and preventative. I learned in college that medicine is "to give and not to take". The philosophical truth is that if it is not to be taken by one it should not be given by another. This philosophy is pertinent and is congenial to the teachings of the great metaphysician, Jesus. Delving a little into the American past, the author is reminded that two of his revolutionary ancestors were *surgeons* in the Continental or Revolutionary Army under the immortal and never-tiring General George Washington. They took part in the battles of Bunker Hill, Monmouth, Stillwater, Bennington, and Saratoga. These two ignorant, but well-meaning forefathers of mine would bleed a soldier to heal his wounds, as was the custom in those times and in most cases the solider would die after bleeding.

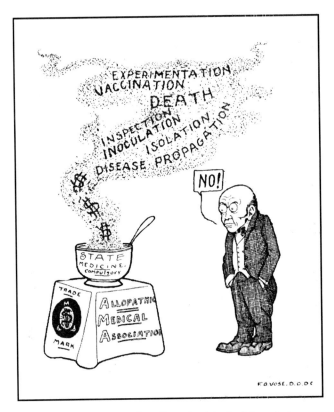

Cartoon lampooning the Allopathic Medical Association.

The patriot needed more blood instead of less to cure his wounds. But, dear reader let an American author and scientist tell you just what happened to General George Washington at the hands of the surgeons in the evening of his eventful life. He had caught a heavy cold while riding around Mt. Vernon on the evening of December 12, 1799, and it developed into pneumonia, but the medical men did not know just what his trouble was. The *surgeons* agreed that the "Father of his Country" was a very sick man, and they at once proceeded to bleed him "copiously". They next gave him calomel. Thrice did they bleed him, and thrice did they give him calomel, but he grew worse.* These strong arms of medical society then caused their patient to inhale the fumes of vinegar while the *head surgeon* gave him six grains of tartar of emetic. In the meantime, the "surgeon's mate" poulticed his throat with bran and blistered his feet. At

---

*Mortality was inevitable for George Washington, who was bled three times and given a total of 68 grams of Calomel. —*Ed.*

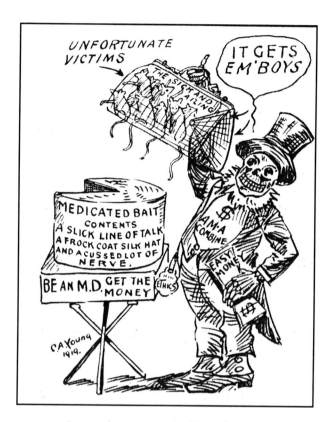

Cartoon lampooning the Allopathic M.D.

last General George Washington who had held the camp at Valley Forge "gave up the ghost" and died. The *surgeon* made this report, "The powers of life seemed to yield to the disorder". In plain words, there were no Chiropractors or Naturopathics in those days and the sharks of *Materia Medica* had killed George Washington. The family or neighbors made no protest, and his brethren in free-masonry followed him to the grave. The medical men of the world in most branches of their so-called science are as much in the woods of civilization as they were in George Washington's day. *Materia Medica* is like the creeds of men in that it is not built on a scientific basis. What many medical men themselves say is enough to wake up the rational and thinking mind to the real science of life and to what kind of treatment the sick should receive.

The great Bismarck has a very learned physician, Dr. Schweninger, who said in part, relative to the drug game as played by medical physicians of his day, "The practice of medicine is a farce; the so-called curing by drugs is a fraud." Prof. L. W. Edwards, M.D., of Omaha, Nebraska, of our day is honest enough to say, "The Allopath, the giver of drugs, wonders why people turn from medicine to Chiropractic, the drugless science. It is because of its great help to suffering humanity. Judge Chiropractic or Naturopathy by their results and one is bound to give them the approval of reason."

This great gigantic trust, the American Medical Association, now secretly working in the politics of the nation, is beginning to see its own funeral assemble. I have attended several institutions of learning and have received many degrees in Science and Letters, but the greatest degree that has been conferred upon me is that of Doctor of Chiropractic. My student and compatriot, look up and learn. Be diligent in your studies, remember the fate of the "Father of his Country", watch the concerns of the American Medical Association, and see to it that the drugless physician has his or her place in the world of science. These political experts working in the name of medicine *are dangerous to the liberties of the masses. They will soon reach the ends of their ro*pes. Why the Allopath is becoming unpopular is a question asked only by those in our midst who are densely ignorant of the trend of popular thought among the children of men. The final passing of the Allopath will be the greatest victory for society since the immortal Sermon on the Mount.

> *They can kill you with medicine and the law protects them, and then after you are dead, they can sign your death certificate, and you nor any of your kith or kin have any redress, and still they want further protection by the passing of more medical laws.*

# 1920

## The Restoration Of Impaired Function
William F. Havard, N.D.

# The Spirit of the Work

*By William Freeman Havard*

*A great work of any kind lives by the spirit which animates it.*

*Its individuality which distinguishes it from everything else must be radiant and always in evidence.*

*The work is carried forward to successful accomplishment by the enthusiasm of the workers.*

*When the spirit wanes the work lags and it fails in its mission.*

*Naturopathy is a great work, a worthy cause and one which requires all the enthusiasm and devotion of its adherents.*

*The world needs these great teachings as it never needed them before. It needs them to point the way to health, happiness and personal endeavor. It needs them to offset the vicious teachings and practices of "medicine."*

*If you believe in the great truths of Naturopathy, get into the work with heart, hand and mind. Show the proper enthusiasm for this cause.*

*Raise the spirit of the movement until it radiates health, happiness and hope to all that are capable of understanding.*

*Realize that you have the knowledge that can be employed to heal, to relieve suffering. What are you doing with it?*

*Put your very soul into carrying the message. It never grows old and there are many who are thirsting for knowledge of health.*

*Rekindle your enthusiasm, unleash your spirit and you will live to hear many shower their blessings on you and your work.*

William F. Havard wrote many poems that were published in *Herald of Health and Naturopath*.

# THE RESTORATION OF IMPAIRED FUNCTION*

## by William Freeman Havard, N. D.

*Herald of Health and Naturopath, XXV (5), 234-237. (1920)*

Symptoms, when traced to their source, are evidences of impaired function. They indicate that the body or some of its parts are struggling to maintain their activity while working against some obstruction. In other words, there is an increased resistance to be overcome. All schools of healing have recognized this fact, and their various theories regarding the character of the obstruction form the basis of their methods of treatment. These theories may be summarized as follows:

## THE ALLOPATHIC THEORY

The "Old School" of medicine has accepted the theory that disease is caused by the presence of germs within the body. The germs elaborate certain poisons or toxins which constitute a chemical irritant interfering with the normal activity of cells. The nature of the disease depends primarily on the kind of germ which has gained admission to the body and the tissue or organ which it has selected for its breeding place. The therapy which this school has evolved consisted of (a) measures to inhibit the activity of the germ and to neutralize its toxins; (b) measures to counteract the effect of the toxins upon the body's functions. Where such measures have proved of no avail surgical removal of the part or organ infected is recommended.

Class A measures consist of germicides, antiseptics, specific serums and antitoxins—all poisons in themselves. Class B measures consist of drugs, counterirritants, heat, cold, electricity, etc.

## THE HOMEOPATHIC THEORY

This school of medicine came into existence as a protest against the drastic medicine of a century ago—before the discovery of the germ. Its founder discovered that every foreign substance introduced into the body gave rise to certain symptoms and that when such symptoms were discovered in an individual they could be overcome by the administration of the drug which would cause them, provided that that drug were given in infinitesimal doses. On this ground Hahnemann gave out his law *Like Cures Like*. Many explanations have been offered for the almost miraculous manner in which this law apparently works, but none of them have

---

*This article was one of a series entitled, "A Course in Basic Diagnosis". —*Ed.*

been satisfactory enough to give Homeopathy universal recognition as a science.

## THE MECHANICAL THEORY

The complexity of the arrangement of the anatomical structure suggested the possibility of obstruction to function arising from pressure of slightly displaced bones upon softer tissues, particularly blood vessels and nerves. This theory, which was first elucidated by Peter Heinrich Ling, a Swedish masseur, later came into greater prominence with the advent of Osteopathy, and has since been elaborated upon, giving rise to numerous systems of mechanical treatment. This theory has been very favorably received, since even the layman now knows that all disease manifestations involve changes in circulation and it is easy for the mind to grasp the relationship between abnormal pressure and disturbed blood supply. The therapy likewise exerts a certain appeal because it immediately goes about correcting what is asserted to be the cause.

## THE NATUROPATHIC THEORY

This theory is more fundamental than any of the ones previously mentioned, because it goes back beyond the germ, beyond the symptoms, beyond the mechanical pressure; in fact, beyond all immediate and apparent causes to the initial deviation from normal function. It declares disease to originate with an accumulation of waste material in the blood and gives as the cause for this condition heredity plus abuse of the body through unnatural methods of living. Its methods of therapy consist of any and all measures which will relieve the body of its encumbrance, purify the blood and assist in the restoration of normal function.

Naturopathy pays little or no attention to the germ because it recognizes him as a product of disease rather than a cause. Its therapy is not directed to the counteraction of symptoms or to the suppression of effects, but to the eradication of the fundamental cause. Naturopathy is built on the foundation of sciences of Anatomy, Physiology, Physiological Chemistry and Pathology, and is the only system of healing which respects the facts of life brought to light by the study of these subjects.

With this introduction we may proceed to a discussion of our subject, "The Restoration of Impaired Function". Were we to consider the body as an assemblage of unrelated parts, we would be justified in employing any measure which came to hand to stimulate a failing organ or member to greater activity. Thus, if we discovered that the liver, for instance, were failing to perform a sufficient amount of work to relieve the blood of all the protein wastes generated by cell metabolism, we might content ourselves by administering a dose of calomel, or by mechanically or electrically stimulating the nerves to the liver. Or if the heart, being overburdened, were showing signs of failure, we might call it scientific therapy to give a heart stimulant, and as the heart responded to the whip, rub our hands and be well content that we have performed an admirable deed. But if we stop for a moment to consider that the body is not an assembled machine but a growth from one cell, we will realize that every part of the organism is related to every other part, and related in such a way that no one part can become disordered without affecting every other part. It should then be readily recognized that the part showing signs of fatigue is not always the part at fault. The failure of one organ can invariably be traced back to reduced function in some other organ; consequently it is not advisable to stimulate the organ which is showing evidence of failure until the added strain placed upon it has been removed.

That there is no system of symptomatic treatment that will eradicate disease is well proven by the failure of all methods of treatment that have not gone deep enough into the etiology of disease to discover the underlying cause or causes. When a case is diagnosed Nephritis (Bright's disease), how many physicians see anything in back of the diseased kidneys? And how many think of the effect of treatment on anything but the kidneys? Nine out of ten physicians will stimulate the kidneys to greater effort, thus hastening their ultimate failure to perform even a part of their function. Provided no foreign substance such as lead has gained entrance to the system, the function of the liver must have been considerably impaired before a condition like Nephritis could be possible. Is it not wrong judgment then, to stimulate the kidneys in this instance? But after tracing the failure back to the liver, shall we stimulate this organ?

Let us examine its condition. If a means could be provided to enable us to watch its operation, what would we see? Two streams of blood pour into the liver, one the venous blood from the digestive organs through the portal circulation, and the other the arterial blood through the hepatic artery. Both systems of vessels break up into capillaries in the liver tissue. From the portal circulation, the liver cells select certain digestive products and arrange them for cellular consumption. From the hepatic circulation the liver cells receive their nutrition and also select waste products of cell metabolism which they rearrange for elimination by the kidneys and sweat glands.

A liver which is overburdened with material brought to it in the portal circulation demands more blood through the hepatic circulation. This follows the physiological law that cells demand nutrition in proportion to the amount of work they are called upon to perform. But the more digestive material the liver handles, the greater becomes metabolism throughout the body and the more waste is created for the liver to rearrange for elimination. After a certain period the liver undergoes hypertrophy, then fatigue and congestion. The liver action now becomes sluggish and much of the waste material is passed out in a half completed form. These partially converted wastes are violent irritants, and the organs whose duty it is to eliminate them suffer irritation, inflammation, congestion and disease as a result.

To return to our question, "Shall we stimulate the liver in this case?" If the liver were capable of greater activity, yes; but unfortunately the liver is not. There is only one solution to the problem, and that is rest, relief from its overworked condition. We now come to the first essential in the restoration of impaired function, whether the organ be the heart, the liver, the kidneys, the generatives, the lungs, the nervous system or the muscles; when its function is impaired the first requirement is rest. There is no therapeutic procedure that can take the place of rest for a fatigued organ or fatigued body.

Is it not strange that after all our scientific study and research, we must come back to the very thing which Nature and common sense dictated to use in the first place?

But how may a man rest his liver? By rational fasting and dieting. There is no procedure that can equal the fast for affording rest to all organs of the body. During a fast the stomach and intestines enjoy almost absolute rest; the liver rests from its creative labors and has opportunity to concentrate on its work of arranging the accumulated wastes for elimination; the heart is relieved of excess strain caused by overloaded vessels and congested tissues; the nervous system rests, particularly the sympathetics; the lungs have a greater opportunity of removing accumulated carbon from the blood, and the multitude of cells throughout the body are given a chance to cleanse their protoplasm.

*The "Old School" of medicine has accepted the theory that disease is caused by the presence of germs within the body.*

*Many explanations have been offered for the almost miraculous manner in which this law apparently works, but none of them have been satisfactory enough to give homeopathy universal recognition as a science.*

*[Naturopathy] declares disease to originate with an accumulation of waste material in the blood and gives as the cause for this condition heredity plus abuse of the body through unnatural methods of living. Its methods of therapy consist of any and all measures which will relieve the body of its encumbrance, purify the blood and assist in the restoration of normal function.*

*But if we stop for a moment to consider that the body is not an assembled machine but a growth from one cell, we will realize that every part of the organism is related to every other part, and related in such a way that no one part can become disordered without affecting every other part.*

*That there is no system of symptomatic treatment that will eradicate disease is well proven by the failure of all methods of treatment that have not gone deep enough into the etiology of disease to discover the underlying cause or causes.*

*The point to be made is solely this, that a lack in mineral combinations is bound to be followed by disturbed vital functions of more or less importance.*

*This theory [Naturopathy] is more fundamental than any of the ones previously mentioned, because it goes back beyond the germ, beyond the symptoms, beyond the mechanical pressure; in fact, beyond all immediate and apparent causes to the initial deviation from normal function.*

**1921**

## CHROMO-THERAPY
GEORGE STARR WHITE, M.D.

## VIOLET RAYS PROPERTY CALLED HIGH FREQUENCY
DR. E. A. MARTIN

# AMERICAN SCHOOL OF NATUROPATHY
# AMERICAN [SCHOOL OF CHIROPRACTIC

## 119 West Seventy-fourth Street
## New York City

NATUROPATHY has become so well known and understood as a "Healing Art" that it is not necessary to give its history. Suffice it to say that all branches of Drugless Therapy are thoroughly taught. A graduate of this School will know all facts first and then may go out and practice, as his conscience dictates, one or all therapies without restraint.

The American School of Naturopathy was founded by Dr. Benedict Lust in the year 1896 and duly incorporated and chartered under the laws of the State of New York in the year 1905. The School has charters in three other States.

### Location

The School is most centrally located. A couple of blocks from the 72nd Street "Express" stations of the West Side Subway or the Ninth Avenue Elevated.

### Courses and Degrees

The School offers the following courses of study:

A resident course of two academic years of nine months each leading to the degree of N. D. (Doctor of Naturopathy.)

A resident course of one academic year of nine months leading to the degree of D. N. Sc. (Doctor of Natural Science.) Open to graduate students only.

A resident course of one academic year of nine months leading to the degree of N. Ph. D. (Doctor of Natural Philosophy). This course includes original research work by the applicant and the presentation of a thesis on some subject assigned by the faculty. This course is open to graduate students only.

The American School of Chiropractic offers a three year course of six months each, leading to the degree of D. C. (Doctor of Chiropractic.)

Special courses in any therapeutic branch are open to students, graduates or laymen. On passing satisfactory examinations a certificate of attendance, but no diploma, will be given to the candidate.

### Clinics

Private clinics will be conducted during the afternoons for advanced and graduate students. Class clinics are for undergraduates.

### Advanced Standing

Undergraduates of recognized colleges will be given advanced standing upon presentation of proper credit.

No credit will be given for work done by correspondence.

### Matriculation and Admission

The student must furnish a certificate of good moral character signed by two reputable men or women. He must exhibit to the Dean evidence of education equivalent to graduation of high school. Lacking such evidence, he may be admitted on examination. Until further notice the trustees reserve the right to admit mature, well qualified students without examination.

### Curriculum

The curriculum will consist of lectures, demonstrations and practical work in the laboratories and clinics. All elementary and advanced subjects of a standard medical college are taught. The greatest advantage is offered to the students by this college, as it teaches all therapies for one tuition.

### Fees and Tuition

Matriculation fee, payable but once $  5.00
Tuition Undergraduate course..... 350.00
Tuition Graduate course............ 200.00

A number of students will be given the opportunity to earn their tuition and expenses while they are taking the course. For full particulars apply to the Dean or President.

### The Faculty

Is composed of the most eminent practitioners in the drugless and medical professions. Each member of the faculty is a recognized authority in his particular department.

Special lecturers will be invited by the trustees from time to time.

### Opening of Session

The School opens its regular school year of instruction on the first Monday of October, every year.

*A cordial invitation is extended to all students of health and natural living to visit the school where they may interview the dean or secretary.*

## FOR FURTHER INFORMATION ADDRESS THE SECRETARY

In 1921, Lust moved his schools of Naturopathy and Chiropractic from near Central Park to 119 W 74th St, New York City. The area where this building had resided, now long gone, is surrounded by exquisite architecture.

# CHROMO-THERAPY*

## by George Starr White, M.D.

*Herald of Health and Naturopath, XXVI (4), 180-183. (1921)*

Chromo-Therapy means treatment of disease by radiant colors and should not be confused with Foto-Therapy which signifies treatment of disease by means of radiant light.

The difference between Chromo-Therapy and Foto-Therapy is similar to that between Homeopathy and Allopathy. Homeopathy treats with finely divided remedies and Allopathy treats with the crude drug.

### CHROMO-THERAPY AND HOMEOPATHY COMPARED

Chromo-Therapy cures by contrasts just as Homeopathy cures by contrasts. Hahnemann says, "Burns are cured by approaching the fire, frozen limbs by the application of snow, etc." Why? Because the reactive law of heat is cold and the reactive law of cold is heat.

A universal law in Nature is that likes repel while opposites attract. The positive pole repels the positive pole. In harmony lies the secret of Homeopathy and Chromopathy or Chromo-Therapy.

By finely dividing an element, for example sulfur, it produces the very opposite effect that the crude mineral does. Crude sulfur will cause a diarrhea while the 200th attenuation of sulfur will cure diarrhea. Why? Not because it is Homeopathy but because it is a natural law and Homeopathy follows a natural law.

Sulfur, like every other element, has an affinity for its opposite. In the crude form it is like an elephant while in its attenuated form it can be compared to a flea. You could dodge an elephant, but if the same weight of fleas were liberated, you could not dodge them.

**Any element subdivided has greater attraction for its opposite than the same element undivided.**

Thus, light subdivided into colors has greater attraction for its opposite than white light.

Colors possess polarity the same as metals. For example, red is irritating and excitative, similar to negative electricity; while blue is soothing and resting, similar to positive electricity.

Colors, however, belong to the finer forces of Nature and the term, "polarity", is not broad enough. For example, metals have two opposite

---

*Benedict Lust selected from Dr. White's latest book, *Think* and reprinted in the phonetic system of spelling, which the author uses throughout his works. When reviewing this article, I found hundreds of errors of spelling and decided to remove these errors so that the article could be read easily. Examples of the words used by White include: wer [were], exampl, hav, negativ, oxigen, robd, littl, cigaret, and many, many more. —Ed.

poles while colors have subdivisions of energy as numberless as the stars in the Milky Way.

### THERAPEUTIC ACTION OF RADIANT COLORS

Chromo-Therapy for Radiant Color Treatment has been used for ages in treating disease. Whether it were used empirically or not, the fact remains that different colors were painted on the skin upon which the sun radiated, or some other method was used for giving color emanations to the body.

We know that the blood selects oxygen from the air which we inhale and in which we are engulfed, because it has an inherent affinity for it. Is it not rational to believe that the tissues change light emanations to meet their special requirements?

Has not the skin the property of selecting from the spectrum such colors as the body needs and for which it has an affinity? Does not the natural call for colors depend upon the normal processes of the body?

I believe and can prove that when there is any lesion or abnormal process going on in the body, there is an affinity at that location for a neutralizing energy—a rate and mode of motion which it seems perfectly natural should be selected from light.

Nature calls for colors the same as it does for light. As long as we are covered by clothing only a small part of our bodies can obtain it. Hence there is a limitless field for light and color therapy.

We, in our uncivilized manner of living, have robbed our bodies of the light and color intended for them. Had we needed clothes, we would have been born with them. We have smothered the skin with clothes; and little by little the barbarous man is trying to smother our respiration by means of tobacco smoke, cigarette smoke, and other filthy, demoralizing fumes.

Recognizing the barbarous surroundings in which we move and have our being, Nature, ever ready to help, tries to right our metamorphosed conditions; but she often has to call for aid.

As we are surrounded by a sea of oxygen we can, if fortunately situated, flee from polluted air and find such air as will give our hungry organism the oxygen it needs; or we can by artificial means make oxygen that meets our requirements.

### COLORS AND HOW TO USE THEM

In the first place, color does not pass thru clothes, so in giving color treatment the body must be natural—that is nude. The skin, when given an opportunity, revels in light and color as a bee revels in blossoming clover.

The skin of the entire body craves light and color; and the more "civi-

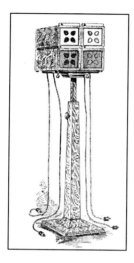

This chromotherapy projector allowed different colors to be mixed to create new color combinations.

lized" we become the more we long for the colors that paint the splendors of the universe.

In general terms, red, orange and yellow are "primitive" colors that is animating, stimulating and warming. Red is especially indicated for the blood, yellow for the nerves, and orange—partaking of both red and yellow—is stimulating and animating to both blood and nerves.

Green has a double action, being nerve animating and blood cooling, that is, sedative in febrile conditions.

Violet, indigo and blue are cold electrical colors that is, cooling, soothing and antiseptic; blue having a special action upon the blood while violet has a special action upon the nerves. Indigo partakes of the nature of both blue and violet and is soothing to both blood and nerves.

Remedies that are anti-febrile are soothing, cooling and anti-inflammatory and have blue predominating; while nervines and heart depressions have much violet.

## RED COLOR

Red color is the warm element of sunlight with especially stimulating effect upon the blood and to some extent upon the nerves. It is indicated in tuberculosis, anemia, physical exhaustion, paralysis, and all debilitated conditions.

Red is **injurious** when there is already too much of an inflammatory condition in the system, or where a person is in a feverish or excitable condition generally.

## YELLOW AND ORANGE

Yellow and orange are nerve simulants and are valuable in constipation, impaired digestion, and many abnormal pelvic conditions peculiar to women. A reddish orange is valuable in cancer and all malignant growths.

Yellow is **injurious** to an over-excited system.

## GREEN

Green is a quieting color if not too green. The color should have no suggestion of yellow. True green has a quieting and soothing effect upon the nerves and also upon the body.

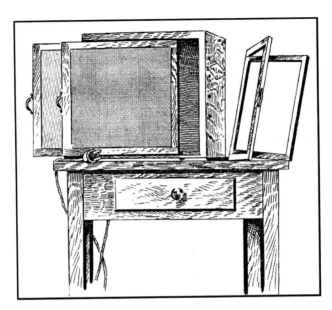

The Bio Cynamo-Chrome with openings for multiple Chromatic Screens.

### BLUE AND VIOLET

Blue and violet are nervines, astringents, refrigerants, febrifuges and sedative; soothing to nerve and vascular systems, especially where inflammatory and nerves conditions predominate.

They are indicated in sciatica, hemorrhage, cerebrospinal conditions, neuralgia, rheumatism, general nervousness, etc.

### GENERALITIES

In general, if a person is working in dark rooms the contrast of being in yellow-orange light is very beneficial. This is especially true during the rainy season when there is a great deal of cloudiness. A person's system is naturally more or less depressed and therefore treatment by means of yellow-orange is very helpful. This also applies to the lighting of the home.

On the other hand, if one is out a great deal in the bright sunlight the contrast of going into a subdued light, such as violet or blue, is restful.

Generally speaking, a person with red hair, or rubicund complexion, does not care for high colors such as red, orange or yellow; but likes green, blue or violet.

There are also countless shades of these various colors. Therefore one must be particular to pick out the colored silk best adapted for the purpose when making shades or screens. The grade of silk made under the trademark name of **Faile-Matinee** I have found to be about right for

Chromo-Therapeutic screens or shades. This special weave of silk is made in many colors and can be procured from almost any of the large dry goods stores.

## Silk vs. Glass For Screens Or Shades

Although I formerly used colored glass as the media thru which light was radiated, I have found many objections to it. It breaks easily, the proper colors often cannot be obtained, and it is expensive and cumbersome.

Silk and linens (and some parchments) of the proper color are the best materials thru which to shed light. They give a softness to the light that glass never can, especially when using artificial lights back of the screen.

## Practicability Of Silk Screens

There is no patent on silk screens. Anyone can make them. All that is required is a wire frame that will surround an electric light globe. This wire frame can be covered with suitable silk for giving the radiation desired.

If the physician is not fitted for giving Chromo-Therapeutic treatments in his office, he should at least be informed as to the colors indicated in any given condition. He is then in a position to instruct his patients intelligently for carrying on the Chromo-Therapeutic treatments in their own homes.

## Therapeutic Action Of Colors

Sunlight shed thru color glass was very much in vogue a few years ago for the treatment of diseases. Probably the reason for its going "out of fashion" was because it was not taken up in a scientific way by the medical profession.

Another reason probably is that color therapy belongs to the finer forces, and commercialism seems to have stunted the finer natures of many people, and grosser methods, such as crude drugs, vaccine and serum therapy, have taken the place of the finer forces.

I have often asked physicians why they did not do more with Chromo-Therapy, and the answers generally have been that it was not practical and did not bring in enough money to make it pay. It seems as though these physicians were ignorant of the true therapeutic value of color light.

Of course, charlatans have taken up Chromo-Therapy the same as they have taken up drugs, surgery, vaccines and serums. In fact the charlatan will take up anything that is popular. Quacks have used hydrotherapy, but that is no reason why any legitimate physician should not prescribe baths.

It seems as though the rank and file of the medical profession condemns any agency that is natural, simple, above-board and easily understood. It seems as though the "old-school" medical fraternity seeks mysterious aids for treating their patients, that is, vaccines, serums and "prescriptions written in an unknown tongue".

That the public has been aroused to the point of breaking loose from such methods is evidenced by the great number of physicians that are carrying out drugless methods. According to actual statistics, more people are being treated by natural methods than by any other.

Chromo-Therapy is so easily handled that any physician can readily fit up rooms for this treatment. He can at least give advice to his patients for carrying it out in their own homes.

Some physicians have said that if they educate their patients too much along the lines of health, they will care for themselves and thereby not need professional care. Any physician who reasons along these lines is deserving of defeat and "war bread" the rest of his life. If a physician cannot be a true physician, he should not be a physician at all.

## A PHYSICIAN MUST BE ALTRUISTIC

That goes with the profession and is included with the name physician. It is true we all have our "rent and taxes" to pay, but the physician who is a true physician and educates the people to live better, is the one who often receives the largest income and has the largest circle of honest friends.

A lawyer who advises his clients in such a way that they will have to go to law is soon out of business.

The public should be educated to pay the physician well for good, sound, wholesome advice rather than for a box of pills. They should be taught that being made sick to get them well is not economy.

In Color-Therapy we have a means for satisfying Nature's needs in a way that is more subtle and far-reaching than by crude drugs of other coarse agencies.

Disease means lack of harmony in the system, and "harmony cannot be brought about until Nature's affinities are satisfied".

One well-known writer has said that without claiming everything for any specific mode or sentiment, it is truly reasonable to contend that such beautiful natural methods as light and color are certainly far more commendable than needless operations and the use of disgusting vaccines and serums, which still hold the fort in many scientific strongholds.

Light-and-Color treatment deserve world-wide attention, and unless we wish to prove fanatics, it well becomes us to employ to the fullest extent possible, all those benignant and agreeable healing agencies which are freely at the disposal of all humanity, if we will but devote some serious thought and attention to the practical utilization of Nature's own delightful remedies.

Although mental suggestion acts powerfully in unison with all modes of treatment, there are no valid grounds for denying or even questioning the demonstrable ingredients of chemical light and color.

Light and color are in themselves highly efficacious healing agents and worthy of the most serious consideration, and as we are living in the most beautiful world which, if shorn of light and color, would instantly become a dreary wilderness and as Nature persistently employs colors in a regularly systematic manner, we are surely acting in concert with the Universal Mother if we study her actions and appareling and array ourselves and our belongings in harmony with the great example set by that unfailing Nature which never deviates from a divinely appointed pathway.

Read by the author before the California State Homeopathic Medical Society, 1918.

*The skin of the entire body craves light and color; and the more "civilized" we become the more we long for the colors that paint the splendors of the universe.*

*Red is especially indicated for the blood, yellow for the nerves, and orange—partaking of both red and yellow—is stimulating and animating to both blood and nerves.*

*Green has a double action, being nerve animating and blood cooling, that is, sedative in febrile conditions.*

*Violet, indigo and blue are cold electrical colors that is, cooling, soothing and antiseptic; blue having a special action upon the blood while violet has a special action upon the nerves.*

*There is no patent on silk screens. Anyone can make them. All that is required is a wire frame that will surround an electric light globe.*

## VIOLET RAYS PROPERLY CALLED HIGH FREQUENCY

**by Dr. E. A. Martin**

*Herald of Health and Naturopath, XXVI (9), 442-449. (1921)*

### ITS USE IN THE TREATMENT OF DISEASES AS APPLIED BY THE MEDICAL PROFESSION

Some few years ago when electricity was discovered, it was so little understood that it was accredited with all kinds of power or force and some medical men went so far as to state that "electricity was life" and their assumption was consequently carried to extremes, this being too much to expect. With the advent of electric lights and electric power motors, the medical profession set to work toward applying this electric force to the human system and with their then crude knowledge, they made machines known as static, galvanic and faradic because of the various currents produced and patients (otherwise victims), were taken for treatment and notwithstanding their contortions and resistance against receiving these violent currents, the more those applying them persisted, under the impression that results were being obtained. It did not take long, however, to discover the error of these methods, the medical profession having become satisfied, by their investigation along these lines, that it was unscientific and contrary to common sense or reason, hence should not be employed as a curative agent because of contrary effects, doing more harm than it did good. Some unscrupulous men, known as advertising doctors, took up this system and by advertising extensively in newspapers that they were able to cure by electrical treatments, obtained many patients and extorted large fees. Needless to say, some patients were benefited, probably from the psychology produced by the appearance and action of the instrument.

In 1900 Nickola Tesla, the greatest man in electrical research work, that this or any other country has ever known, directed his attention to investigating the reasons why electricity had proved a failure in the treatment of disease and though not a physician, he approached the subject as a scientist. He realized that in the human system vibration was the greatest factor and that the sense of hearing, smelling and seeing are due to vibration of the ether, also that these organs of the senses responded in proportion to the number of vibrations that were received per minute. Therefore, if electricity was to be introduced into the system in an acceptable form, it was necessary to harmonize by raising the vibrations in the body. Tesla also found that the optic nerve, taking it as an example of all other nerves in the system, had its limits in which it could visualize objects in proportion to the vibration present, this being proved by an experiment of sitting in a train going at a moderate speed. It was found that provided

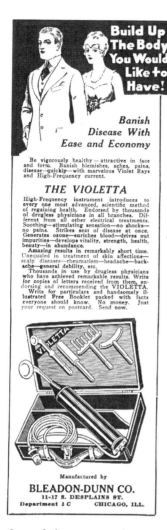

One of the many Violet Ray appliances advertised.

this speed was maintained, it was very possible to distinguish fence posts very readily along the way but as soon as the train increased to express speed, these posts immediately appeared as one or like a continuous fence. This experiment gave the key to the situation, indicating that vibrations of high degree were beyond the ability of the sensory nerve to trace; also determining the necessity for raising the vibrations of voltage of electric currents intended to be introduced into the system in order that it might be accomplished successfully.

Electricity applied to the body at a low voltage or speed has the effect of violently contracting muscular tissue. If introduced in a large volume it has the effect of shocking the nervous system to such an extent as to produce death. Should ten to fifteen amperes be allowed to come into contact with any person at high voltage, he will immediately be electrocuted; therefore, electricity at high amperage is used in most of our penal institutions. By increasing the voltage from 110 to 40,000 volts, such as is now delivered by a Violet Ray instrument, it is impossible for sensory nerves to detect the source from which these currents come nor are there any muscular contractions produced. To overcome danger of shock Tesla also found it was necessary to give electricity in very small doses (homeopathically it might be expressed), and therefore, he reduced the amperage to practically a negative quantity in the Tesla coil with which Violet Ray is equipped. To illustrate the last proposition mentioned, let us compare a fire hose projecting water in large volume at great speed or force against a man. Just as it comes from the hydrant, it doubtless would pierce a hole clear through his body or at least would lift him off his feet and throw him several yards, this because of the quantity of water which would strike him with such force. But if the same hose had several screens placed before it, each of the smaller mesh than the others until it finally had, we will say, 20,000 screens, the same volume of water could be projected against a man at close range and all that he would feel would be mist or spray. This is just what Tesla accomplished by changing the construction of former electric instruments into Violet Ray machines with Tesla coils. He increased the voltage to practically nothing. Therefore, by this change of method, electricity is sprayed into the system in such a manner that it cannot resist, the quantity being so small that it is imperceptible, nevertheless produces most beneficial results; such is a perfectly constructed Violet Ray machine of today.*

Electricity administered in this form acts as a stimulus to blood circulation and also to nerve action, combined with which is the beneficial effects obtained from light and heat produced by the electrode used in conjunction with Violet Ray instrument. Light Therapy has become popular of late because of the study made by taking the sun as an example; it has been found to produce seven colors in its spectrum which have wonderful healing properties. Each and every color, which can be distinguished separately when passed through a prism of glass produced various effects. These having been noted by using them separately artificially, red being exciting, blue and violet very quieting or soothing, yellow still more so to the organism and to the nerve system likewise curative to diseased tissues, particularly in skin diseases. Light Therapy enters as a part of Violet Ray treatment because it is produce in the vacuum tube when in operation. The tube exhibits Violet Rays. It also contains the other colors of the spectrum, but the violet, which are produced by the many ions of electricity discharged in the vacuum tube bombarding molecules within the tube are most predominant and result in the phenomena of exhibiting a violet light. That is why a High Frequency instrument is called Violet Ray. But though Violet Rays have soothing and quieting effects, they have little curative properties. However, Violet Rays after they leave the electrode and are projected against the body, produce innumerable sparks which contain Ultra-Violet Rays, invisible to the eye, yet particularly destructive to the micro-organism. In laboratory tests, it has been shown that micro-organisms subjected to Ultra-Violet Rays are immediately destroyed. Therefore, this is an additional feature which makes Violet Rays of value as a therapeutic agent. The thermic effects resulting from the electrode getting hot while being used removes congested conditions by inducing a greater flow of blood to the affected area.

The medical profession is using a glass electrode which has a silver inner coating—this because electricity has a great affinity for metal and thus the electrode heats considerably, making it similar to the heat reflect-

---

* Dr. Letitia Dick-Kronenberg continues in her father's footsteps and uses the Violet Ray in her Naturopathic practice. —Ed.

ed by a Therapeutic Lamp. While the Violet Rays are invisible in this kind of electrode, since it is obstructed by the silver lining, nevertheless it does not hinder the passing out of Ultra-Violet Rays which is the true germ destroyer. Plain or clear glass electrodes are sold at 75¢ while non-vacuum silver lined electrodes sell for $7.50. Yet the medical profession, because of the added advantage of the heat they obtain from it, use the coated electrode, notwithstanding their greatly increased price, inasmuch as this electrode does not interfere with the passage of Ultra-Violet Rays.

Dr. Noble M. Eberhart states in his textbook that,

High Frequency current is an alternating (oscillating) current in which the frequency is beyond the point of producing muscular contraction. If we apply a low frequency current to a muscle we find that the muscle contracts; this is powerful and may be strong enough to be painful. As we increase the frequency of the current the painfulness decreases, but more than a single muscle tends to contract. These are currents of medium frequency of which the sinusoidal current is a type. At a frequency of about 10,000 cycles, these tetanic contractions disappear and above that frequency there is neither pain nor gross muscular contraction. The absence of pain is supposed to be due to the inability of the sensory nerves to comprehend such rapid alternations just as we have vibrations that cannot be recognized by the auditory nerve as sound or by the eye as light. In these higher frequencies the contractile effect is expended upon the individual cells making up the tissues instead of on individual muscles. This is called cellular massage and it is one important reason why High Frequency currents produce such a marked benefit on nutrition and metabolism.

Metabolism of course includes anabolism and catabolism, the phenomena which makes the continuation of life possible in our bodies, the building up and the tearing down of tissue. The effects of High Frequency as they are presented in Violet Ray instrument passing through the system materially aid in this direction. They also favor oxidation.

Martin's *Anatomy of the Human Body* states, "Oxidation and burning have been used as equivalent phrases in accordance with the teachings of chemistry. To the chemist, a substance is burned when it is combined with oxygen, whether this combination takes place slowly or rapidly. If the combination occurs rapidly, the burning or oxidizing mass becomes very hot and also gives off light. Such a rapid and vigorous oxidation is called combustion; no combustion takes place in our bodies. It has however been proven that whether the combination of oxygen with an oxidizable or burnable substance takes place rapidly or slowly, at the end of the process exactly the same amount of energy will have been set free in each case. When the oxidation occurs in a few seconds, the oxidizing mass becomes very hot; when it occurs slowly, in a few days or weeks the mass will never be very hot because the heat set free in the process is carried off nearly as fast as it appears. As an illustration, if a piece of magnesium wire be ignited in the air, it will become a white hot flame and leave at the end of a few seconds only a certain amount of incombustible rust or magnesia, which consists of metal combined with oxygen. Under these circumstances it has been burned or oxidized at high temperature. The heat or light evolved in the process represents the energy which is set free by the union of the metal and oxygen. We can, however, oxidize the metal in a different way. If, for instance, we leave it in damp air, it will be gradually turned into magnesia without having even been hot to the touch or luminous to the eye. The process takes days or weeks but in this slow oxidation just as much energy is liberated as in the former case, although now all take the form of heat. The slowly oxidizing magnesium is in consequence at no moment noticeably hot, since it loses its heat to surrounding objects as fast as it generates it.

The oxidation occurring in our bodies are of this slow kind. Wet wood or wet coal we know will not burn easily, but other kinds of oxidation which takes place in the presence of moisture are well known. The rusting of iron, for example, is an oxidation of the metal and takes place faster in damp air than in dry; during the slow rusting in moisture just as much heat is set free as if the same compound of iron and oxygen were oxidized in a more rapid way. Such experiments throw great light on the oxidation which takes place in our own bodies. All of them are slow oxidations, which never at any one moment give off a great amount of heat and all occur in the wet tissues.

### CELL NUTRITION

Each cell has work to do for the body as a whole; it has also to look after its own well being in order to be able to do its work. This means that each cell of the bodies of the higher animals must take food materials in the form of serum albumin or globulin, sugar, oxygen, etc., must combine them into a compound which is capable of ready oxidation for the liberation of energy, must then be prepared to liberate this energy under the stimulation of nerve impulses, must direct the energy into useful channels and get rid of the waste products of oxidation. It must appropriate substance and build it up into its own protoplasm for growth or repair. Again, up to a certain point an increase of exercise for the cells of the body means an increase of power, and apparently their full power is not reached unless this opportunity for practice and exercise is given them, meaning the cells. When thus exercised they become larger as well as more effective. Other tissues than those exercised also feel the stimulus. This is especially true of the exercise of the muscles, which seem able, by making indirect demands upon the other cells of the body, to bring about the full development of all. Even the passive tissues, such as bone and tendon, are influenced through muscular exercise.

Violet Ray treatment has a marked effect in producing cellular as well as muscular massage acting as a stimulus on the motor vaso system.

We are informed in this connection that "the amount of blood in the body is not sufficient to allow a full stream of blood through all its organs at any one time. The muscular fibers controlling the diameter of the arteries are used to regulate the blood flow in such a manner that parts hard at work shall get an abundant supply, and parts at rest shall get just enough to keep them nourished. Usually when one set of organs are at work and their arteries dilated, others are at rest and their arteries contracted. For example, when the brain is at work, its vessels are dilated and often the whole head flushed; when the muscles are exercised, a great portion of the blood of the body is carried off to them; during digestion, the vessels of the alimentary tract are dilated and absorb a large share of blood. This control of the amount of blood which any organ receives is accomplished by nerve control through the branches of the sympathetic nerve system upon the muscle fibers in the walls of the arterioles. These branches are called vaso-motor nerves and the control is called vaso-motor action. Contraction of the arteriole is vaso-constriction, and relaxation of walls vaso-dilation. Vaso-motor action makes it possible to give any organ the amount of blood it needs at any time without calling upon the heart for extra work."

We can, therefore, understand how hard thought or violent exercise soon after a meal, by diverting the blood from the abdominal organs, is apt to produce an attack of indigestion.

By applying gentle electrical stimulation to nerve or muscle tissues, they are exercised to the end of producing accelerated circulation in the body with consequent greater nourishment for rebuilding tissues, such is the effect of Violet Ray treatment when introduced into the system.

Young persons whose organs have a super-abundance of energy, which enables them to work under unfavorable conditions, are less apt to suffer in such ways as their elders. One sees boys running about after eating, when older people feel a desire to sit quiet or even sleep.

"Sunlight is split into seven distinct color or rays which are visible to our eye or as seen in the colors of the rainbow: red, yellow, green, blue, violet, indigo and orange. This color picture of the solar rays is called the spectrum.

"The wave lengths of the different rays decrease from red to violet, the red having the longest, the violet the shortest wave lengths. Beyond the red and violet of the visible spectrum are the rays which are invisible. These rays are infra-red, to the left of the red, and ultra-violet, to the right of the violet. The long-waves red and infra-red rays diffuse heat and penetrate deeply. The shorter-waves, the violet and ultra-violet, give little or no heat and are called cold rays. These rays are easily absorbed and do not penetrate as deeply as the heat waves.

"Since light-therapists have learned to distinguish between the specific effects of the different qualities of light, special attention has been directed to the long waves of the red rays and to the short waves of the blue rays. The Ultra-Violet Rays especially possess decided chemical properties which are employed successfully for varied medical purposes.

"When Finsen laid the foundation for light therapy in certain local affections, he attributed his success with his concentrated cold light to the blue-ultra-violet side of the spectrum.

"The general treatment with Ultra-Violet Rays from artificial light sources did not gain a foothold until Dr. Rollier of Lesyn, and before him Dr. Bernhard of Samaden, had found that a sun bath given in the Alps had achieved a great success. These were effective principally because of the abundance of Ultra-Violet Rays obtained from the sun in the higher Alps."

In the use of the Violet Ray, while at no time is it dangerous or can a person injure themselves with it while using a closed electrode, the machine can be used with an electrode which has an open end to it where the spark comes off a wire which is called a live spark. In this manner it is used to remove warts or blemishes from the surface of the skin. It is usually accomplished painlessly and without leaving a scar, but there is one warning which has to be given where this machine is used in hairdressing establishments, where it has obtained considerable popularity because it has been found to be very useful in the treatment of dandruff conditions, falling of hair and restoring the color of the hair by returning the pigment or coloring matter to the follicle of the hair.* It is proper that I should give this warning. There is danger of using the High Frequency spark on the scalp in connection with lotions containing a high percentage of alcohol or other readily inflammable material. The High Frequency spark must be used first and the lotion applied afterwards, as there is danger of igniting the alcohol contained in such tonics or lotions. It is understood of course that the closed electrode, not the one with open end, is being mentioned in connection with scalp treatment since it gives off sparks also. A closed or open end electrode will light a gas jet. Another very valuable

---

*Violet Ray continues to be used by estheticians with no or little training. I had attended a Spa trade show and was surprised to see so many modern Violet Ray machines for sale. —Ed.

thing that I wish particularly to call your attention to are the curative properties of Violet Ray treatment in cases of X-Ray burns. Many of our best scientists, investigating the phenomena of X-Ray, have sacrificed their limbs and even lives by exposing themselves to these dangerous X-Rays. X-Ray is destructive in character because of the intensive penetrative light rays of higher potentiality. It penetrates any substance except lead and it destroys or burns tissue by arresting circulation. Therefore, in cases of cancer or abnormal growths it has been found useful. It is also used in taking photographs of the viscera or internal portions of the body because it goes clear through all tissue. But frequent exposure to these rays is dangerous, yet the very opposite maintains when speaking of Violet Ray which brings blood to the part instead of driving it away and therefore, builds up and nourishes tissue. Dr. Eberhart tells us in this connection, "The ultimate action of the application of X-Ray is to cause a decreased amount of blood in the part treated through the action of the ray in thickening the cellular lining of the arterioles and thereby producing a diminution in their caliber. It is well known that in deep X-Ray burns we have a condition of starvation and death of tissues, resulting from insufficient nourishment. As far as the action of High Frequency current on the vessels is concerned, it is diametrically opposite. It increases the blood supply to the part treated and to this extent it tends to offset the anemia produced by the X-Ray. Otherwise the two methods usually act in harmony with one another in a large number of diseases, particularly those affecting the skin, and by combining the two, a greater amount of X-Ray may be safely used, while its action is hastened by the complementary effect of the High Frequency current bringing the blood to the parts and allowing the ray to drive it away. This must not confound the reader with the action of strong sparks, which, as in fulguration, destroy arterioles, or produce an endarteritis similar to that caused by the X-Ray."

It is possible to burn with Violet Ray if you use a special electrode for the purpose called a fulguration, before referred to in this article, this electrode having an open end with wire projecting.

## PHYSIOLOGICAL ACTION OF HIGH FREQUENCY CURRENTS

Dr. Eberhart says: "When vacuum tubes are applied locally there is soon produced redness and hyperemeia or erythema with all of the resultant benefits on nutrition. In short, the fundamental value of high frequency currents is their beneficial effect on all nutritive processes. Incidental to this is produced increased oxygenation of blood and tissues, increased leucocytosis and phagocytosis and increased elimination." We have stimulated the eliminative organs of the body to depurate and get rid of the waste product made by oxygenation of the tissues. "There is no painful sensation produced by the vacuum when held firmly in the hand;

ordinarily there is sensation of heat. Removing the tube produces a spark which increases in sharpness as the tube is drawn away; up to a full length spark it is capable of emitting. The longest spark which may be drawn from the tube has been my method of roughly calculating the strength of the current and the regulation of the dosage."

Unscrupulous manufacturers have been making Violet Rays machines not in true accordance with the Tesla principle and Tesla coil. In other words, they have tried to cheapen the instrument to the extent that they have been satisfied for example, to produce an instrument that would give Violet Ray but lacking the 38,000 vibrations per minute which a properly made machine should give and producing 40,000 volts of electricity, raising it from 110 at the socket to 40,000 when passed into the system. It therefore behooves everyone, in buying a Violet Ray machine to guard against being deceived by the appearance of Violet Rays in the tube or glass electrode because there have little virtue or benefit in themselves where other more vital conditions are absent in such machines. To obtain results a machine must be scientifically constructed, such as are sold by the Guarantee Electric Products Co., who employ an expert who has had many years' experience in Europe making X-Ray and High Frequency Machines. The instrument in order to give satisfactory results must have reserve force, give one inch and a quarter spark and vibrate at the rate of 38,000 vibrations per minute, while the condenser, resonator and coils must be so constructed and attuned as to insure perfect harmony in all working parts.

"In a general way the action of the current when applied by means of the glass vacuum electrode is as follows: a mild current with tube in the contact is sedative. As the current is increased, or the electrode removed from the surface, allowing the spark to pass, it becomes first mildly stimulating, then stronger and finally caustic or destructive. The whole gradation of effect from sedation to cauterization is essentially a question of current intensity and length of sharpness of spark. With this is the effect of hyperemia and the germicidal action of the spark and the ozone which it liberates.

### Summary Of The Vacuum Tube Effects

Summary of the vacuum tube effects from Oudin resonator or Tesla separating coils:

1. Increase blood-supply to a given area. (Hyperemia).
2. Increase oxidation and local nutrition.
3. Increase oxygenation of blood.
4. Increase intake of oxygen.
5. Increase output of carbon dioxide.

7. Increase elimination of waste products.

8. Liberate ozone, with the resultant benefit of more or less of this ozone being inhaled by the patient, and also probably carried directly into the tissues.

9. Increase bodily heat, without a corresponding rise in temperature.

10. Locally germicidal.

11. Mild and medium sparks stimulate or soothe according to length and character of application.

12. Strong sparks are caustic.

13. Sparks to spine increase arterial tension.

14. Promote absorption of plastic exudates or adhesions.

"These effects of vacuum tube applications while essentially local, are not absolutely so. The current traverses the body in all direction, from the point of entry but is of course, most intense and pronounced at the latter point. Prolonged applications of vacuum tubes will give systemic effects but these are obtained more easily by auto-condensation."

Violet Rays are now generally used by physicians in their private practice as well as in hospitals in the United States because these High Frequency currents were used with such success in hospitals in Europe during the late war in treating soldiers who had developed neuro-psy-chic afflictions brought about by fearful shock to their nervous system, through exploding shells and the horrors which they witnessed around them. The medical profession stood aghast—helpless and with hands up when the war ended having nothing in their armamentarium that could possibly help these boys and there were thousands who would have been sent to insane asylums and sanitariums for the rest of their lives as incur-ables had it not been for Violet Ray treatments. Some great psychologist and an electro-therapist conceived the idea of treating these soldier boys by Violet Ray applications and talks on psychology, the object of the sug-gestions was for the purpose of making them realize that they were men and that they had nothing to fear; that they could restore their health by self-confidence; that nothing could harm them, and that most of their ills were in their imagination. The Electro-Therapist using a Violet Ray machine accomplished the final cure, this by adjusting balance to the ner-vous system and restoring normal circulation. The combination of Vio-let Ray treatments and wholesome talk on psychological lines resulted in returning thousands of these soldiers in perfect health to their dear ones at home. Under these circumstances one must have the most profound confidence in High Frequency currents or Violet Ray since proof in abun-dance is available of what it has accomplished in thousands of hopeless cases among our soldiers and those of other nations during and after the end of the late Great War.

There are textbooks written on the subject of High Frequency; one by Dr. Snow of New York and by Dr. Noble M Eberhart, M.D., Ph. D., D.C.L., of Chicago, references from which have been quoted in this article and those who wish complete information on this subject or obtain copies of these textbooks, may do so by applying to the author of *Herald of Health*, New York City.

In conclusion, it must be stated that there is no case on record of any injury having been sustained by anyone using Violet Ray properly or improperly, that to say with or without experience. Nor is there such a thing as an overdose or over application, the rule set down, however, being that ten minutes is the limit that any one should apply the current as no good can be accomplished by a longer treatment, the system having absorbed all it will receive in this period of time. Two or three applications may be given in the course of twenty-four hours, if required; ordinarily one a day is sufficient.

It must be thoroughly understood that while Violet Ray treatments are beneficial in a great number of afflictions or diseases because of the fact that it is a powerful nerve and fluid movement stimulant, due to the tremendous amount of vibrations it is capable of producing, nevertheless it is by no means a cure-all. There are a number of diseases in which Violet Ray would have no effect and doubtless contraindicated in such cases, for instance, where there is already too great an accumulation of blood or where bringing blood to the parts would encourage malignant growth of abnormal tissue. Therefore, those unacquainted with the proper uses of Violet Ray should be guided by the information obtainable from good textbooks on High Frequency treatment or from instructions received from someone thoroughly practical in this therapy. Full instructions are, however, always sent with every Violet Ray Machine sold.

The papers in an article published May 9th state that Dr. Albert H. Hess, head of the Medical Department of the Home for Hebrew Infants, reports that Violet Rays are a cure for Rickets and that six months' treatment with Violet Rays had proven successful. Rickets is a malnutrition disorder which is said to affect a high percentage of the poor children of this and all other cities.

I cannot conclude this article without again referring to the importance attached in using and selecting a thoroughly scientifically constructed Violet Ray machine, already touched upon in a previous paragraph. There is an old adage which states that "Neither wise men nor fools can work without tools," which would seem to apply fittingly to this subject inasmuch as no matter how skillfully a Violet Ray treatment may be given, results would be impossible unless the machine delivered the right amount and quality of current in the way prescribed by the inventor,

Nikola Tesla. Price is not a factor which should enter into the selection of a machine from which results are required because those who pay fees for treatment in search of health have a right to expect full value for their money. Anyone, therefore, employing any but a dependable, scientifically constructed instrument would be guilty of fraud and deception thereby losing patronage and reputation, both essential to all aiming for a successful career. The same rule applies to Violet Ray machines as does to all other commodities, one cannot obtain high grade material at too low a price and the higher the grade of the article, necessarily the greater in price, therefore, where the most essential requirement in the production of an article is expert labor which is not easily obtainable, the greater the reason for a corresponding high price. Therefore, beware of instruments offered at such prices as can only indicate that the seller has ulterior motives in offering same, regardless of results or consequences to the buyer.

*If electricity was to be introduced into the system in an acceptable form, it was necessary to harmonize by raising the vibrations in the body.*

*To overcome danger of shock Tesla also found it was necessary to give electricity in very small doses (homeopathically it might be expressed), and therefore, he reduced the amperage to practically a negative quantity in the Tesla coil with which Violet Ray is equipped.*

*Violet Rays after they leave the electrode and are projected against the body, produce innumerable sparks which contain Ultra-Violet Rays, invisible to the eye, yet particularly destructive to the micro-organism.*

*In short, the fundamental value of high frequency currents is their beneficial effect on all nutritive processes. Incidental to this is produced increased oxygenation of blood and tissues, increases leucocytosis and phagocytosis and increased elimination.*

*It must be thoroughly understood that while Violet Ray treatments are beneficial in a great number of afflictions or diseases because of the fact that it is a powerful nerve and fluid movement stimulant, due to the tremendous amount of vibrations it is capable of producing, nevertheless it is by no means a cure-all.*

_1922_

## Animal Magnetism, Curative Magnetism
### Benedict Lust

—

## Spinal Concussion
### Benedict Lust

Electrotherapies were used by the early Naturopaths and today there is a resurgence in their use.

# ANIMAL MAGNETISM, CURATIVE MAGNETISM*

## by Benedict Lust, N.D.

*Herald of Health and Naturopath, XXVII (4), 168-171. (1922)*

Ray magnetism, the inner sense of the word, means the peculiar property of certain bodies of attracting iron. Those which already possess this power in their natural state, as the magnet stone, are called natural magnets. Those, which have acquired it through artificial treatment, are termed artificial magnets. In early times, natural magnets, especially the magnetic stone, were used as curative agents, very frequently in the treatment of cramp.

The magnet is placed on the affected part of the body for from fifteen to thirty minutes, the part affected being at the same time turned toward the north, while the south pole of the magnet is placed in such manner that its north pole is directed towards the north. In other cases, on the contrary, the magnetic stone was constantly carried about on the body. It was bound to the chest in large flat pieces, or to the abdomen, limbs, etc., or worn in the form of necklets, bracelets, etc., these being inlaid with minute portions of the stone. This curative treatment was founded on mineral magnetism. Analogous to the laws by which iron is attracted to the magnet, the attractive power which draws all bodies towards each other was already, in primitive times, connected with magnetism. For maintaining a harmonious balance between the organic and inorganic worlds, some common power was supposed to exist, as connecting medium between body and soul, light and matter, motion and rest. This magnetic influence worked between organic bodies, men, animals and plants and especially in perfection, between man and man. The attraction existing between living bodies was termed animal magnetism. Paracelsus, who reintroduced the science, was the first to connect magnetism with physics, and he held that all mutual attractions were magnetic. He speaks of magnetism, magnetic power and magnetic mysteries. "Man," he says, "possess a hidden power, which, in one way may be compared to a magnet, for by it he draws from surrounding chaos the possibility of infection through the air. Man possesses a magnetism, without which he cannot exist, and they said magnetism exists on account of the man, not vice versa; and further, it is of stellar descent."

So for Theophrastus Paracelsus, everyone thus possesses the power of influencing, either voluntarily or involuntarily, those with whom he comes in contact. This power is developed in different grades, according to individual constitution. Some possess more, others less magnetic

---

*This article was one of a series written by Benedict Lust entitled, "Natural Treatment of Diseases". —Ed.

power, but, as experience shows, it may be increased by practice. To prove the certainty of this existing power, one has only to commence experimenting with himself. The nerves are, without doubt, the carrying medium of this power, and in the emanation of this nerve fluid lies the peculiar magnetic influence exerted by one individual over another.* Anyone then who possesses a surplus quantity of this nerve fluid, or "life power" or at least possess it in a high degree, may exercise an extraordinary influence on others in what way he chooses to direct it and most of all in the curative direction. Those who are most susceptible to this influence, magically exercised over them by others, are of course those of delicate health, or those who possess the peculiar fluid only in a very small proportion. The magnetically-strong man imparts to a weaker one some of his surplus "life power" by manipulating his body and hereby magnetism emanates from the operator and produces a wholesome effect on the physiological course of his patient's organism. For the performance of this, "many are called but few chosen". He only is capable of it who possesses a strong will and mental powers, religious feelings, benevolence and love in harmonious combination. The born magnetiser must seek to show his psychic powers by deep-rooted, constant exertion for their perfection. He must be morally pure and harmoniously disposed. Strength of will cannot stand alone. Many persons of strong will power exercise a fascinating influence over their neighbors, but their curative influence would be nil. The healer must be inwardly convinced of his calling and his healing powers, the highest and best work of his life. Only a pure-minded magnetiser can impart a pure magnetism. The immoral and uncalled lives a life of discord, and so suppresses any magnetic influence he may be possessed of. How true, then, are the words of Justin Kerner, in his work, *The Prophetess of Prevorst*, "For God's sake let no one try his hand here in whose heart true religion and earnestness do not rest."

In the next place, a sympathetic bond must exist between the healer and his patient for successful magnetic treatment. Should the magnetiser be in doubt as to his ability to help the patient, he should stand behind him and smell his hair. If the smell is disagreeable, his magnetic influence has been of no effect, for the nerve fluid imparted by a magnetiser is, as Professor Jäger states in his work entitled *Discovery of the Soul*, only carried to the diseased cells in a patient's body when a physical affinity exists between himself and his subject. In magnetic treatment, this mutual sym-

---

*The present conception of magnetic power is of course opposed by men of more antique views. In former times, a fine, ethereal, generally pervading matter was supposed to be dispersed everywhere penetrating animal matter generally and indifferently and predisposed towards sick people. The older theories on animal magnetism have been utilized by Professor Oscar Korschelt, in his invention of the Sun Ether Ray Apparatus which has opened up a new era.

One of many books on Magnetism.

pathetic attraction, the mutual interchange of physical sympathy, is called "magnetic rapport" (relation). The peculiar Curative Treatment consists, firstly, in posture, that of the subject corresponding to that of the magnetiser; secondly, in the manner of placing one or both hands, or the finger tips, to the patient's body, or in laying hands on the body; thirdly, in blowing or breathing upon the patient or on certain parts of the body; fourthly, in words spoken; fifthly, in the magnetiser's look. The patient's eye under operation should be directed towards the south, to facilitate this, his comfortable bed or easy chair should be, top end, facing the north. Dr. Anton Mesmer (born 1734, at Weiler, near Constance, on the Lake of Constance, who founded animal magnetism and from whom the name originates) prescribes as follows for magnetic treatment:

1. For successive mesmeric cure it is absolutely essential that the manipulant be physically sound, his influence, in the other event, would be more injurious than beneficial; and it is a fact, testified by experience, that in weakly-administered mesmerism the symptoms of the patient have been transmitted to his operator.

2. Mesmeric strength depends upon individual peculiarities. Apparently, weak persons, women, even children work in certain cases far more

efficiently than men and as a general rule, it may be said that opposite sexes produce better effect upon each other than one sex upon the same.

3.  The morning hours are best fitted, when animation of the organism is the end in view. The evening being best when it is tranquility and sleep.

4.  A quiet spot should be selected for the operation and all curious folks and on-lookers kept at a distance because strangers always have a disquieting influence and they would probably hinder the proper development. Added to this are the finer antipathies, which nature, suspicion of moral influences, set in motion.

5.  The clothing should be kept light, certain materials, as silk, are to be avoided; and it is not necessary, although beneficial, to uncover the body, or even parts of it.

6.  The magnetic sitting should begin with ten minutes and gradually increase to twenty minutes, rarely reaching the outside figure—half an hour.

So much for Dr. Mesmer. I must, in view of restriction, consent in such an article as this, forego a closer view of the minute details of a magnetic sitting, and will only mention that two treatments, a positive and a negative, are distinguished. In the former the magnetiser works in the full extent of his will power. He looks fixedly at the patient, turns his palms towards him, holds up all his finger-tips, or thumb alone, before him, and strokes all his body—by long, slowly-drawn strokes and from different points of view, from head to foot, then backwards to the head in an upward and curved direction. He should also blow strongly on the patient. In the negative form the magnetic operation takes the form of short quick strokes from head to foot. Affected or painful parts are not blown upon, but breathed over. Therefore, analogous to the principles of the water cure treatment, a stimulating, lowering, soothing, anti-inflammatory method may be spoken of, or a distinction between an imperative or receptive magnetism drawn.

Magnetic treatment is further divided into a general and local one. The former generally precedes the latter. The hands, *par eminence*, take the first place in magnetic treatment. The nerve fluid streams from the finger tips, where the seat of the odic [sic] bio-magnetic principle is most in evidence.

According to the manner in which the hands are placed on the body, or parts of it, the effect is modified in its extent; and, according to the effect—weak or strong—desired, the hands should be placed at a corresponding distance from the body. The farther the distance, the stronger the effect. Manipulation may take place with one or both hands, with one or several, or all the fingers. The strongest effect is produced by the thumb, and then, in order, the middle, index, ring, and little fingers. The inner edge of the hand—applied locally—has a positive effect, the outer, negative.

For the completion of the direct magnetic manipulation, intermediate bodies in many cases are chosen, which are then the conductors of the odic biomagnetic principle. For example, drinking or bathing water, wadding, flannel, paper, wood, glass, etc., are magnetised either positively or negatively, and applied in corresponding manner. The method of magnetising water, positively, is as follows: The magnetiser holds a glass of water in his left hand. The finger tips, drawn to a point, are held at a distance of one to two inches over the surface of the water. In about one to one-and-half minutes they are loosened and held horizontally at the same distance. After a short time they are raised from five to seven inches pointed, and retained there for about a minute, when they are again lowered to the original distance of one to two inches, where they are horizontally maintained over the surface of the water. Those manipulations are repeated once or twice, when the drinking water has become positively magnetised. Its curative powers may then be applied in the case of diarrhoea, when it should be swallowed in little sips, at intervals from four to five hours. Little children have a teaspoonful off and on, perhaps every one or two hours.

When water is to be magnetised negatively, the glass is held in the right hand and the magnetiser carries out minutely the above-mentioned prescription with his right hand. Negatively magnetised water is an antidote for constipation. Woman—as representative of the negative principle—magnetises water positively with her left hand and negatively with her right. As in all other curative methods striving for the true health of the body, not the suppression—at the expense of the collective organism—of the symptoms of disease; so it is in the application of curative magnetism which brings about a crisis. But it is possible to decrease the crisis in its intensity, the remedy being to hand in the magnetisers finger tips. Curative magnetism is, without doubt, one or the most effective Natural Cure Treatments known, and has a great future awaiting it.

*The magnet is placed on the affected part of the body for from fifteen to thirty minutes, the part affected being at the same time turned toward the north, while the south pole of the magnet is placed in such manner that its north pole is directed towards the north.*

*In the next place, a sympathetic bond must exist between the healer and his patient for successful magnetic treatment.*

*When water is to be magnetised negatively, the glass is held in the right hand and the magnetiser carries out minutely the above-mentioned prescription with his right hand.*

# Spinal Concussion

## by Benedict Lust

*Herald of Health and Naturopath, XXVII (11), 526-529. (1922)*

A general rule is that slow strokes are soothing in nature, while the rapid are exciting and more stimulating. If, therefore, some center is to be concussed for sedative effects, make the strokes in an interrupted manner. If some center is to be concussed to stimulate, let the strokes be rapid and interrupted at the proper periods. Nerve pressure, also, will stimulate for about thirty seconds and will then begin to act the other way.

If we wish to stimulate some center by concussion, we should make the strokes rapidly, say ten to twenty per second, continuing for thirty to forty seconds at that center. Then either cease for a like period or pass for concussion to some center needing the concussion. If several centers all need the concussion, pass alternately from one to the other. For instance, if we want to strengthen and regulate a weak but rapidly beating heart, we should make rapid concussion over the seventh cervical segment or vertebra for thirty to forty seconds, after which pass, say, to the twelfth dorsal to concuss for some trouble of the prostate gland. Then return to the seventh cervical for rapid concussion to that region for another period of thirty or forty seconds. Several centers may come in for concussion before returning to the seventh cervical. However, remember that if we are concussing for a bad heart, we should return to the seventh cervical more often than to other segments.

Concussion is always better if applied after the spine has received proper adjustments. Much good may be accomplished by spinal concussion alone, but a much greater good may be accomplished by first adjusting the spine and in a shorter period of time.

### Origin And Exit Of Spinal Nerves

The spinal nerves all have their origin somewhat above the point of exit from the spinal cord. The following rules will lead you to this origin very accurately:

- For the upper four cervical nerves, subtract 1 from the number of the nerve. Thus the root origin of the third cervical nerve is at the second cervical segment.

- For the nerves from the fourth cervical down to the sixth dorsal nerves subtract 2 from the number of the nerve. Anywhere in this region the root origin will be found to be two segments above the point of exit.

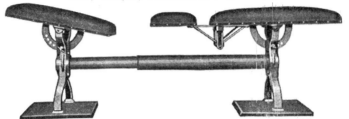
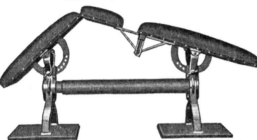
Ad for the Spears Stationery Adjusting Table.

- For the lower six dorsal nerves subtract 3 from the number of the nerve, making the root origin three points above the exit of the nerve.

- The lumbar nerves have their root origins at the region of the tenth and eleventh segments of the dorsal region of the spine.

- The sacral nerves originate at the segments of the eleventh dorsal to the first lumbar segments.

## Concussion Of The First And Second Cervical Segments

This stimulates the centers of origin of the upper four cervical nerves and has a very powerful effect on the Pneumogastric nerve [Vagus nerve] and the Phrenic nerve, as well as upon all the Cranial nerves. As the viscera of the body are reached by the Pneumogastrics [Vagus nerve] and Phrenics, these viscera all reached in some measure by concussion of the first and second cervical vertebra.

Concussion of this region will have a powerful effect upon the eyes and the ears, will affect the action of the heart, making it regular and rapid. Will brighten the memory, nourish the brain, cure vertigo, tone up most of the internal organs of the body and cure pain in the viscera as well. A very important point for concussion.

## Concussion Of The Third Cervical

Concussion of this segment gives strength to teeth and gums and will assist in the cure of any disease of those organs. Will stimulate and quicken the action of the heart. Will also, strengthen the action of the lungs.

## Concussion Of The Fourth And Fifth Cervical

Concussion of this region will prevent and check hemorrhage of the lungs in consumption and other troubles and tone the lungs and speaking apparatus, helping some forms of asthma. Is an aid in the treatment of exophthalmic goitre. Will also stimulate the adrenal glands through the Phrenic Nerves. Nose bleeding of any origin whatever may be stopped either by adjustment or concussion of this region.

## The Sixth Cervical Vertebra

A great aid to the voice and speaking apparatus and goitre of any kind. Stimulates the heart also, as well as the stomach and the lungs, gives steadiness to the head and strength to the arms. Increases the general temperature of the body.

## Seventh Cervical Vertebra

Concussion of the seventh cervical vertebra is very important for all heart weakness. Overcomes dilation and leaky valves of the heart very quickly, making the organ steady and strong. The most important heart strengthening center of the entire organism. Greatly constricts the blood vessels throughout the organism. Will abort many bad colds, stop sneeze, cure la grippe [flu] and kindred troubles. A great aid in most forms of asthma, in connection with cervical region up to middle. Has a very marked effect in the reduction and cure of exophthalmic goitre. Will resuscitate drowning or fainting person very quickly. Will relieve angina pectoris. Will give warmth to cold extremities. Prevents and cures aneurism, hardened arteries and tones up the entire circulatory system. For any heart trouble whatever this center must not be neglected.

### FIRST AND SECOND DORSAL VERTEBRAE

Spinal concussion or pressure in this region will inhibit and strengthen the action of the heart, stimulate the action and substance of the lungs, contract the muscles of the eye and seems to give tone to the sigmoid flexure of the colon. Will strengthen the action of the heart, as in case of seventh cervical, but not in so marked a degree.

### THIRD DORSAL VERTEBRA

Concussion or pressure of this region, as in the proceeding, will inhibit the action of the heart. Will stimulate the solar plexus and the stomach and the throat. Will dilate the cardiac orifice of the stomach and contract the pyloric orifice, relieving any choking sensation in the throat. Of considerable importance to all the organs mentioned above.

### FOURTH DORSAL VERTEBRA

Concussion or pressure properly applied to this region will stimulate the entire central nervous system; strengthen the heart muscles, making that organ beat more steadily and more slowly. Stimulates the spleen and enriches the blood. May be safely given for the heart, though not so strengthening as concussion of the seventh cervical for that organ.

### FIFTH DORSAL VERTEBRA

Concussion of this region will very greatly affect the solar plexus and all organs receiving smaller plexus branches from this great plexus. Will stimulate the liver and the pancreas in particular. Will greatly dilate the pyloric orifice of the stomach, enabling that organ to more readily drain the digesting substances into the duodenum. Under this action the stomach will assume a position more nearly vertical and its walls will contract more than otherwise in its peristaltic action.

### SIXTH, SEVENTH AND EIGHTH DORSAL VERTEBRAE

Concussion of this region will stimulate the Lesser and the Least Splanchnic Nerves and will therefore increase the vital forces of all the organs supplied by these nerves and will constrict them. Will dilate the lungs and will be useful in some forms of lung troubles, where dilation of those organs is desired. Will increase the action of the kidneys, particularly if tenth and eleventh segments are alternately percussed.

### Ninth Dorsal Vertebra

Concussion of this region will dilate the gall bladder and the gall duct and becomes a very important treatment for gall stones and troubles of either the gall bladder or duct. Will tone and constrict the bladder. Concussion and adjustment of this region is a powerful treatment for some stubborn cases of asthma, as well as lung and bronchial troubles.

### Tenth And Eleventh Dorsal Vertebrae

Concussion of these vertebrae will dilate the blood vessels throughout the body and all the viscera, making internal digestion more active, will make the blood richer in red corpuscles and will overcome constipation. A very powerful treatment for the viscera of the body, but fraught with danger in cases where aneurism exists or where heart is weak and dilated. In such cases, the seventh cervical should be alternately concussed with this if it be desired to concuss this region.

### Twelfth Dorsal Vertebra

A most important segment for concussion, as enlarged prostate will reduce very rapidly from it. Old cases of enlarged and painful prostate gland will become normal in size and function in so short a time as to amaze you. Concussion of this region will also stimulate all the viscera of the pelvic cavity and by constricting the sphincter muscle at the neck of the bladder will go far toward curing incontinence of urine.

### Third To Fifth Dorsal Vertebrae

Concussion of this region as a whole will contract and stimulate abdominal viscera, including the stomach, liver, spleen, pancreas, intestines, and will increase the amount of blood to the lungs, and make the circulation more perfect.

### Fifth To Eighth Dorsal Vertebrae

Concussion of this region will stimulate and contract the kidneys, mesentery, omenta, increase the circulation to and through the lungs, will dilate the pyloric orifice of the stomach and contract the cardiac orifice and become important for some kinds of stomach trouble.

### Third To Eight Dorsal Vertebrae

Concussion of this region will dilate the lungs, contract the viscera of the middle and lower abdominal cavity, give more blood to the lungs, will prevent and overcome hernia in the inguinal region. A peculiar effect of concussion of this region is the reduction of fat or adipose to the organs of the abdominal region. It becomes important in the reduction of fat.

Concussion here, with the proper adjusting, will rapidly reduce flesh where there is too much adipose.

### Ninth To Twelfth Dorsal Vertebrae

Concussion of this region will dilate the heart and the aorta, and should not be made where aneurism exists, or where there is weakness of the heart in any way. Will dilate the stomach, spleen, intestines and kidneys. Always concuss cervical seven before and after concussing this region where any heart weakness exists. Take no risk and no harm can follow.

### First, Second And Third Lumbar Vertebrae

Concussion of this region will constrict all the abdominal viscera. Will correct or allay hemorrhage of the uterus, will contract and strengthen the sphincter muscle at the neck of the bladder, and will contract the stomach, liver, spleen and the intestines, and tone and strengthen the walls of the colon. Concussion of the second lumbar vertebra will elicit all these phenomena more decidedly than the other segments here named. Marvelous results sometimes follow concussion of this region.

### Fourth And Fifth Lumbar Vertebrae

Concussion of this region will give tone to the bladder and give strength to the legs and will greatly aid all rectal troubles where there is too much weakness of sphincter muscles, pile [anal] tumors and similar troubles or disorders.

### The Sacrum

We know from experience that concussion over the sacrum has a most decided effect on the rectum, bladder. It should not be overlooked in the treatment of rectal disorders of all kinds. Very excellent results are often obtained through concussion of this region.

*For instance, if we want to strengthen and regulate a weak but rapidly beating heart, we should make rapid concussion over the seventh cervical segment or vertebra for thirty to forty seconds,*

*However, remember that if we are concussing for a bad heart, we should return to the seventh cervical more often than to other segments.*

*As the viscera of the body are reached by the Pneumogastrics [Vagus nerve] and Phrenics, these viscera all reached in some measure by concussion of the first and second cervical vertebra.*

*1923*

## The Effects Of Drugless Treatments: Light, Chiropractic And Mechanotherapy
Henry C. Sperbeck, A.B., D.C., M.T.D.

---

## The Blood Washing Method
Benedict Lust

---

## The Physiology Of Curative Movements
Benedict Lust

---

## Nature's Method Of Curing Diseases
Charles H. Duncan, M.D., D.C., D.N.

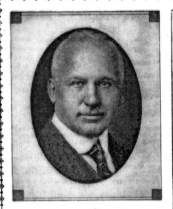
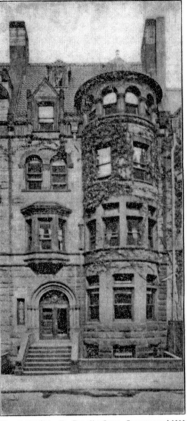
Benedict Lust moved to this building that was a couple of hundred feet from Central Park in 1923.  Today, this magnificent building is gone and replaced with a parking lot.

# The Effects Of Drugless Treatments:
# Light, Chiropractic And Mechano-Therapy

## by Henry C. Sperbeck, A.B., D.C., M.T.D.

*Naturopath, XXVIII (2), 63-69. (1923)*

No drugless treatment can be given with intelligence without knowing its effects upon the patient. Dual effects may and often are produced. Some of them are good while others are not good. The undesirable effects are to be corrected by other treatments. Most Chiropractors think of the vertebra to be adjusted and give no more thought to their work. But no one can work on the spine with any degree of intelligence without knowing the spinal reflexes. Chiropractic is more than the work of adjustment. The thrust will increase the blood in the spinal column and in the organ supplied by the nerves of that area.

Is this a good thing to do? The same effect will be secured as the concussion of that vertebra. Take a few examples: suppose the liver is in a hyperemic condition, would it be wise to send more blood into it? If the bowels are in a dilated and flaccid condition a thrust on the eleventh dorsal would increase the dilatation and the effect would be bad. One who uses concussion would not make this mistake because he would take into consideration what effect he wished to secure. Or suppose the appendix was much inflamed and a thrust was given on the second lumbar, the organ might be ruptured. To ignore the spinal reflexes may lead to such bad results as to exhaust them and so make the patient a helpless invalid. Nature must work by reflex action. I have known of cases where chiropractic simply put the man out of business. Too often the chiropractor will think that any bad symptoms are due to the patient re-tracing. Better look into the therapy. It may be bad. If a thrust must be given on a vertebra and bad effects are produced there must be other treatments or the vertebra treated that will overcome the undesirable effects. If the liver is already congested and you thrust the second dorsal better follow that up with a thrust that will contract the organ. Or concuss the one, two and three lumbars.

Consider the effects of color treatments. Color treatment has long been used as being of value in certain conditions. Red is known for its stimulating effects. But to know nothing more than its general effects is to work in the dark. And some drugless doctors who use light do work in darkness because they do not know the results of their therapy upon the patient. Red has a specific effect when used upon the abdomen, chest or back. It contracts the heart, increases blood pressure, increases the rate and force of the heartbeat.

The same effects can be secured by concussion of the seventh cervical. Another very important point is: the light should not be used continually, but should be shut off every half minute and then turned on again for the same time during the whole treatment. This will give the light vibration a better chance to secure their results. It will be more acceptable to nature. This rule must be followed with the use of all color treatments.

In the use of both red and violet lights the condition of the vagus nerve must be known. We have symptoms of decreased vagal tone in the dilatation of the heart and liver, in diabetes, in neurotic temperament and in gastric and intestinal neurosis. In these conditions we would endeavor to increase the tone of the nerve and could do so by the use of the red light. But if one did not know these facts and used the violet light he would make the patient worse. Or again the vagus tone may be increased as in such diseases as—asthma, phthisis, emphysema and in angina pectoris. The object now is to decrease the tone of the vagus. The treatment would be the violet light. There will often be cases where the effects will be what we are after, but other effects will be produced that will not be good for the patient and to get the very best results we will have to use other treatments that will overcome the bad effects. This we will take up under the subject of blood pressure. Color is a very interesting subject in therapeutics and unless we know how it acts upon the patient we will do more harm than good. The reason some have better success in their work is due to the fact that they know what bad therapy is. Few think that they can make any mistakes in their method of treatment. They work upon the general rule that not the disease but the patient is to be treated. But there is a bad blunder. The disease must be known. The effect of the treatment upon it must be known. The reflexes must be mastered. We must "prove all things and hold fast to that which is good". If a patient has been doing brain work during the day and we treat him with the yellow light at night the effect will be over stimulating to his nerve system. Violet is the color he should have in such a case.

But other facts must be known also, such as the blood pressure and the vagus tone. If any color is offensive to the patient no treatment with that color should be given him. Yellow light will increase the respiration more than the red or green colors. In red the respiration will be fifteen a minute. In yellow it will be nineteen. Tonics like iron and strychnine have the yellow principle. Yellow is a laxative and this is true both in the drugs that have the yellow principle and in the light. The same thing holds true in other drugs. Color in medicine and color in light produce like effects in the body, but the light color does not have any of the ill effects that drugs produce. The treatment by color-vibrations is more in accord with nature and gives us every advantage over the drug method. The lungs, kidneys and the bowels respond well to yellow. Blue is valuable for deaf-

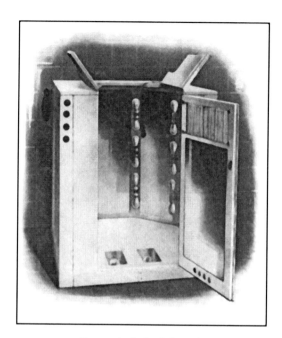

Electric Light Bath (open).

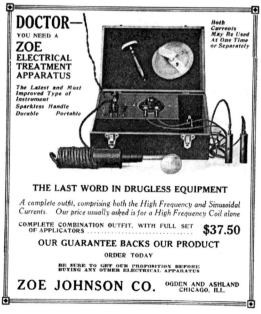

High frequency current was used in electrical devices.

ness, flatulency, gastritis, insomnia and is a stimulant to the venous blood. But like the red it has a specific effect which must always be remembered or bad effects may be produced by it. This specific effect is as follow: dilates the heart, lowers the blood pressure, dilates the bronchial tubes. It has the same effect as concussion of the third and fourth dorsals. The red increases the tone of the Vagus nerve. The blue decreased its tone. You must know then, if the treatment of the Vagus is to be increased or decreased. The "Vagal Reflex" can be ascertained by the proper diagnosis which I cannot give here. But without this diagnosis you would be working in the dark. Blood pressure will help you to use the red or blue with some degree of intelligence as you would not use the blue in a case of low blood pressure. But again in a nervous subject the blue would be very valuable and if you used it the treatment would have to be followed by overcoming the effects of the low blood pressure. Hence you will proceed to raise the blood pressure by other means. This holds good in many forms of treatment and is always to be kept in mind in all light treatments. We will have more in this line in a few minutes. For a general tonic treatment I have found the orange light very useful. It is to be tried out in all cases of paresis, lymphatic treatments, kidney trouble, bronchial affections, and low vitality.

Orange can be used with white, red, or blue. In cases of paralysis the red and the orange may be used with excellent results. But in such cases if the blood pressure is already high the red should not be used. Do not use the red in syphilis, but the blue; because in this disease the Vagus nerve is increased.

In some diseases both the orange and the blue lights may be used such as: cramps, diabetes, and where tonic and sedative effects are desired. The white light followed by the blue may be used in nervous exhaustion, in all forms of pain, and in sciatic rheumatism. The white light is used first over the part to be treated and then the blue one third as long as the white. But if the blood pressure is low use another treatment to increase it.

A drugless doctor made the remark that we should treat the patient not the disease and that a general treatment was the best. But in such a method we must know the effects of the general treatment. Suppose the general treatment is manipulation of the body. You will increase the circulation, stimulate digestion, aid assimilation and increase respiration. But suppose the patient has high blood pressure and you do not know it— you will increase it with such a treatment. Or suppose you give a general massage in the form of kneading and the patient has low blood pressure— you will make it still lower. Light percussion of the chest will reduce the blood pressure and heavy percussion will raise it and yet you are working in the same area. But if you know that the patient has high blood pressure and you use movements, better combine them with kneading so as to not raise the blood pressure.

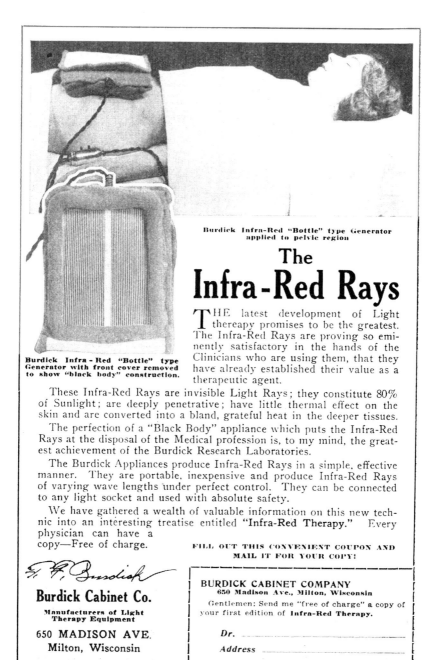

Burdick Infra-Red "Bottle" type Generator applied to pelvic region

# The
# Infra-Red Rays

THE latest development of Light thereapy promises to be the greatest. The Infra-Red Rays are proving so eminently satisfactory in the hands of the Clinicians who are using them, that they have already established their value as a therapeutic agent.

Burdick Infra-Red "Bottle" type Generator with front cover removed to show "black body" construction.

These Infra-Red Rays are invisible Light Rays; they constitute 80% of Sunlight; are deeply penetrative; have little thermal effect on the skin and are converted into a bland, grateful heat in the deeper tissues.

The perfection of a "Black Body" appliance which puts the Infra-Red Rays at the disposal of the Medical profession is, to my mind, the greatest achievement of the Burdick Research Laboratories.

The Burdick Appliances produce Infra-Red Rays in a simple, effective manner. They are portable, inexpensive and produce Infra-Red Rays of varying wave lengths under perfect control. They can be connected to any light socket and used with absolute safety.

We have gathered a wealth of valuable information on this new technic into an interesting treatise entitled "Infra-Red Therapy." Every physician can have a copy—Free of charge.

FILL OUT THIS CONVENIENT COUPON AND MAIL IT FOR YOUR COPY!

## Burdick Cabinet Co.

Manufacturers of Light Therapy Equipment

650 MADISON AVE.
Milton, Wisconsin

BURDICK CABINET COMPANY
650 Madison Ave., Milton, Wisconsin

Gentlemen: Send me "free of charge" a copy of your first edition of Infra-Red Therapy.

Dr. ........................................

Address ........................................

The early Naturopaths explored light therapy using Infra Red appliances.

The same—knowing the effects of your treatment—holds good in the use of the electric light bath. I have heard men say that they could not stand this bath because the heart action increased rapidly and the temperature run up to 126° F. [52° C.]* in a few minutes. There is something wrong with this treatment. I take the temperature in a part of the cabinet where the heat is the strongest—near the top and I have had patients in there for twenty minutes and could not get over 100 degrees. I may add that I use the Fellwock cabinet. I do not want any better one and I have used it for six years. What are the effects of the electrical light bath? Do you know them? Are they all good for the patient? Should they be followed by some other treatment to keep the good effects of the light bath and eliminate the bad effects? These are vital questions. Let us take up the good effects of the light bath.

Dilates the surface vessels. This will relieve internal congestion and increases the activity of the skin. Excellent for elimination. Increases metabolic activity—fine for all constitutional disorders. Acts upon the blood and increases the circulation. But it also depresses the nerve system. They may be good in some cases of over nerve activity, but in a weak subject it would not be so good. Lowers the blood pressure when the bath is prolonged. Quickens and weakens the heart action and respiration. The patient should have a cold compress on the head and one on the heart. If a bath follows the light bath and the water is cool, re-action will take place that will overcome the bad effects. Or the patient may be given a treatment after the light bath as mechano-therapy and so raise the blood pressure, and secure other good effects that will give an ideal treatment. Kellogg shows that light is one of the best tonics we have, but to get the tonic effects of light you must know how to give the treatment.

One author heats the light bath to 110° F. [43° C.] and then puts the patient in for one to three minutes and that constitutes an excellent tonic effect. But in all these treatments you must know the effect upon the patient and make all treatments short until the effects are known. Bath should be always followed by water or some other form of treatment. In my cabinet the temperature never goes up in a sudden jump. I cut down the number of lights or give more air in the cabinet to regulate the temperature. No patient ever complained of ill effects and I always make it a point to ask them the next time they come for treatment. I have kept them in for twenty minutes treatment with no ill effects. And many of them while in the bath enjoyed the sensation of the heat rays.

CLINICAL REPORTS

Mrs. K—came to me suffering with an itching sensation all over the

___
*The author is referring to the temperature in the electric light bath cabinet.   —Ed.

body and had tried everything she heard of with no results. I used the violet (Blue) light all over the body and made treatments three times a week and she responded to the treatment from the first. In a few weeks she was cured. No return of the trouble and it has been now six years since she took treatments.

Male 49 years old, came to me in a depleted condition. Unable to work for over a year. Vitality was very low and low blood pressure. I gave him the orange light on the spine, mild manipulations, and in some treatments used the violet light followed concussion of the seven cervical. His progress was slow but sure and he was able to return to work in a few months. Later I found that he improved under the arc light treatment.

Female 31 years old suffered from indigestion. Her husband sent her to her mother's home which was in my town. She had been taking medicine for three months and was in a rundown nervous condition when I was called to treat her. I used the blue light over the stomach and down the spine and then followed that with a mild vibration. She responded to the treatment and was able to return home in three weeks.

Female had been operated for cancer of the breast. The organ was removed. I was called to treat her for her nerves. She was in a bad condition. Unable to do any work, could not rest at night and was very weak. I used the blue light over the 3rd and 4th dorsals and I was surprised how soon her heart decreased in its beat. She began to breathe with more ease and after the treatment could sleep. On account of her condition little could be done for her and so I could do no more than to give her some relief and put her in a condition to rest at night. Cancer was doing its deadly work and the muscles of her spine were set so that I saw she was in a bad condition. About a month later she passed away. But the blue light gave her the comfort that nothing else could have given her. She expressed her satisfaction with the relief.

Case of Tabes [emanciation]. Male 39 and confined to bed. Given up by the best M.Ds. in this part of the country. Used chiropractic, concussion, arc light and general massage. Made excellent progress and feels good but has not fully recovered at this time.

Male 45, a case of lumbago. Used the 500 lamp over the lumbar region followed with vibration and the blue light with concussion of the seventh cervical. He went south and felt no more of the trouble.

Case of eczema; male age 50 suffered for a number of years. The best treatment that I gave him was the arc light. He has recovered.

Case of neuritis, male, a painter by trade, age 45, pain in the right arm suffered so that he could not rest or sleep and walked the streets at night. I gave gentle massage of the arm, used the blue light for fifteen minutes and in a little over a week he was back to work and felt no pain in the arm.

## OUTLINE OF TREATMENTS FOR DISEASES

### ASTHMA

1. Vibration of the chest.
2. Pressure on the head of the first rib (during an attack).
3. Manipulate the cervical region.
4. Asthma may be due to general neurasthenia.
5. Examine the nose.
6. Vigorously knead the muscles of the chest and back.
7. Adjust between the two vertebrae—9th and 10th dorsal (during an attack).
8. Electric light bath.

### BRIGHT'S DISEASE

1. Electric light baths.
2. Kneading and percussion of the back and chest (ulnar percussion).
3. Kneading of the colon.
4. Circumduction of the legs and arms.
5. Arc lamp to the spine 12th [thoracic] to 1st lumbar.
6. Chiropractic.

### NEURASTHENIA

Inquire into the habits of the patient.

1. Loosen the muscles along the spine.
2. Abdominal massage for 10 minutes.
3. Vibrate from the 6th to 12th dorsal—stimulate.
4. Arc lamp to whole spine and to abdomen.
5. Begin with short arc light treatment and increase.
6. Keep the bowels open.
7. Breathing movement to close every treatment.

### PLEURISY

1. Improve the respiration.
2. Arc light for any painful parts.
3. Circumduction of the trunk and of arms.

4. Kneading and percussion of the chest. (If patient has T.B. omit percussion as may cause bleeding from the lungs).

5. Chiropractic—3rd dorsal.

## MENOPAUSE

1. Give a general treatment.
2. Examine spine and adjust according to findings.
3. Respiratory movements.
4. Circumduction of legs.
5. Abdominal kneading.
6. Mild spinal vibration.
7. Arc lamp to spine for tonic effect.
8. Light bath—tonic.
9. Treat symptoms as they appear.
10. Keep out in the air.
11. Be regular in habits.
12. Use no stimulants.
13. Look for heart, kidney, stomach, and uterine disease.
14. Massage of abdomen will quiet the heart.

## NEURITIS

1. Massage the parts.
2. Vibrate over the involved muscles.
3. Radiant heat.
4. Blue light.
5. Inhibit over painful area in spine.
6. Adjust vertebra.
7. Treat the bowels.
8. Electric light bath.

## HIGH BLOOD PRESSURE

1. Adjust 2nd, 4th cervicals.
2. Lamp to spine 15 minutes (500 C.C. power).
3. Kneading of muscles.
4. Blue light on abdomen or spine.

5.  Massage of abdomen will lower the blood pressure by reflex.

6.  Stimulate the vasodilators (action of the Vagus).

NOTE: In each treatment select what will be the best for each case. Any one full treatment as given above would be too much.

## FOR LOW BLOOD PRESSURE

1.  Manipulation.

2.  Red light on chest or abdomen or back.

3.  Adjust the 1st, 2nd, 4th cervicals.

4.  Concuss 1st, to 3rd lumbar, 7th cervical.

5.  Stimulation of vasoconstrictors.

## BLADDER TROUBLES

1.  Concuss 5th lumbar.

2.  Hot fomentations over the organ.

3.  Vibrate from the 9th dorsal to end of spine.

4.  Treat the lymphatic in groin.

5.  Adjust 10th dorsal and 1st lumbar.

6.  Arc lamp over the bladder or blue light for pain.

## UTERINE DISEASES

1.  Stimulate 3, 4, 5 lumbars.

2.  Congestion of uterus will require the vasoconstrictors.

3.  Local treatment over the abdomen.

4.  Examine the coccyx.

5.  Hip circumduction.

6.  Abdominal massage.

7.  In ovarian neuralgia inhibit with pressure from 8th dorsal to 2nd lumbar.

8.  For hemorrhage use shave grass tea [Equisetum arvense].

9.  Vacuum cup treatment on the lower spine.

10. Flex the thigh upon the chest.

## INSOMNIA

1.  Arc light to the spine in the early part of the day.

2.   Massage of the back.

3.   Rectal dilatation.

4.   Massage of the head.

5.   Stroke the whole spine.

6.   Use the blue light.

7.   Examine the atlas.

8.   Circumduction of the feet, legs, and head.

## ARTERIOSCLEROSIS

1.   Take the blood pressure.

2.   See under blood pressure.

3.   Electric light bath-short observe effects upon subject.

4.   Arc light.  Give it so as to cover the whole body in a week.

5.   General massage.

6.   Regulate the diet and habits of the subject.

## HEMORRHOIDS

1.   Stimulate the spine from the 8th dorsal, to the coccyx.

2.   Ulnar percussion over the liver.

3.   Massage abdomen for 10 minutes.

4.   Beating of the sacrum.

5.   Rotation of the body.

6.   Rectal dilatation.

## RHEUMATISM

1.   Give a general treatment.  Manipulate the neck, shoulders, chest muscles and knead the tissues.  Begin where the soreness is absent.

2.   Treat the kidney, liver, and intestines.

3.   Electric light bath.

4.   Use the arc light over joints.

5.   Vibration of the joints.

6.   Circumduction of the joints.

7.   Regulate the diet.

8.   Use heating compress.

NOTE: Dr. Nenton N. Higbe of Chicago gave me the information as to the effects of the electric bath and of the red and blue light.

## HEART DISEASE

A diseased organ is a weak organ and rational therapy would indicate that rest was the ideal treatment. Movement constitutes the best treatment for all forms of heart trouble, but they must be given within the limits of the patient's strength. If the patient is very feeble the treatment must be limited to kneading and stroking of the extremities alone. Treatment must be discontinued if there is fatigue, hurried breathing, dilatation of the nostrils, pallor, palpitation of the heart and yawning (Despard's *Book on Massage*). Ostrum says that at first the séance should last but ten minutes. The aim is twofold: 1st to rest the heart, 2nd to strengthen its muscles. To accomplish the first we give passive movements only.

After this has been done for some time we go to resistive movements in which the patient resists the operator and the operator resists the patient. Since the hand is about the size of the heart and we employ both hands in kneading we act as a pump at the other end and so take off the labor of the heart.

## OUTLINE OF TREATMENT

1. Stroking movement in the centripetal direction. This peripheral pressure will produce a suction—so aiding venous flow.

2. Kneading of the extremities.

3. Abdominal massage (this will slow the pulse by reflex action of the vagus.

4. Deep inspiration which will create a "negative press [sic] in the big trunks of the venous system. Be careful about raising the arms above the head at first.

5. Rotation of all the joints—passive. If the patient can stand it, use quick rotatory movements.

6. Flexion and extension of the thigh.

7. Hip rolling.

8. Rapid ulnar percussion along the spinal column. But if the patient is a neurasthenic omit this as it is very stimulating to the nervous system.

9. By this time we can take up the resistive movements with the object of strengthening the heart muscle.

10. Have patient resist in such movements as flexion and extension of the legs. Separating and closing of legs.

11. Same of the arms.

12. Short electric light baths with compress over heart. Make this a tonic bath as given under electric light treatment.

13. Study the Schott system of movements* and select from them the best for your individual case. Begin with the mild movements and increase them.

14. Concussion may be of service in some cases of weak heart, but if you use it make it short and do not use it too often.

15. Chiropractic can be used as needed, but there is nothing better than the above outline as it is so comprehensive as to include the whole circulation. Chiropractic would not rest the heart.

Concussion would not do this. It would stimulate and if the heart is weak it would help along some, but to rest the heart you would not use concussion as a system of treatment.

You must work on the circulation to take over some of the work because already the heart has more work than it can do and the fact is the operator can do some of that work.

## THERAPEUTIC EFFECTS OF TREATMENTS

### CHIROPRACTIC

1. Increases the activity of all the parts supplied by the posterior primary nerves.

2. Increases the blood supply to the spinal tissues.

3. Sends more blood to the organs supplied by the spinal nerves.

4. Stimulates the spinal nerve centers and so has the same effect as concussion of that vertebra.

5. The thrust will stretch the ligaments and so move the bone.

6. In chronic conditions it will be a long time to move the vertebrae and if there were no other effects—as some Chiropractors think—how could one account for the improved condition of the patient? These other effects are the only way to account for them.

### MECHANO-THERAPY

1. Increases the chest capacity.

2. Raises the blood pressure.

3. Increases the co-ordination.

4. Raises the vital resistance.

5. Stimulates the nerve activity.

---

*Dr. Theodor Schott developed strengthening exercises for those suffering from heart ailments which he combined with the Nauheim bath. —Ed.

6. Relieves the congestion of organs.

7. Improves nutrition and digestion.

8. Increases nutrition and digestion.

## Kneading

1. Lowers the rate and force of heart beat.

2. Lowers the blood pressure.

3. Increases elimination and metabolism.

4. Stimulates the nerve system (deep).

5. Kneading of the abdomen will increase the activity of the stomach, liver, bowels and pancreas. Also will tone up the intestinal walls and the abdominal muscles.

## Light Treatment

1. Increases general perspiration.

2. Increases oxidation.

3. Lowers arterial tension (white light to spine 15 minutes or light bath).

4. Acts upon the metabolism.

## Arc Light

1. Is rich in ultra violet rays.

2. Light that passes through glass except the quartz—do not have ultra violet rays (we refer to the electric globes).

3. The arc light is good for pathological conditions.

4. T. B. of the lymphatic glands [Tuberculosis lymphadenitis].

5. Skin diseases.

6. Pain and congestion.

7. Does not depress the nerve system.

8. Can be used after the electric light bath.

9. Is excellent for the blood and nerves.

## Electric Light Bath

1. Depresses the nerve system.

2. Lowers the blood pressure (if prolonged).

3. Raises the temperature.
4. Dilates the surface vessels.
5. Increases the skin activity.
6. Relieves congestion of internal organs.
7. Acts on all the spinal centers.

The patient should have a cold compress upon the heart and one upon the head. Some other treatment should follow the bath.

## WHY DO YOU PUT THE PATIENT IN THIS BATH?

1. Is it for a tonic effect? Heat it up to 110° F. [43° C.] and put patient in for one or two minutes.
2. Do you wish to have a sedative effect? Put him in and keep the temperature to below 90° F. [32° C.] but not long enough to sweat.
3. Is the object elimination? Low temperature not over 90° F. [32° C.] for 15 minutes. Have him drink warm or hot water before going in and apply the necessary treatment after the bath.

*Another very important point is: the light should not be used continually, but should be shut off every half minute and then turned on again for the same time during the whole treatment.*

*Color is a very interesting subject in therapeutics and unless we know how it acts upon the patient we will do more harm than good.*

*The lungs, kidneys and the bowels respond well to yellow. Blue is valuable for deafness, flatulency, gastritis, insomnia and is a stimulant to the venous blood.*

*The red increases the tone of the Vagus nerve. The blue decreased its tone.*

*For a general tonic treatment I have found the orange light very useful. It is to be tried out in all cases of paresis, lymphatic treatments, kidney trouble, bronchial affections, and low vitality.*

# THE BLOOD-WASHING METHOD

## by Dr. Benedict Lust

*Naturopath, XXVIII (10), 521-526. (1923)*

### A RESTORATIVE AND CREATIVE REVELATION FOR IDEAL PERFECTION

Motto: "Glorify, and bear God in your body."—St. Paul.

The subject of this communication is the most vital subject in the world; it treats about the possible and sure and true transformation of the 80, 100, 60 or 50 year old person in every way, while being in possession of the wonderful experiences of the 100 years. This statement should not bring any unpleasant excitement to anybody, but comfort and joy to everybody, and the gratitude belongs only to our Lord. Old age does not exist. But something like it exists and it is noticed that bright old people always declare that their heart is as young as ever. This, in fact, explains that there is something which drives them and keeps them away from youth and life, but their thoughts are the same as ever before. It will be admitted that every person in the world has the right to be young. Youth is a natural source of good will. Now, this may seem to come from an unexpected source and way, but in fact it does not. The discoverer of the method below has been an athlete in general from childhood.* He is a self-educated man and a very profound student of nature. He has been, and very successfully, his own doctor and now with this method he has uncovered deceit and learned the secret of nature. Thanks God. The method is practical, easy and so simple, that if the hows and whys and wherefores are not explained first, it would not be able to attract the attention and interest and the realization of the reader.

To explain the method we must first find out what old age is substantiated. Old age is the worn out, run down, weak and unhealthy state and appearance of the whole body. Second, what is it that causes old age? Old age is caused by a chemically analyzed lifeless matter in the flesh, stuck to the flesh and growing into the flesh every day in the year for not being met with practical opposition, just as the dust would penetrate and grow into a brown sponge, changes its color to grey and makes it a nest of unhealthy microbes if the sponge is left in a damp place and out of the way of an air-current. Now, this lifeless matter grows upon the body automatically, through unavoidable carelessness, because it exists everywhere, including the air, the liquids and the food. It goes into the body, stays there and

---

*The originator of the Blood Washing Method was Christos Parasco who shared with Benedict Lust his discovery. Lust was so impressed that he became very active in promoting the Blood Washing Method in his publications, schools and clinics. —*Ed.*

grows because no successful way is used to drive it out, also ignoring the correct way of breathing, drinking, eating, sleeping, working, playing and, on the other hand, worrying, excitement, exhaustion and exposure and all wrong ways assist this lifeless matter to deprive the blood of its strength and its purity. Sooner or later the blood will be unable to produce any opposition to the growth of this lifeless matter, which keeps on growing, till around the first 20 years it causes the growth of the body to stop gradually and then it begins to fight against unprotected life. In the coming years it begins to be felt by producing in the body various weaknesses and inefficiencies, thus discouraging the mind and as if by mystery, making the mind thinking that the body begins to grow old. Thus the mind is doing injustice to the body and is beginning to put various barriers between the body and life, while terribly neglecting it. And all the while this lifeless matter continues to grow until it becomes an invincible enemy of life, producing old age, so that in later years it completely dominates the body, takes possession of it and drives away martyred life.

To rid the body of the lifeless matter must not be done by any other way except by washing it out from the flesh with pure water; but none of the known ways of washing the body can do such cleaning. The lifeless matter cannot be washed away in one hour or two or ten, but it takes about as much time as it would for a big burn or a wound upon the aged body to heal and if any of the known ways were used, sooner or later the system would get exhausted and would badly discourage the mind. The body gets quickly exhausted by the known ways, because it is at the same time overtaken from everywhere either by too much heat or by too much cold, too much vapor or lack of pure air for breathing or by the lack of the free and joyful ways of exhausting the nervous system. In other words, by the absence of the right way of washing, without which the lifeless matter cannot be reached; also terrible and fatal exhaustion would follow if attempted to resist the required time with the known ways.

But here is the method by which the lifeless matter can be taken away from the body, so the body will again become young and will stay young. In our especially constructed and patented shower bath the continuously shooting and showering water has the virtue to harmlessly penetrate the flesh and to produce stimulant-electricity, with the aid of which the water molds and shakes the flesh, dissolves and washes away the lifeless matter, thus enabling the blood to overcome it and to thoroughly supply the relieved flesh and all parts of the body with new life, like the water fills up the sponge. In this special shower bath the temperature of the water can be changed and regulated at will and according to the pleasure with our patented regulator, to suit the variously and periodically changing temperature of the body. These changes happen because some parts of the body and of the flesh are more sensitive than others and they become a little more harmlessly uncomfortable, while all parts have been treated

# Technic of The Blood-Washing Method

**(Use always our Special Patented Shower Head as otherwise you will not have real results.)**

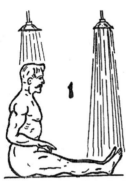

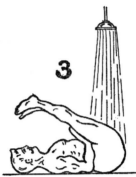

*Shower top of head only a minute when starting or when feeling dizzy, with cool water. Always put a plug of cotton in your ears to prevent inflammation. Shower face, sides and back of head longer, especially over ears in congestion. Feet from every angle repeatedly. Shower every part of the body at least 15 to 30 minutes at one place or as long as agreeable and repeat.*

*Shower lower abdomen and thighs, pelvic region for a long time. Turn over and shower all of back from neck to heels thoroughly, also sides, then raise legs and let shower strike over rectum, lower back, groins and inside the legs.*

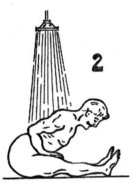

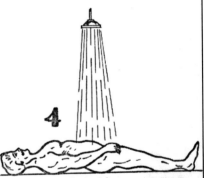

**Shower back and neck in sitting and lying position, also sides of arms and shoulders for a long time. Repeat.**

Shower over chest, abdomen, sex organs, legs and feet repeatedly for a long time. Turn to right and left sides and shower for a long time all the way up to shoulders.

The first four steps in the Bloodless Washing Method.

with the same, the whole system affecting power, consequently changes of temperature of the body occur. While hopeless exhaustion would follow if the whole body was to be treated at once from all sides in this shower bath, with this method one part of the body at a time is to be treated; in the meantime the other parts are resting and enjoying the charming ben-

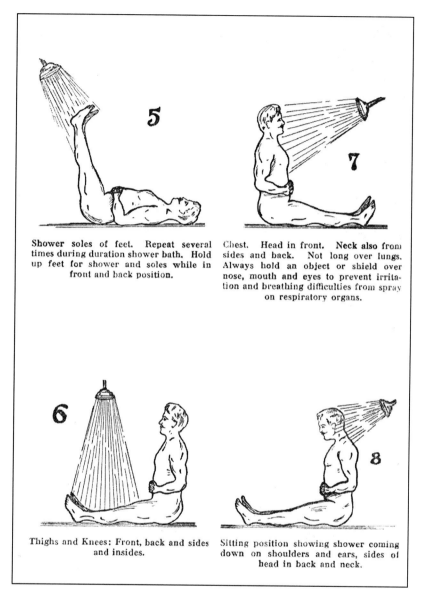

Shower soles of feet. Repeat several times during duration shower bath. Hold up feet for shower and soles while in front and back position.

Chest. Head in front. Neck also from sides and back. Not long over lungs. Always hold an object or shield over nose, mouth and eyes to prevent irritation and breathing difficulties from spray on respiratory organs.

Thighs and Knees: Front, back and sides and insides.

Sitting position showing shower coming down on shoulders and ears, sides of head in back and neck.

Keep in mind the shower head is raised up to 14 or more feet above the patient.

efits of the treated parts making up for it. Then the next part is treated, while the one already treated makes up tenfold. By treating all parts this way, a feeling of great relief and a very pleasant sensation are created. Following this method the body can stand the shower bath the full required time and instead of getting exhausted, it acquires every minute more strength and more power of resistance, a feeling of joy and happiness; in other words—youth.

## THE TREATMENT

The treatment is as follows: put up this special shower head of our own invention to a height from 8 to 14 feet and let the hot water fall upon a cork matting, wood crating, air-mattress or just a porcelain or tile floor, whereon the body, with extended arms and legs, head and feet, can comfortably spread out or may assume any other position. Start by showering the lower parts of the body, the lower joints, the knees, then going upwards all over the body, front, back and sides, from the toes up to the top of the head, then the same showering all over again and again, or according to the pleasure. Forty percent of the showering more or less is to be applied upon and around the stomach and the intestines, also upon the sexual parts, the rectum and surroundings and all over the most sensitive parts of the body. Also plenty of showering must be applied upon all parts which during many years have acquired an old look, but not much showering to be applied to the chest and ears on the first three hours of the eight hour unit. The temperature of the bath room must be mild and comfortable and it must be without vapors; the air must be pure and wholesome. During the treatment no food of any kind should be taken, but soft warm water as much as desired, as it helps very much the cleansing of the internal body. During the treatment everyone will be able to stand the shower bath individually for himself and will be convinced and will realize that he is able to stand it and in fact, will enjoy very much the hot water for long hours. Instead of getting pneumonia or rheumatism, as some people may imagine, this treatment will drive away these diseases forever from them and they will realize and will become convinced that with the help of this method they will not have to submit someday to old age and to its misfortunes, but they will thank God for this blessing. After the shower no towel should be used to dry the body, but the water should be gently rubbed from the body with one's own hands until the body is well dry by the cool air.

After the bath the one who is treated ought to take a rest for 45 minutes. Then, whether the call of nature has been answered or not, an internal bath should be taken with a regular syringe and with pure heated water. This application promotes greatly the process of cleaning. Any time after this, vegetarian food may be taken and if it is wholesome, fresh and finely chopped, to save much valuable energy of the stomach, or if it is liquidated in the form of a vegetable soup or vegetable cream soup, so much the better. After the meal, rest comfortably for two hours. The rest of the times may be utilized according to pleasure, but it must be enjoyable. Sleeping in bed at night should be kept up not less than 10 hours, whether sleep comes or not. This is one of the most important factors of this treatment. Also let it be known that the shower for rejuvenating should be applied each time at least for 8 hours. Internally take every night with one-third glass of water "Inner-Clean" or eat one-half teaspoonful with each meal. Follow Ehret's Mucusless Diet, as outlined in

Ehret's Specific Healing and Body Renewing Eating Systems.* You may read or do something else of the sort which is interesting and enjoyable to you. After this do some physical exercise for 15 minutes, but not so strenuously to cause perspiration. Every part of the body should be exercised. Therewith the treatment ends, except with possible modifications in special cases. Otherwise for staying young, healthy and efficient follow strictly the natural method of living as so wonderfully explained in detail and so easy to follow by Adolf Just's book, *Return to Nature*.

This true and real natural and common-sense treatment for rejuvenating must necessarily last about twice as many days as it requires for the healing of a large wound upon the aged body, and according to the age and the percentage of the existing quantity of lifeless matter upon the body more days are required for older people than for the younger. In order to regulate your daily habits and to practice the natural life for permanent youth, the highest efficiency and happiness, follow the methods of Kuhne, Just, Kneipp, Bilz, Ehret and Engelhardt. Read and follow also Dr. B. Lust's ten Health and Success Lessons, the so-called Vitalisme Series.

---

*Old age is caused by a chemically analyzed lifeless matter in the flesh, stuck to the flesh and growing into the flesh every day in the year for not being met with practical opposition, just as the dust would penetrate and grow into a brown sponge, changes its color to grey and makes it a nest of unhealthy microbes if the sponge is left in a damp place and out of the way of an air-current.*

*The treatment is as follows: put up this special shower head of our own invention to a height from 8 to 14 feet and let the hot water fall upon a cork matting, wood crating, air-mattress or just a porcelain or tile floor, whereon the body, with extended arms and legs, head and feet, can comfortably spread out or may assume any other position.*

*Forty percent of the showering more or less is to be applied upon and around the stomach and the intestines, also upon the sexual parts, the rectum and surroundings and all over the most sensitive parts of the body.*

*Also, let it be known that the shower for rejuvenating should be applied each time at least for 8 hours.*

*Follow Ehret's Mucusless Diet, as outlined in Ehret's Specific Healing and Body Renewing Eating Systems.*

---

* Arnold Ehret died in 1922 from a fall on a slippery curb in Los Angeles as he was leaving one of his lectures. His book, *Mucusless Diet Healing System* is still popular. —*Ed.*

# THE PHYSIOLOGY OF CURATIVE MOVEMENTS

**by Benedict Lust, N.D.**

*Naturopath, XXVIII (11), 647-652. (1923)*

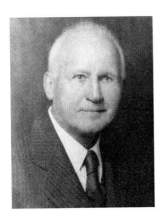

Benedict Lust.

In prehistoric ages man lived a predatory life, a life of continual terror and nearly always met a violent death. Nowadays man has advanced to the larval stage of civilization and is more or less controlled by moral law, but his physical life is sedentary and through lack of exercise his poisoned body endures a miserable existence and dies an early death.

Physically speaking, what man needs is the physical activity of prehistoric times combined with a willing obedience to moral law to give him physical and moral happiness and security.

But the highly organized condition of modern society, rendered necessary by the competition of thousands of economic enterprises, compels myriads to undergo a sedentary existence whether they are killed by such an existence or not.

Sedentary life is hard on muscles, heart and lungs. Mental as well as physical ills follow physical restraint and inactivity. It is better to live an active life and be poor than to grow wealthy in a sedentary occupation.

Exercise, when employed within the reactive powers of the patient, has a wonderfully restorative power on the enfeebled organism. It increases the circulation of the blood, develops the muscles, counteracts emaciation and development of adipose tissue, strengthens the action of the heart and other internal organs, invigorates the metabolic processes, stimulates the activity of the bowels and all other excretory organs to the end that poisonous waste matters may be rapidly expelled from the system.

Curative exercise further stabilizes nervous energy, quiets the emotions, prevents mental confusion and indecision, invigorates the will, and creates that pleasurable feeling caused by the integrity that our tissues are maintaining against the destructive agencies of time and the wear and tear occasioned by those functional activities common to all animal organisms.

Exercises of a military character and those of purely physical culture, while not intended for the cure of disease, yet are preventive of disease and minister to a very large extent in maintaining the organism in a condition of health.

General exercises produce to a considerable extent those chemical and physical changes which accompany muscular contraction with the resulting prophylactic effects on the muscle itself and the general environment of blood and lymph.

They exercise and train the heat-regulating mechanism and tend to relieve congestion in the internal organs by bringing the blood in larger quantities to the skin.

They increase the ventilation of the lungs, train the heart and increase the flow of blood in the arteries and veins, and also the flow of lymph in the lymphatics. They exert a favorable influence on the digestive apparatus.

Exercise is the best stimulant to the lungs, to the digestive organs, to the liver and kidneys.

Seeing that the muscles are the principal mechanism for the supply of oxygen to the blood, and for the removal of carbonic acid and water therefrom, their activity reduces to innocuous forms all surplus noxious materials, whether entering the body from without or the product of waste in the system.

Such exercises, when indulged in primarily for the cure of disease, can be made to yield surprising results. They can be intelligently directed so as to improve both the quality and circulation of the blood.

They can be used to strengthen the heart, stimulate the functions of the bowels and of all other excretory organs and in conjunction with massopathy are of the greatest service in promoting and establishing the health of the patient.

The chief aim of curative gymnastics is to accelerate the current of the blood and lymph so as to aid the nutrition of the tissues and eliminate morbid products. The nutritive and mechanical processes of the body cannot be carried on in the absence of motion. The muscles require good blood to function properly and develop strong tissue in proportion as they are reasonably exercised.

This very exercise is productive of good blood, whose nutritive properties make the muscles stronger and larger. Not only the muscles benefit, but every organ in the body partakes of the nutrition that is so lavishly supplied. Blessed are they who hunger and thirst after muscular activity, for by such movements they shall be made strong and happy.

## The Physiology Of Massopathy

In chronic ill health, when the energy due from the muscles for developing vital energy fails in amount, mechanical energy can be derived from other sources, that is, from the passive exercises known as massopathy and mechanopathy. In being imparted to the vital tissues, it follows the same channels and is largely transformed in the same manner to those physical processes on which the vital tissues utterly depend. Such exercises endeavor to produce the same physical conditions, promote the same physical changes, evolve the same products and enforce a restitution of losses sustained through muscular insufficiency.

Motion with pressure can be communicated by another individual called a masseur and the operation of which the patient is the recipient is massopathy.

Any communicated motion in which the will power of the patient is not engaged is massopathy, while the vibrations that proceed from the mechanical source of motor energy are known as mechanopathy.

Massopathy is a method of transmitting energy in the form of motion to the organism or its parts, which energy, acting in conjunction with the physiological processes, aids in perfecting their functions so as to produce the condition of health.

Massopathy is a manipulation of the tissues of the body by movable pressure in the form of stroking, rubbing, pinching and kneading. Massopathy, whether active or passive, counteracts atrophy of the tissues, increases the circulation, promotes the absorption of pathological elements and improves the general nutrition.

The purpose of massopathy is that of inciting, reinforcing and regulating the nutritive activities whereby functional power is maintained throughout the vital organism and involves the resolution and dismissal of the materials that yield functional energy. It is, therefore, a method of super-inducing the self-sustaining processes of health. It has power to destroy local impediments, whether chemical or physical, by oxidation, and coincident production of heat by the necessary interchanges of matter by which heat is developed.

But it must be admitted that passive movements have a far less extensive physiological role than active movements. They only exercise the muscles to a limited extent, but its power to change by its own work chemically stored vital force into movement and heat is only limited by the physiological limits of the organism.

For a certain number of ailments hygienic gymnastics must be combined with massopathy, and it may be employed in advance of gymnastics to remedy obstructions of blood and lymph circulation; to prepare for absorption new growth and exudations and to stimulate the functions of the skin, nerves, muscles, glands, etc., before the active and resistance exercises can act effectually. Following massopathy, gymnastic exercises support the acceleration of the circulatory fluids already started by the masseur.

In massopathy the exercises are:

- Passive exercises given by the masseur.

- Complex or resistance exercises.
- Simple active exercises that are taken by the patient alone.

Besides the operations carried out by the hands of the masseur, there are other passive exercises that are given by mechanopathy or the employment of mechanical means adopted to affect the deeper regions of the body. Such vibratory force does not primarily affect the skin, as the pressure is applied through the skin and not to the skin.

In complex or resistance exercises, the contraction of certain groups of muscles on the part of the patient is either opposed by an external force on the part of the masseur that offers more or less resistance or else the external force endeavors to effect a contraction by pressing against it with varying force, or to overcome it.

The larger number of active gymnastic exercises starting from lying, sitting, kneeling, standing, or hanging; starting points enable us to set in motion certain groups of muscles by themselves. The beneficial effects of such exercise are only limited by the power reaction to same on the part of the organism.

With regard to those operations that are purely passive, the skin is the medium through which the masseur acts upon the organism. The skin cannot respond to any impression other than those adapted to its powers. The skin can only exclude such products of waste as are conveyed to it by the blood in a state prepared to exclusion, just as bladder, lungs and rectum discharge waste matters confided to their depurative functions. Although the normal products of waste excreted by the skin are carbonic acid, urea, water and salts, it is not as a depurative agent that it concerns massopathy. In feeble health there is always a deficiency of voluntary energy, hence the molecular vibration supplied by massopathy is a positive addition to the system of transformable energy available for physiological processes.

The object sought for is to aid all forms of physiological activity, so that embarrassments of all kinds may be dissipated and the organs allowed to function in perfect health.

The intravascular fluids that are intermediary between the vital acting cells that develop vital energies and the sources of their nutritive support in the contents of the blood vessels as well as the contents of the cells are equally amenable to the influence of massopathy.

In massopathy the vital system is relieved by transmuted motion of serious disturbances that cause ill health and regains power, which is the chief aim of all mechanical vibration.

All races have had some idea of kneading, rubbing, stroking, clapping and beating. Hippocrates practiced massopathy 400 years B.C. Asclepiades was the father of mechanopathy, and Galen, the most eminent doctor of the Roman Empire, was a great authority for the use of passive exercises. The ancient Romans were extremely fond of baths and continual rubbings of their bodies by their slaves.

Later the Arabs became adept in massopathy. In modern times Dr. Metzger of Amsterdam and Wiesbaden won public confidence to a high degree in demonstrating the cure of disease by his manipulations. Langenbach and Billroth pointed out the importance of massage. Heuter, Esmarch, Barbieri, Volkmann, Gussenbauer and many others in Germany began to use it and when its effects were sufficiently demonstrated, people in Germany and Austria began to see that massage and medical gymnastics had the same claim to be examined as other branches of therapy and that their misuse by charlatans bore no relation to their proper use by men of scientific attainments.

## METHODS IN MASSOPATHY

Manipulations in massage are classified as:

1. Friction or rubbing with pressure.

2. Petrissage or pinching and rolling.

3. Effleurage or stroking.

4. Tapotement or blows, slapping, tapping, hacking, clapping, shaking and vibration.

## FRICTION

Friction is the form of massage most often employed because it is chiefly employed in sub-acute and chronic affections. It consists of circular and centripetal rubbings executed at times with considerable pressure over such regions of the body as require treatment which have been well rubbed in with fat [massage oil]. Respiration, oxidation and heat production are controlled by the varying impressions made on the exterior nerves by touch and variations of temperature. The mechanical impulse imparted by the muscles of the operator blends directly and becomes an addition to the pre-existing motion of the body fluids. Any pressure upon an artery or vein which narrows its caliber displaces and pushes forward a corresponding amount of the contents of these vessels. Their fluid contents cannot go back on account of their anatomical construction. The oftener the motion is applied the greater the gain in circulation.

In the case of synovial effusions, in chronic synovitis either in special muscles or in the synovial sheaths, friction massage is very beneficial. It is also of great value in hastening retrogressive changes in products of inflammation, infiltrations and exudations, and to press into the outlying lymphatics the products of disintegration.

## PETRISSAGE

Petrissage is a form of massage which consists in grasping part of a muscle between the hands and lifting it apart from the surrounding tissues, and kneading it between the hands. An alternate treatment consists in rubbing with the flat of the hand with pressure that part of the muscle being treated. This is done to reduce inflammatory swelling that affects muscles either singly or in groups, as in acute or chronic muscular rheumatism or in sciatica, where the muscles in the vicinity of the nerves are affected. Petrissage is frequently employed to remove the matter that produces fatigue in overstrained muscles due to competitive sports or from severe labor. It is also used to rejuvenate paretic and atrophic muscles.

## EFFLEURAGE

Effleurage consists of centripetal stroking of the skin that has also been well rubbed in with fat. These are performed with a much lighter pressure than friction movements with the flat of the hands over a larger section of the affected part, the direction being from the periphery to the course of the lymphatic vessels and veins. The object is to hasten the removal of the lymph and inflammatory products by the circulation. It is principally employed in severe acute cases where the tissues are hot and inflamed and painful. The time during which the stroking as well as the other methods of massage are applied will depend on the pathology of the case. In certain ailments, as in paralysis, motion may be applied without sting. Other ailments require slower treatment, the demeanor of the patient being a guide to the degree of application.

## TAPOTEMENT

Tapotement means a tapping, beating, hacking, or clapping of any part of the body to arouse the circulation and stimulate nervous energy. When done with the closed hand it is for the purpose of influencing the nerves and blood vessels of the deeper tissues and when done with the flat hand it is to influence those of the skin itself. Another method is to hold the hand in a concave shape so as to strike the skin with the cushion of air that is held in the hand. Tapotement is frequently used as a preventive for baldness or to relieve neuralgia of the face. In such cases an electric percussor is often employed or the fingers of the masseur are rapidly agitated by being connected with an electric vibrator.

It will be seen from such operations as are above referred to that massopathy is a direct means of refreshing and renewing local nutrition in a normal manner. No medicament whatever can become the alter ego of a defective operation of the physical properties of vital tissue.

In giving gymnastic treatments, not only should the patient's ailment be taken into consideration, but also the age, strength, constitution, when prescribing the movements to be made.

Weak persons should have at first only passive movements.

The passive movements of massopathy are divided into those performed by the masseur or mechanical agent, in particular joints, the muscles of the patient not being used, and those movements of resistance in which the masseur and patient act in conjunction with each other, and finally those operations of friction, petrissage, effleurage and tapotement, already described, which are conducted by the masseur alone.

Very weak persons are only given at the onset wholly passive movements. As vitality is being restored, the passive movements are alternated with active movements and the restfulness of this method permits the fullest strength of the patient being put into the active movements.

The best results follow a certain order being observed in conducting the several movements, so that operations on the arms, legs, head and trunk movements should follow each other in a regular daily program. Interspersed with such movements, are those of a depleting character, an abdomen treatment, a nerve treatment, etc. All programs should begin and end with special respiratory exercises.

As to the number of movements to be given in each exercise it has been found not to give more than eight movements at the outset and increase to twelve movements produces the best results. After each movement there should occur an interval of rest during which the patient should walk about slowly. The fatigue that follows active manipulation of the tissues at the beginning of a treatment is only a physiological result that will pass away and gradually disappears entirely after the patient gets accustomed to the exercises and is replaced by a feeling of energy and *bien aise* that is most agreeable.

In case a patient should exhibit an unusual degree of fatigue during treatment, great caution must be observed not to push the program to extreme limits at such a séance  It may be necessary to agree with the patient to suspend all treatment until he is in a state to resume the cure. Where the patient suffers from shortness of breath, from heart or lung disease passive respiratory movements, such as chest-lifting or arm-rolling, leg-rolling, trunk-rolling and circle-rolling. In any case, no séance should last longer than one hour.

## Mechanopathy

Mechanical power is a more prolific source of energy than that possessed by any human organism, hence its economic value in the cure of disease. There is no difference between the mechanical vibration furnished by the muscles of the masseur's arms and those generated by a machine designed to make the same movements, the principle of massopathy and mechanopathy being absolutely alike, that is, to generate in the tissues of the patient interior molecular and chemical motions. The advantage lies with the machine in the fact that it never grows tired, and the smallest machine made can sustain a greater and longer vibration than any one masseur can impart, however vigorous he may be.

In feeble health there is always a deficiency of voluntary vibration which furnishes heat and chemical activity to the system, hence the vibration supplied by an exterior force, as well as that generated by curative gymnastics, provides a positive addition to the system of transformable energy available for physiological purposes. The intravascular fluids that are intermediary between the vital acting cells and the source of their nutrition in the blood are equally amenable to the influence of massopathy and mechanopathy.

Massopathy or mechanopathy supplies to the muscle-cell all the physical conditions for the chemical and nutritive changes to which it is adapted, for the mechanical energy from exterior forces is substituted for the ordinary exercises that depend on the action of the will.

Blood is supplied to the muscles in proportion to the artificially exaggerated demand. This is a principle of the greatest physiological importance. The purpose of massage is that of reinforcing and regulating the nutritive activities whereby functional power is maintained.

*Massopathy is a manipulation of the tissues of the body by movable pressure in the form of stroking, rubbing, pinching and kneading. Massopathy, whether active or passive, counteracts atrophy of the tissues, increases the circulation, promotes the absorption of pathological elements and improves the general nutrition.*

*Petrissage is a form of massage which consists in grasping part of a muscle between the hands and lifting it apart from the surrounding tissues, and kneading it between the hands.*

*Effleurage consists of centripetal stroking of the skin that has also been well rubbed in with fat. These are performed with a much lighter pressure than friction movements with the flat of the hands over a larger section of the affected part, the direction being from the periphery to the course of the lymphatic vessels and veins.*

*Tapotement means a tapping, beating, hacking, or clapping of any part of the body to arouse the circulation and stimulate nervous energy.*

## NATURE'S METHOD OF CURING DISEASES

**by Charles H. Duncan, M.D., D.C., D.N.**
(Discoverer and Founder of Autotherapy)
*Naturopath, XXVIII (12), 774-778, (1923)*

### I.

What a monotonous world this would be if we all thought and acted alike. If we all whistled the same tunes and the admiration of all men were centered on the same women and vice versa. If all the world employed chiropractic and nothing else, or if all the world were practicing some pathy or cult to the exclusion of other methods of known value. Denying truth is not convincing. It may be misleading.

Let us understand at the outset that there is some truth in all established methods of treating diseases. To assert that chiropractic is a failure would be stating what we know is not so. To say that the use of drugs is ineffective in some instances, displays ignorance, as homeopathic physicians are curing patients every day and let us not forget that people are cured by methods that are unknown to many of us. When a method of treating disease is considered all sufficient and we do not know or care to use other methods of known and accepted value, we are not doing justice to our patients. But with all the various ramifications of the healing art let us remember with humility that Nature is the healer and the physician or practitioner, her servant. Our efforts in treating the sick should be directed in assisting Nature in her efforts at restoration.

All changes in the human body, whether it is in life or death, are governed by natural laws. We do not break natural laws; they break us. Science is the classification of established facts. All theories that do not agree with established facts are false.

The above observations were made recently at a meeting of practitioners by the complacent self-satisfied, shall I say the "Plaster of Paris" smile of approval that went over the audiences when the medical procession was slammed good and hard by some non-medical speakers. This is not as it should be for, while there is bias among medical men, who can say that bias is confined to them alone. We are all seeking the truth by whatever highways and byways it may lead, so, in bringing to your attention in a series of articles which I proposed to write for Doctor Lust's paper, let us receive with an open mind anything that appeals to our common sense and judgment, especially if it is a new natural process of treating the patient—namely autotherapy.

Doctor James Law, ex-Dean and Professor Emeritus at Cornell University says, "Medicine has passed through many and varied experiences; any endeavor to trace its history would lead us into paths that would be anything but complimentary to its doctrines and its practitioners. But when we come up against autotherapy, we are at once reminded of certain truths as venerable as the race of man, and in some sense a matter of common knowledge. First, who has always been the great Healer? Is it not the great Creator? Before medicine had a name or a substantial reality sick and wounded men and beasts largely recovered from their morbid condition by what would be called the defensive action of Nature. No thinking man can close his mind to the obvious fact that every recovery is a triumph of the living being over the malign conditions and cause that besets it."*

"Had the evil influence continued with unabated force in a system that could get up no greater resistance than at first (immunity), a fatal outcome would have been inevitable. The repair of the wounded tissues has been expected and looked for." **Immunity** is but another word for resistance to disease or the tendency to cure. Give a dog a good name and you can introduce him into respectable society, but give him a bad name and you can hang him.

Second. Contagious diseases even in the gross ignorance of the dark ages produced an explanation of the transference from one victim to another of the morbid agent which in place of losing its power through dilution from a sequence of victims constantly measured its evidence of increase by the number of its martyrs and added to its strength as it met victims that had lessened the power of resistance." I am tempted at present to throw the force of this entire thesis in straightening out chiropractors regarding immunity, but time and space and the interest of the reader I fear would be encroached. It seems, however, to be a fitting time to warn all seekers after truth to refrain from criticizing a subject with which they are more or less unfamiliar. Ignorance in action is indeed pitiable. No one can deny that a patient who has had smallpox becomes immune to the disease and no one will still further deny that the dog, in licking his wounds immunizes or cures himself quickly to an infection of the foot. These are but samples of many other similar conditions that could be mentioned with much interest, but it is possible only to refer to them briefly in an article of this nature. Now there must be some principle that underlies immunity in the two instances above mentioned—first, the methods Nature employs in healing and preventing a recurrence of the disease, and second, the method of assisting Nature to quickly immunize the patient by outside influences as does the dog in licking and curing his sore foot. Whether immunity is established by chiropractic or autotherapy, it makes little difference. It was this last animal method of treating

---

*Thus Nature immunizes the patient and on account of this immunization he may not again contract the disease: he becomes immune.

disease by the introduction into the mouth of the pus from the wound by the dog that led the writer to further investigate this method of treatment and to place autotherapy on a sound scientific and clinical basis. No one can deny that the act of licking the wound by the lower animals and the instinct for the human animal to place an injured finger in the mouth is a natural method of healing.

With this introduction the writer hopes that he may be able to hold the attention of the readers of the *NATUROPATH* in subsequent articles that will appear under the title of "Nature's Method of Curing Disease".

## II.

The thought uppermost in the mind of those who read the writer's former article under the above title is: First, what is Autotherapy? "Autotherapy is the physician's method of treating the patient with unmodified poisonous substances elaborated within the latter's body during the course of his disease, against which the tissues react in a curative manner." In other words, by means of autotherapy the patient is treated with his own unmodified poisons. This is what Nature attempts to do and does when a spontaneous or nature cure occurs with no outside assistance; "**Nature tends to restore the tissues**". Not everyone who contracts a common cold dies, yet many have died and are dying all around us from this disease. When a person becomes sick he develops poisons within his body peculiar to and corresponding with his disease but also these poisons are as different as each individual is different from any other. When a patient recovers without assistance it is because he develops resistance to his own individual unmodified poisons which has been generated within his body during the course of his illness. Literally speaking, *Auto* means self, and *Therapy* means cure, so the two words combined means self-cure. Autotherapy is the word the writer coined to fit this new natural method of treating the patient with his own parent poisons.

Observing the dog licking and invariably curing his sore foot, led the writer first to investigate and then to develop this method of treatment till at the present time autotherapy covers the whole range of curative medicine and much that lies entirely without its borders.

In a subsequent paper the writer will show the close relationship between autotherapy and chiropractic and how Naturopathy supports it by its slogan of "Sane Rational Living", to keep well and rigid diet, hygiene, etc., to get well. There is a medical axiom, old and venerable with age, which states "Every disease carries with it its own cure", and like all other sayings that persistently appear in medical literature, it contains some truth. Autotherapy picks out this grain of truth and utilizes it by proving that it is the **patient** and not necessarily the disease that carries the remedy. We physical therapeutists know this well! We are all so different in this world that when we attempt to treat a patient with vaccines, that is, with poisons or micro-organisms from another, we are taking a chance and often a long chance of not curing him with the added potentiality and possibility of injuring him. But it is different with autotherapy. It is difficult to injure a patient by placing back into his body that which came out of it, unless we are grossly careless. The principle on which autotherapy rests is everlasting and immutable. It is based on Nature's first law—"Self Preservation"! Autotherapy throws a new light on this law, for it proves that **"the remedy comes from within the patient's body"**. The human body is a self-regulating mechanism. It automatically restores normal equilibrium; restoring normal equilibrium is the all important factor in the treatment of the disease. When the writer in his initial tests of autotherapy gave that first drop of pus by the mouth to cure disease in 1909, it registered the dawn of a new era in healing. Another milestone in the century's old search for health was reached; while thousands of practitioners in all parts of the world are using autotherapy successfully and everyone who uses it is enthusiastic about it, the rank and file of physicians is skeptical. It has ever been so in medicine regarding things that are new and medical history in this instance repeats itself, running true to form in its oppositions to truth. But "one by one science is curing the links in the chain that binds the human mind to the rocks of ancient unbelief, until now one of the most ancient and cherished relics of the past, our ideas of medicine has been smashed by the conception of new thought, embodied in autotherapy" and I may add chiropractic.

It would be extremely interesting the readers of the NATUROPATH to analyze the objections that are made by physicians, to the use of autotherapy for they would probably recognize in these some of the artillery that has been unsuccessfully employed against Naturopathy. Truth is a stubborn thing. It would take too much space in this valuable journal at present to more than state that the opposition to autotherapy is due to ignorance, jealousies, false doctrines and medical money changers, of whom there is not a few. I may add at this point a brief account of that celebrated Austrian physician, Dr. Semmelweiss, who, over a century ago, called the physicians of his day to task for the death of so many women during confinement. He bluntly told them that they, the physicians, were to blame for these deaths, on account of their dirty hands. Of course, they did not like this, and their august body, in conclave assembled, arose and adjudged him insane and he was locked in the lunatic asylum for the remainder of his life. Nearly a century passed before his writings were reviewed sanely and it was then found that instead of being insane he was a century ahead of his time, and a monument now stands in Vienna in testimony of his wisdom, and lack of wisdom and jealousy of his contemporaries. The persecutions of Hahnemann are too well known to be more than mentioned at present. History is replete with incidents of this nature. Our own Doctor Lust could furnish us many incidents of persecutions of this kind. When autotherapy was discovered this jealousy and persecution were expected, looked for, and the writer was not disappointed, but in this advanced age the average physician likes to pose as an advanced thinker and is more inclined to accept anything that appeals to common sense than formerly. Be encouraged, therefore, you Naturopaths and Chiropractors! The good in your work will live; the chaff will be driven away! This fervid grasping after notoriety of our present-day physicians has led many egotists, quacks and charlatans to pose as discoverers and almost every year brings forth a new crop of men who try to steal openly the crumbs that fall from the autotherapeutic table. This is one of the greatest proofs, if any were needed, of the great value of autotherapy.

Let us return briefly to the history of this Great Truth. "The remedy comes from within", the **Magna Charta** of the Healing Art, as it percolated on down thought the ages; for I hope to show in this series of articles that the trend of all ancient and modern healing thoughts drift unmistakably in but one direction, and that is towards autotherapy, or Nature's method of healing. Those who prefer the older methods of therapy may find some solace in the following paragraph from the historical account of Aesculapius,* the God of Greek medicine: "The sick visiting his temple has to spend one or more nights in the sanctuary, after which time remedies to be used were revealed and given to him in a dream. Those who were cured offered a sacrifice to Aesculapius."

The readers of the NATUROPATH easily conceive that the old rascal discovered autotherapy over twenty-four centuries ago, faked the divine element for profit and praise and got away with it. How else could he have cured his patients so quickly except by obtaining the patient's remedy from the patients' bodies and giving it to them in ways that have never been known until the discovery of autotherapy; for with the knowledge of autotherapy anyone can now do this self-same thing, cure their patients often as if by magic. Being more or less familiar with his miracles and writings, philosophers and wise men since then have ever sought the secret spring of life and its relation to disease. They sought it in the boiling pot and magic powders of the alchemist; in the stars, in mysticism and in incantations. Scientists delved into the bowels of the earth in search of new minerals (radium) and life-giving waters. Ever and anon they seemed about to grasp it and almost every generation has heard the cry— "Eureka", but the main secret has ever been illusive and has evaded us. Achilles gave his name to the little flower—the Yarrow—that grows by the roadside, for, with its medicinal virtues, it was said to heal the wounds

---

*Asclepius, Greek god of medicine; Latin: *Aesculapius*. —Ed.

## What Is Auto-Hemic Therapy?

It is a system of treatment originated and developed during the past seven years by Dr. L. D. Rogers, of Chicago. It consists in giving the patient a solution made by attenuating, hemolyzing, thermolyzing, diluting and potentizing a few drops of his or her own blood, and administering it according to a perfected and refined technic developed by the author. The remarkable results that he himself has obtained have been duplicated and paralleled by scores of other physicians whom he has instructed in the technic. They report cures little short of the miraculous.

During the medical conventions held in Chicago in September and October, 1917, some sixty physicians formed a national League for the Study of Auto-Hemic Therapy, and agreed to report their successes, their failures and their discoveries in the North American Journal of Homeopathy.

Judging from the reports already published, it would seem that there was scarcely any limit to the applicability and practicability of this new treatment. Some of the most obstinate cases of anemia, insomnia, nervousness, constipation, eczema, diabetes, goiter, hay fever, rheumatism, mental and physical debility, ulcers, insanity, morning sickness, high blood pressure, and other conditions too numerous to mention, have been benefited, if not permanently cured, by Auto-Hemic treatment in an incredibly short time, after all other methods had failed.

Dr. A. B. Collins, of Linesville, Pa., writes, "I regard Auto-Hemic Therapy the king of therapies. Brings more cures with gratitude, and more money than all others ——to me as good as $5000 in five months."

Dr. O. W. Joslin, Medical Director of Pine Grove Sanitarium, Dodgeville, Wis., says, "The latest and most wonderful of all serums known to progressive physicians is the Auto-Hemic, discovered by Dr. L. D. Rogers, of Chicago."

Dr. P. C. Jensen, of Manistee, Mich., writes: "I would rather abandon all my other medical knowledge and resources than to be without my knowledge of Auto-Hemic Therapy."

B. Lust, N. D., M. D., President and Manager of the American Naturopathic Association, 110 East 41st St., New York City, under date of January 8, 1918, writes as follows: "Naturopathy and homeopathy work together to a large extent, the underlying principle being essentially the same. Dr. Rogers' new system, Auto-Hemic Therapy, should be introduced to every drugless doctor in the country. * * * It looks to me a real nature cure and a valuable addition or auxiliary to the different systems of therapeutics. As there are no drugs or "bugs" used with it, it should be incorporated in the treasury of drugless medicine."

These express the sentiment of scores of other physicians who have taken the course of instruction under Dr. Rogers and thus properly prepared themselves to administer this new treatment correctly.

Copy of a journal containing reports of the surprising results obtained by many physicians, also particulars regarding Dr. Rogers' book and course of instruction, sent on application to

### North American Journal of Homeopathy
2812 North Clark Street
CHICAGO, ILL.

Homeopathy included safe and effective potentized remedies made from the patient's own blood.

of his soldiers. Ponce De Leon sought the fountain of youth in unknown lands across the sea. Modern medicine has ever teemed with prophecy as yet unfilled with desires unsatisfied, with hopes deferred, with prayers unanswered and still the riddle is unsolved.

Our modern laboratories with inexhaustible funds have promised much, but as yet the truth, like the rainbow's end or the will-o'-the-wisp has never been fully grasped. Hippocrates taught that "Nature is the healer and the physician her servants". And his expectant treatment is often now the best we know. Bouchet aptly says, "After two thousand years of observation, experience and controversy, the Naturism of Hippocrates stands upright."

We seek to,
"Pluck the luster from the stars,
And loose the jewels at our feet."

The wise men no longer have to search the heaven above nor the earth beneath nor the waters under the earth for a remedy to cure a patient with a localized infectious disease, for autotherapy proves, "The remedy the patient needs lies within his body." This is the remedy we long have sought and mourned because we have found it not. The scales are fast falling from our eyes. Formerly we saw through the glass dimly, but now face to face we see naked, natural truths taking form and outline.

Autotherapy is natural therapy. The cures made by its use are based upon the first laws of Nature—self-preservation. Old Dame Nature is the pharmacist supreme, and an unalterable trust may be reposed in her therapeutic preparations. On the other hand, autotherapy agrees with much that we know to be true and may easily be scientifically demonstrated. All science is based on natural laws or phenomena, and if science did not agree with autotherapy we would strongly suspect that our science has been too finely spun or has been misnamed and led us astray, but from the fact that clinical observation affords abundant proof of the operation of the first law of Nature, and it is proven scientifically that "the remedy comes from within", we can safely rely on autotherapy and not be disappointed.

To Hahnemann we owe the discovery of homeopathy or the fact the remedy that will tend to cure the patient will develop a similar set of symptoms in the healthy human subject, to those from which the patient suffers. To autotherapy must be given the credit for a simple, safe and satisfactory method of treating the patient that is a big advance of homeopathy, for autotherapy treats the patient with the substance that causes the symptoms. The homeopathic or similar remedy is a good substitute for the natural or exact remedy. The question may be asked—what is the use of discussing a subject of this nature in a distinctly naturopathic journey? The answer to this question may be made in various ways. First of all, every Naturopath desires to have his patient cured. This can often only be done by natural methods. Since autotherapy is a natural drugless system of therapy and Naturopaths, who employ only natural methods of healing, cannot know too much about another natural method of healing that is so wide in its application, and whose results are so dependable. Then again we do not know when the State laws will be so amended that all people may choose the method of treatment they desire; and then, not to know autotherapy, the truly natural method of healing, would be a calamity. Again patients come to you from time to time suffering with diseased conditions that are difficult to cure by the means at your command. Everyone who has practiced Chiropractic and Naturopathy for but a few years has seen many, we regret very much, turning our patients over to men who employ the drug treatment of disease when there is a superior method of natural healing at hand that would tend to cure their patients in the quickest and best manner possible, even though as individuals we may not be now able to employ it ourselves.

Let us hear the conclusion of the whole matter. "Revere Nature and sustain her laws, for this is the whole duty of the practitioner."

*Autotherapy is the word the writer coined to fit this new natural method of treating the patient with his own parent poisons.*

*The human body is a self-regulating mechanism. It automatically restores normal equilibrium; restoring normal equilibrium is the all important factor in the treatment of the disease.*

*To Hahnemann we owe the discovery of homeopathy or the fact the remedy that will tend to cure the patient will develop a similar set of symptoms in the healthy human subject, to those from which the patient suffers.*

# References

Arledge, P. (2008). Study reveals evidence of the healing properties of clay. *Natural News,* January 9, 2008, http://www.naturalnews.com/022475_clay_healing_bacteria.html.

Bieri, R. (1909). The healing power of clay. *The Naturopath and Herald of Health,* XIV (10), 620-622.

Boller, G. (1901). Osteopathy and its relation to nature. *The Kneipp Water Cure Monthly,* II (10), 269-271.

Brown, G. P. (1919). Why the Allopath is unpopular. *Herald of Health and Naturopath,* XXIV (9), 441-442.

Collins, F. W. (1914). The science of kinesiology. *The Naturopath and Herald of Health,* XIX (1), 14-16.

Collins, F. W. (1920). Nomination of Dr. F. W. Collins for President of the U.S.A. *Herald of Health and Naturopath,* XXV (5), 221-223.

Czeranko, S. C. (2009). Biological blood washing. *Naturopathic Doctor News and Review,* VIII (8), 27-28.

Duncan, C. H. (1923). Nature's method of curing disease. *Naturopath,* XXVIII (12), 774-778.

Erieg, S. T. (1908). The early morning walk. *The Naturopath and Herald of Health,* IX (6), 179.

Goettler, M. (1911). The "nature cure". *The Naturopath and Herald of Health,* XVI (4), 199-201.

Gowenlock, T. R. (1912). Vibration and health. *The Naturopath and Herald of Health,* XVII (11), 713-715.

Havard, W. F. (1915). The science of cure. *The Naturopath and Herald of Health,* XIX (10), 600-604.

Havard, W. F. (1916). A comparative analysis. *Herald of Health and Naturopath,* XXI (7), 479-482.

Havard, W. F. (1916). Neuropathic diagnosis. *Herald of Health and Naturopath,* XXI I (3), 151-153.

Havard, W. F. (1916). The restoration of impaired function. *Herald of Health and Naturopath,* XXV (5), 234-237.

Hoegen, J. A. (1916). Nauheim treatment, carbonic acid baths. *Herald of Health and Naturopath,* XXI (1), 61-62.

Ioannidis, J. P. A. (2011). An epidemic of false claims. *Scientific American,* 304 (6), 16.

Jaquemin, T. (1909). The sanitary power of the climate of high altitude. *The Naturopath and Herald of Health,* XIV (7), 416-420.

Just, A. (1903). Return to nature. *The Naturopath and Herald of Health,* IV (3), 44-47.

Just, A. (1906). The value of earth as a remedy. *The Naturopath and Herald of Health*, VII (1), 23-25.

Kabisch, K. (1902). Naturopathy. *The Naturopath and Herald of Health*, III (2), 65-68.

Kaim, L. E. (1916). Narcotics and the osteopath. *Herald of Health and Naturopath*, XXI (6), 390-391.

Kneipp, S. (1904). Snow. *The Naturopath and Herald of Health*, V (2), 37-39.

Knoch, H. (1906). The Kuhne cure. *The Naturopath and Herald of Health*, VII (2), 53-58.

Lindlahr, H. (1910). The correct diagnosis. *The Naturopath and Herald of Health*, XV (1), 28-30.

Lindlahr, H. (1910). The scurf rim. *The Naturopath and Herald of Health*, XV (5), 263-266.

Lindlahr, H. (1910). Itch or psora spot. *The Naturopath and Herald of Health*, XV (8), 449-454.

Lindlahr, H. (1918). How I became acquainted with nature cure. *Herald of Health and Naturopath*, XXIII (2), 122-130.

Lust, B. (1900). Hardening. *The Kneipp Water Cure Monthly*, I (9), 152-153.

Lust, B. (1901). Prospectus of the New York Naturopathic Institute and College and the Sanitarium Jungborn. *The Kneipp Water Cure Monthly*, II (7), 197-199.

Lust, B. (1901). Mechanical massage, how it is applied. *The Kneipp Water Cure Monthly*, II (9), 245-248.

Lust, B. (1903). Internal irrigations. *The Naturopath and Herald of Health*, IV (11), 330-331.

Lust, B. (1903). Hypnotism in surgery. *The Naturopath and Herald of Health*, IV (11), 339.

Lust, B. (1904). Pneumathotherapy, breathing cure. *The Naturopath and Herald of Health*, V (3), 52-53.

Lust, B. (1904). Heliotherapy (sun cure) and thermotherapy (heat cure). *The Naturopath and Herald of Health*, V (4), 87-90.

Lust, B. (1905). How shall we live? *The Naturopath and Herald of Health*, VI (1), 3-5.

Lust, B. (1907). The spring cure. *The Naturopath and Herald of Health*, VIII (5), 139-140.

Lust, B. (1908). The science of nature cure. *The Naturopath and Herald of Health*, IX (1), 1-3.

Lust, B. (1908). Prevention is better than cure. *The Naturopath and Herald of Health*, IX (3), 82.

Lust B. (1910). The art of living. *The Naturopath and Herald of Health*, XV (4), 228-229.

Lust, B. (1910). Is medicine behind time? *The Naturopath and Herald of Health*, XV (12), 749-750.

Lust, B. (1911). Rules of bathing in the air-light bath. *The Naturopath and Herald of Health*, XVI (5), 288.

Lust, B. (1919). What more? *Herald of Health and Naturopath*, XXIV (4), 166.

Lust, B. (1922). Animal magnetism, curative magnetism. *Herald of Health and Naturopath*, XXVII (4), 168-171.

Lust, B. (1922). Spinal concussion. *Herald of Health and Naturopath*, XXVII (11), 526-529.

Lust, B. (1923). Additional fundamental facts on the biological blood-washing method. *Naturopath*, XXVIII (9), 421-424.

Lust, B. (1923). The blood-washing method. *Naturopath*, XXVIII (10), 521-526.

Lust, B. (1923). The physiology of curative movements. *Naturopath*, XXVIII (11), 647-652.

Lust, L. (1902). Provoking people. *The Naturopath and Herald of Health*, III (1), 42.

Metcalfe, R. (1901). The value of physical exercise. *The Kneipp Water Cure Monthly*, II (11), 312-314.

Martin, E. A. (1921). Violet rays or properly called high frequency. *Herald of Health and Naturopath*, XXVI (9), 442-449.

Nelson, P. (1918). Radiant light in naturopathic practice. *Herald of Health and Naturopath*, XXIII (5), 469-473.

Palmer, B. J. (1905). Chiropractic. *The Naturopath and Herald of Health*, VI (10), 284-289.

Peters, R. (1916). The importance of nutritive salts. *Herald of Health and Naturopath*, XXI (5), 304-308.

Purinton, E. E. (1906). Try the laugh cure. *The Naturopath and Herald of Health*, VII (7), 270-274.

Purinton, E. E. (1912). Hints on how to sleep soundly. *The Naturopath and Herald of Health*, XVII (2), 75-81.

Riley, J. S. Zone therapy. *Herald of Health and Naturopath*, XXIII (3), 265-267. (1918)

Schaefer, G. H. A. (1900). Natural therapeutics and electricity. *The Kneipp Water Cure Monthly*, I (7), 110-111.

Severson, R. (2012). NCNM's library collection analysis data overview. February 6th, 2012.

Sperbeck, H. C. (1923). The effects of drugless treatments, light, chiropractic and mechano-therapy. *Naturopath*, XXVIII (2), 63-69.

Staden, C. (1900). The Thure Brandt system. *The Kneipp Water Cure Monthly*, I (2), 23.

Staden, L. H. (1909). The relationship of the inorganic salts in the vegetable and mineral kingdoms. *The Naturopath and Herald of Health*, XIV (10), 618-619.

Stretch, E. K. (1916). Gynecology, minus the knife. *Herald of Health and Naturopath*, XXI (1), 40-42.

Stroebele, L. (1899). Mountain air resort "Bellevue", Butler, New Jersey. *Amerikanischen Kneipp-Blätter*, IV (5), 141.

Van Buskirk, E. (1913). The use of phrenology in medicine. *The Naturopath and Herald of Health*, XVIII (6), 412-414.

Weil, R. (1908). Homeopathy and its relation to Naturopathy. *The Naturopath and Herald of Health*, IX (10), 297-299.

White, G. S. (1921). Chromo-therapy. *Herald of Health and Naturopath*, XXVI (4), 180-183.

Wood, A. L. (1902). Influence of water on health and longevity. *The Naturopath and Herald of Health*, III (2), 74-78.

Young, C. W. (1904). Return to nature. *The Naturopath and Herald of Health*, V (3), 66-69

# Index

## A

Ablution/s, 72, 111, 140, 283
Abscess/es, 80, 178, 325
Air, 73-75, 81, 103, 109, 112, 114, 123-126, 143, 150, 153, 159-160, 180, 185-188, 206, 211-212, 221-227, 242-244, 267, 320, 331, 431; bath, 61, 80-81, 90, 123-126, 146-148, 152, 155, 159, 184, 188, 201, 240, 244, 268, 271-272, 283-284; cure, 150-152, 217, 261-264; fresh, 209, 211, 275, 442; hut, 123-126, 233
Acid, 96, 256, 328; carbonic, 223, 242, 320-321, 445, 447; hydro-chloric, 328; lactic, 326; sali-cylic, 215; uric, 116-117, 235, 242-243, 244, 256, 365
Alcohol, 112, 147, 161, 185, 211, 256, 258, 334, 365, 398
Alkalie/ine, 96, 327, 328
Alkaloids, 256
Allopath/y, 109-110, 215-217, 248-249, 371-374, 377, 385; treatment/s, 79, 246, 369
Anemia/Anaemia, 75, 360, 387, 399
Antidote, 114, 189, 411
Antiphlogistine, 147
Anti-pyrine, 110
Antitoxin, 246, 251, 261, 377
Appendicitis, 112
Appendix, 263, 423
Appetite, 102-103, 132, 187, 223, 225; lack of, 221, 229, 309-310
Arc Lamp, 359, 430-432
Arteriosclerosis, 256, 326, 365, 433
Assimilation, 89, 115, 154, 200, 206, 221, 230, 281, 325, 331, 426
Asthma, 80, 142, 167, 225, 250-251, 254, 356, 415
Barefoot, 34, 72-73, 81, 137-138, 148, 152, 178, 233, 267
Bath, 13, 72-76, 83, 110, 278; carbonic, 320-321; cold, 28, 72, 244, 283, 309; earth, 234-235; foot, 111, 283; internal, 131-132; natural, 123, 146, 148, 150, 155, 159; nauheim, 200, 320-321, 435
Sitz, 29, 111-113, 182-184, 283; Turkish/steam, 26, 61, 116, 182, 239, 248, 283, 302; warm, 73, 350

## B

Bellevue, 22, 26, 28-29, 46, 61-62, 79, 82
Bladder, 132, 418, 432, 447
Blood, 32, 66, 70, 74, 84, 98-99, 102-103, 115, 117, 161-162, 225, 289, 324-332, 335, 340, 386-387, 391, 416, 435, 439, 457; circulation, 46, 51, 53, 70, 84, 89, 91-92, 94-95, 98, 115, 137, 182, 223, 243, 281-283, 286, 347, 350, 363, 379, 394, 397, 399-400, 423, 428, 444-447, 451
Disturbance of, 92-93, 177, 200, 234, 281, 313, 317, 338, 365, 378, 402
Pressure, 242, 244, 346, 348, 378, 423-424, 426-429, 431-433, 435-436
Vessel/s, 94, 109, 249, 256, 345-346, 348, 378, 397, 415, 417, 449
Blood Washing Method, 55, 438
Bloodless surgery, 11, 13
*Book on Massage,* 434
Bone/s, 92-94, 99, 115, 132, 286, 325-328, 351, 378, 397, 435
Bowel/s, 104, 130, 445-456; disorder/s, 80, 112, 130, 131, 200, 244, 252-253, 423;

# INDEX OF NAMES

# About The Editor, NCNM, NCNM Press

Sussanna Czeranko, ND, BBE, is a 1994 graduate of CCNM (Toronto). She is a licensed ND in Ontario and in Oregon. In the last twenty years, she has developed an extensive armamentarium of nature-cure tools and techniques for her patients. Especially interested in balneotherapy, botanical medicine, breathing and nutrition, she is a frequent international presenter and workshop leader. She is a monthly Contributing Editor (Nature Cure —Past Pearls) for NDNR and a Contributing Writer for the Foundations of Naturopathic Medicine Project. Dr. Czeranko founded The Breathing Academy, a training institute for Naturopaths to incorporate the scientific model of Butyeko breathing therapy into their practice. Her next large project is to complete the development of her new medical spa in Manitou Beach, Saskatchewan, on the shores of a pristine lake comparable to the Dead Sea in mineral composition.

NCNM (National College of Natural Medicine, Portland, Oregon) was founded in 1956. It is the longest serving, accredited naturopathic college in North America and home to one of the two U.S. accredited graduate research programs in Integrative Medicine. NCNM is also home to one of North America's most unique classical Chinese medicine programs, embracing lineage and a powerful mentoring model for future practitioners.

NCNM Press, an ancillary venture of NCNM, publishes distinctive titles that enrich the history, clinical practice, and contemporary significance of natural medicine traditions. The rare book collection on natural medicine at NCNM is the largest and most complete of its kind in North America and is the primary source for this landmark series—*In Their Own Words*—which brings to life and timely relevance the very best of early naturopathic literature.

The Hevert Collection: *In Their Own Words*

A Twelve-book Series

*Origins of Naturopathic Medicine*

*Philosophy of Naturopathic Medicine*

*Dietetics of Naturopathic Medicine*

*Principles of Naturopathic Medicine*

*Practice of Naturopathic Medicine*

*Physical Culture in Naturopathic Medicine*

*Herbs in Naturopathic Medicine*

*Water Cure in Naturopathic Medicine*

*Mental Culture in Naturopathic Medicine*

*Vaccination in Naturopathic Medicine*

*Clinical Pearls of Naturopathic Medicine, Vol. I*

*Clinical Pearls of Naturopathic Medicine, Vol. II*

From the NCNM Rare Book Collection On Natrual Medicine.
Published By NCNM Press, Portland, Oregon.

CPSIA information can be obtained
at www.ICGtesting.com
Printed in the USA
FSOW01n1733090915
10721FS

9 780977 143580